Sinusitis

CLINICAL ALLERGY AND IMMUNOLOGY

Series Editor

MICHAEL A. KALINER, M.D.

Head, Allergic Disease Section
National Institute of Allergy and Infectious Diseases
National Institutes of Health
Bethesda, Maryland

1. Sinusitis: Pathophysiology and Treatment, *edited by Howard M. Druce*

ADDITIONAL VOLUMES IN PREPARATION

Eosinophils in Allergy and Inflammation, *edited by Gerald J. Gleich and A. Barry Kay*

Molecular Biology of the Allergic Immune Response, *edited by Arnold I. Levinson and Yvonne Paterson*

Sinusitis

Pathophysiology and Treatment

---

edited by

Howard M. Druce

Hoffmann-La Roche Inc.
Nutley, New Jersey
and University of Medicine and Dentistry
of New Jersey—New Jersey Medical School
Newark, New Jersey

Marcel Dekker, Inc.   New York • Basel • Hong Kong

Library of Congress Cataloging-in-Publication Data

Sinusitis: pathophysiology and treatment / edited by Howard M. Druce.
    p.   cm. -- (Clinical allergy and immunology; 1)
    Includes bibliographical references and index.
    ISBN 0-8247-8845-1
    1. Sinusitis. I. Druce, Howard M. II. Series.
    [DNLM: 1. Sinusitis--physiopathology. 2. Sinusitis--therapy. WV 340 S618
1993]
    RF425.S5   1993
    616.2'12--dc20
    DNLM/DLC
    for Library of Congress   93-20821
                                                                            CIP

The publisher offers discounts on this book when ordered in bulk quantities. For more information, write to Special Sales/Professional Marketing at the address below.

This book is printed on acid-free paper.

Marcel Dekker, Inc.
270 Madison Avenue, New York, New York 10016

Current printing (last digit):
10 9 8 7 6 5 4 3 2 1

Printed in the United States of America

To my wife, Debbie, and sons, David and Benjamin
Their patience with my endeavors made this work possible

Series Introduction

The decision to initiate a series of books on clinical allergy and immunology was based upon the need to create a library of texts useful for both clinicians and scientists in these rapidly enlarging fields. There already are excellent textbooks providing overviews of the fields of allergy and immunology, and the scientific journals attempt to provide concise reviews of selected topics of interest. However, there is no library of books that take relevant topics and expand them into texts, with the express purpose of making them of interest to both clinicians and scientists. Thus, this new series.

Clinical Allergy and Immunology will develop into the premier series of texts for our field. The initial book is directed at sinusitis and represents the type of amalgamation of pathophysiology with treatment that will be reflected in most of the books yet to be published. The series will include books focused on areas of allergy, immunology, specific diseases, and important clinical entities, developing areas of research relevant to clinicians, major changes in therapeutic approaches, and research areas that warrant a text. The beneficiary of this series should be the patient because physicians will now have a series to seek when searching for concise but authoritative summaries of a field. The other beneficiaries will be clinicians. Despite the fact that allergy is the single most prevalent chronic disease, only a small number of medical schools incorporate allergy in their curricula, and medical students are notably deficient in the knowledge of these diseases. As allergy is largely an outpatient specialty, few house officers see allergic patients other than asthmatics and patients experiencing anaphylaxis. To clinicians, this series offers the chance to develop an extensive knowledge about selected topics, each chosen for its clinical relevance.

Immunology is the field of the future. Advances in our understanding of immune processes and their relevance to health and disease are increasing at a breakneck pace. As therapeutic approaches become defined, the new relevant immunological knowledge will become incorporated into texts in this series.

With the publication of *Sinusitis: Pathophysiology and Treatment* edited by Howard M. Druce, M.D., the series begins. At this moment, some 16 additional books are in the planning and development stages, with about four to appear in the next year or so. This commitment involves some 300 scientists and clinicians combining their talents. With such a commitment, the success of the series is nearly guaranteed. This first text represents an extraordinary effort by Dr. Druce, who organized and completed the book in record time. This initial contribution is well written, contains authoritative chapters on all of the relevant aspects of sinusitis, and should become the reference book for this topic. It is a pleasure to have such a stalwart book initiate the series.

I accepted the challenge of producing this series with the hope and expectation that clinicians and scientists will find information that will lead to improved understanding of allergic and immunological diseases and their treatment. I hope the readers of these texts agree that we have succeeded.

Michael A. Kaliner

Preface

What is the need for a specific textbook on sinusitis? Sinusitis is one of the most commonly diagnosed chronic diseases in the United States, yet there is no universally accepted definition of the syndrome. This leads to confusion in diagnosis and treatment. The resulting lack of communication has held back research progress.

Consensus documents have tried to address the problem (1,2). Although they have been received enthusiastically by colleagues, they have failed to impact a wide audience of generalists. This may be because they have appeared in specialist journals. The clinical management of sinusitis overlaps several disciplines. Otolaryngologists, allergists, internists, microbiologists, anatomists, pediatricians, and family practitioners all lay legitimate claims for expertise in this area. This fragmentation can hamper an understanding of the genesis and perpetuation of chronic symptoms. Faced with a patient with long-standing nasal drainage, we are still often at a loss to ascribe it to chronic ethmoid sinusitis, for example, or chronic allergic rhinitis. Many practitioners, having exhausted empirical therapeutic trials, will tell patients that they "have to live with it." Lay publications often advocate unorthodox remedies or are directed toward allergic disease. However, it is expected that this will be remedied by a forthcoming book (3) designed especially for the patient. Its content was provided and reviewed by many accepted experts in the field, including some authors of chapters in this book.

This book does not claim to answer all the problem areas identified above. Its purpose is to collate the state of the art of science and medical wisdom in sinusitis. The chapter authors have been selected for their expertise in sinusitis. They are active in sinusitis research and/or have busy practices that specialize in sinus disease. The content is designed to integrate medical and surgical approaches and to provide relevant background basic science. Advances may be expected in this area when science advances to the extent beyond descriptive studies, for at that point federal funding becomes feasible.

I hope that the knowledge gained from this book by the physician will help in understanding the patient who has to live with this long-standing unpleasant illness.

Howard M. Druce

REFERENCES

1. Kennedy DW. First-line management of sinusitis: a national problem? Otolaryngol Head Neck Surg 1990;103:845–888.
2. Shapiro GG, Rachelefsky GS. Mechanisms, diagnosis, and treatment of sinusitis in children and adults. J Allergy Clin Immunol 1992;90:417–556.
3. Larkin M. Relief from chronic sinusitis. New York, Dell Publishing, 1993. In press.

Contents

Contributors

James N. Baraniuk, M.D., F.R.C.P.(C.) Assistant Professor, Department of Medicine, Georgetown University, Washington, D.C.

William E. Bolger, M.D. Assistant Professor, Department of Surgery, Uniformed Services University of Health Sciences, Bethesda, Maryland

Michael R. Borts, M.D. Assistant Clinical Professor of Internal Medicine and Pediatrics, Department of Allergy and Clinical Immunology, Saint Louis University School of Medicine, St. Louis, Missouri

James H. Boyd, M.D. Assistant Professor, Department of Otolaryngology, Saint Louis University School of Medicine, St. Louis, Missouri

Margaret H. Cooper, Ph.D. Associate Professor, Departments of Otolaryngology and Anatomy–Neurobiology, Saint Louis University School of Medicine, St. Louis, Missouri

Howard M. Druce, M.D., F.A.C.P. Associate Director, Therapeutic Research, Hoffmann-La Roche Inc., Nutley, New Jersey, and Clinical Associate Professor of Medicine, Division of Allergy and Immunology, University of Medicine and Dentistry of New Jersey—New Jersey Medical School, Newark, New Jersey

John H. Gladney, M.D.   Professor, Department of Otolaryngology, Saint Louis University School of Medicine, St. Louis, Missouri

Eliot W. Godofsky, M.D.   Clinical Assistant Professor, Department of Medicine, Polyclinic Medical Center, Harrisburg, Pennsylvania

Jack M. Gwaltney, Jr., M.D.   Professor, Division of Epidemiology and Virology, Department of Internal Medicine, University of Virginia Health Sciences Center, Charlottesville, Virginia

David W. Kennedy, M.D.   Professor and Chairman, Department of Otorhinolaryngology, University of Pennsylvania Medical Center, Philadelphia, Pennsylvania

Alan P. Knutsen, M.D.   Associate Professor, Department of Pediatric Allergy/ Immunology, St. Louis University Medical Center, St. Louis, Missouri

Rodney P. Lusk, M.D.   Surgeon-in-Chief, Department of Pediatric Otolaryngology, St. Louis Children's Hospital, Washington University, St. Louis, Missouri

Richard B. Moss, M.D.   Associate Professor of Pediatrics, Division of Allergy, Immunology, and Respiratory Medicine, Stanford University School of Medicine, Stanford, California

Michael J. Schumacher, M.D., F.R.A.C.P.   Associate Professor, Department of Pediatrics, Steele Memorial Children's Research Center, University of Arizona Health Sciences Center, Tucson, Arizona

Guy A. Settipane, M.D.   Clinical Professor, Department of Medicine, Brown University School of Medicine, and Director, Division of Allergy/Immunology, Department of Medicine, Rhode Island Hospital, Providence, Rhode Island

Russell A. Settipane, M.D.   Instructor, Division of Allergy/Immunology, Department of Medicine, Rhode Island Hospital, Providence, Rhode Island

Gail G. Shapiro, M.D.   Clinical Professor, Department of Pediatrics, University of Washington, Seattle, Washington

Raymond G. Slavin, M.D.   Professor of Medicine and Microbiology, Department of Allergy and Immunology, Saint Louis University School of Medicine, St. Louis, Missouri

Frank S. Virant, M.D. Clinical Associate Professor, Department of Pediatrics, University of Washington, Seattle, Washington

Ronald G. Washburn, M.D. Associate Professor of Medicine, Section on Infectious Diseases, Wake Forest University Medical Center, Winston-Salem, North Carolina

S. James Zinreich, M.D. Assistant Professor, Division of Neuroradiology, Department of Radiology, Johns Hopkins Medical Institutions, Baltimore, Maryland

John J. Zurlo, M.D. Assistant Professor of Medicine, Division of Infectious Diseases and Epidemiology, Hershey Medical Center, Hershey, Pennsylvania

1

Introduction: Scope and Epidemiology

HOWARD M. DRUCE
Hoffmann-La Roche Inc.
Nutley, New Jersey
and University of Medicine and Dentistry
of New Jersey—New Jersey Medical School
Newark, New Jersey

Sinusitis is an extremely common disease. According to one set of statistics, it is this country's most common health-care complaint. Although primary care physicians treat most of the patients who manifest the symptoms of sinusitis, the syndrome has attracted research and clinical interest from otolaryngologists, allergists, infectious disease specialists, and others. This interest underscores the problem that the diagnosis and treatment currently offered is often unsatisfactory. At a symposium held in 1990, the following clinical areas were outlined for attention (1):

1. Identification of the patient with the clinical signs and symptoms consistent with the diagnosis of acute sinusitis, recurrent acute sinusitis, and/or chronic sinusitis. It is unhelpful to label all patients with head congestion, rhinorrhea, and/or drainage as having "sinusitis." This does not advance the clinical diagnosis beyond a patient's complaints of "sinus."
2. Recognition of sinusitis as a potentially debilitating problem that requires precise diagnosis and specific, effective treatment. The proportion of patients who develop acute sinusitis that is incompletely treated, and develops into chronic sinusitis, is unknown. The adverse consequences of acute severe fulminant sinusitis are well recognized, such as cavernous sinus thrombosis and orbital extension. However, the physical and economic consequences of chronic infections are rarely appreciated.

1

3. Formulation of a management plan based on the pathophysiology of sinusitis, with attention to the relatively new knowledge of the role of obstruction of the ostiomeatal complex. The prescription of antibiotics alone is insufficient therapy for a bacterial infection in a closed cavity. It is equally important for the physician to diagnose and treat the underlying condition that led to obstruction of the ostiomeatal complex.
4. Use of a protocol for first-line medical management of sinusitis, with antibiotic and decongestant therapy as baseline therapy, and adjuvant measures for selected patients.
5. An understanding that antihistamines are indicated only in the management of patients in whom predisposing allergic factors are present. Physicians need to understand the pathophysiology of allergic diseases as well as those syndromes that are part of the differential diagnosis.
6. Prediction of failure of plain x-ray films to yield conclusive information about the ostiomeatal complex in sinusitis. There has been a wealth of new data indicating the limitations of plain radiographs. Physicians need to be aware of other imaging modalities.
7. Differentiation, from among a group of patients, of individuals who may need further evaluation of the ostiomeatal complex by nasal endoscopy and, in select cases, computed tomography (CT) for identification of the underlying cause of recurrent acute and chronic sinusitis. Physicians need to be aware of the potential of specialist referral, including office diagnostic procedures and their indications.
8. Selection of patients who might benefit from early referral for surgery aimed primarily at abnormalities of the ostiomeatal complex. Surgery for sinusitis has undergone significant advances in the last few years. Patients should be referred to surgeons who have particular expertise with the new procedures.
9. Identification of patients previously labeled ''chronic complainers'' for whom new hope may now be available. Many patients have been told that their postnasal drainage or head congestion is not amenable to treatment. It is important to realize that some of these patients may have chronic sinusitis or other upper airway pathology that may be identified only after special tests are done on the upper respiratory tract.
10. Prediction of the economic and social consequences of inappropriate management of the patient with sinusitis.

Answers to some of these questions were addressed at the symposium and a monograph arising from it (1), as well at symposia conducted by organizations such as the American Academy of Allergy and Immunology. Practical strategies on evaluating patients have been described. In a recent paper we advocate more detailed investigation of patients with sinus-associated symptoms under the following circumstances (2):

1. Symptoms are interfering with activities of daily living (e.g., work or leisure pursuits).
2. Symptoms are recurrent, for example, more than three to four severe episodes per year.
3. Symptoms are not adequately controlled by nonpharmacologic measures (e.g., steam inhalations or saline spray) or over-the-counter medications.
4. Symptoms affect more than one anatomical site, for example, sinus and ears, sinus and teeth, sinus and eye, or sinus and brain.
5. Sinus disease associated with distal problems, for example, exacerbations of asthma or chest symptoms perceived by the patient as "bronchitis" or "pneumonia."

Underlying these clinical problems are numerous basic questions regarding the pathogenesis of sinusitis that remain unanswered. For example, the relationship between sinus symptoms and allergic disease, sinus symptoms in the absence of infection, fungal sinusitis, and sinusitis and asthma need additional elucidation.

Many of the epidemiologic and demographic studies that have characterized asthma and other allergic disease have not been performed in patients with sinusitis. There is no generally accepted clinical definition, and thus many research studies are based on arbitrary criteria. The figure of 31 million is widely quoted as the numbers of Americans affected by sinusitis (3). It is impossible to determine if this diagnosis represents an overestimate or underestimate since objective criteria are not required to establish the diagnosis. The problem is common, and 16 million physician visits in 1989 were ascribed to it (4). In the same year $150 million was spent on over-the-counter prescriptions for the upper respiratory tract. This figure includes $100 million for antihistamines. This is an inappropriate expenditure, since the only upper respiratory condition in which histamine levels clearly rise is allergic rhinitis.

The purpose of this volume is to incorporate material that attempts both to address the research questions and to provide clinical solutions, based on scientific information that is currently available. Although the state-of-the art in sinusitis research does not yet approach the molecular biology and genetic research developed in other diseases, significant new knowledge has been added in the last few years. All the authors in this volume are actively engaged in sinusitis research and are intimately involved in patient care. The editor hopes that if improvement in the practitioner's management of sinusitis patients seen in the office or clinic occurs, this volume will have fulfilled its purpose.

REFERENCES

1. Kennedy DW. Overview [of Symposium: First-line management of sinusitis: a national problem?] Otolaryngol Head Neck Surg 1990; 103: 845–6.
2. Druce HM, Slavin RG. Sinusitis: a critical need for further study. J Allergy Clin Immunol 1991;88:675–7.
3. Moss AJ, Parsons VL. Current estimates from the national health interview survey, United States—1985. Hyattsville, MD: National Center for Health Statistics, 1986:66–7, DHHS Publication No. (PHS)86-1588. (Vital and Health Statistics; Series 10;No.160).
4. National Disease and Therapeutic Index. Plymouth Meeting, PA: IMS, Inc. 1988–9:487–8.

2

Anatomy of the Nasal Cavity and the Paranasal Sinuses

MARGARET H. COOPER
Saint Louis University School of Medicine
St. Louis, Missouri

I. NASAL CAVITY

The nasal cavity extends from the face to the nasopharynx. The most anterior openings onto the face are the nares, and the openings posteriorly are into the nasopharynx by way of the posterior nasal apertures, or choanae. The anterior part of the cavity is the vestibule, which extends from the nares to the limen nasi, which corresponds to the upper margin of the alar cartilage. It is lined with skin with coarse hairs. The vestibular skin is continuous with the nasal mucosa at the limen. The rest of the nasal cavity is the olfactory region and the respiratory region. The olfactory region is in the superior aspect of the cavity and includes parts of the roof, septum, and lateral wall. The rest of the nasal cavity is the respiratory region. The space is divided in the midline by the nasal septum. Bones that make up the boundaries of the nasal cavity include the maxilla, palatine, sphenoid, ethmoid, frontal, nasal, lacrimal, inferior concha, and vomer (Fig. 1). The nasal septum is made up of cartilage anteriorly and bone posteriorly and superiorly. The bones include the vomer and the perpendicular plate of the ethmoid. The septal cartilage articulates with the perpendicular plate of the ethmoid, vomer, and the nasal crest of the maxilla in a ''tongue and groove'' manner that allows for movement of the anterior part of the septum. The arrangement of loose connective tissue and the perichrondium and the

5

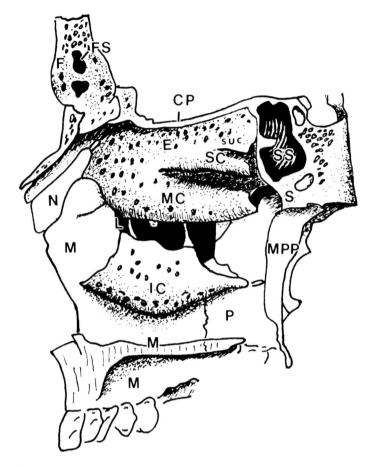

Figure 1 Schematic diagram of the bones of the lateral nasal wall. CP: cribriform plate of ethmoid bone; E, ethmoid bone; F, frontal bone; FS, frontal sinus; IC, inferior concha/turbinate; L, lacrimal bone; M, maxilla; MC, middle concha/turbinate; MPP, medial pterygoid plate; N, nasal bone; P, palatine bone; S, sphenoid bone; suc, supreme concha/turbinate; SC, superior concha/turbinate; SS, sphenoid sinus.

periosteum allows for the mobility of the septum (1). The floor of the nasal cavity is formed by the palatine process of the maxilla anteriorly and the horizontal plate of the palatine bone posteriorly, both of which separate it from the oral cavity. The roof, which is much narrower than the floor, is formed by the nasal, frontal, ethmoid, and sphenoid bones. The ethmoid part of the roof is the cribriform plate, which is dotted with holes through which the olfactory nerves traverse to the anterior cranial cavity (Fig. 1).

The mucosa that lines the respiratory region of the cavity is respiratory. It consists of columnar or pseudostratified ciliated columnar epithelium with goblet cells, serous, and mucous glands. The vasculature is cavernous in nature. The mucosa is closely adherent to the periosteum, causing the term mucoperiosteum to be used.

The lateral wall of the nasal cavity is by far the most complicated wall of the nasal cavity. It is composed of portions of seven bones: maxilla, palatine, sphenoid, ethmoid, lacrimal, nasal, and inferior nasal concha (Fig. 1). The complexity of the wall is caused by bony projections, spaces, and openings. There are three large constant bony projections (Figs. 1, 2, 5, 6, 7). The two superiorly placed projections, which are part of the ethmoid bone, are the superior and middle conchae. The most inferior of the projections is the inferior concha, which is an independent bone (Figs. 1, 2, 5, 6a, 7b). The proper term for these projections is concha, but the term turbinate is prevalent in the clinical literature. Posterosuperior to the superior concha/turbinate there is frequently a small projection of the ethmoid bone, the highest or supreme concha/turbinate (Figs. 1, 2).

As the inferior concha/turbinate proceeds from anterior to posterior it articulates with the lacrimal, maxilla, ethmoid, and palatine bones. It is concave in shape with a free inferior border. The mucosa, respiratory in nature, that covers the bone is similar to erectile tissue in that there are numerous venous spaces that can become engorged. Posteriorly the concha/turbinate ends in the inferior portion of the posterior choana at the level of the auditory tube in the nasopharynx (Figs. 2, 6).

As part of the ethmoid bone, the middle concha/turbinate plays an important part of the ethmoidal sinuses or labyrinth. The attachment of the concha/turbinate to the lateral wall of the nasal cavity is termed the basal or ground lamina (Fig. 6a). The middle concha/turbinate may be composed of numerous air cells and has a medial wall or lamella and a lateral wall or lamella. Anteriorly the medial lamella continues into the roof of the nasal cavity just lateral to the cribriform plate (Fig. 5a, b). Posteriorly it deviates from the cribriform plate and becomes incorporated into the labyrinth itself. The lateral lamella is actually part of the labyrinth (Fig. 5b). The posterior edge of the concha/turbinate lies in the superior part of the choana. At the point where the posterior limit of the concha/turbinate attaches to the lateral wall, it is in the same plane as the anterior wall of the sphenoid sinus. Anterior and somewhat superior to the middle concha/turbinate is a slight projection, the agger nasi (Fig. 2).

The superior concha/turbinate is a small bony projection that lies posterior to the middle concha/turbinate. (Figs. 1, 2, 5e). The sphenoethmoidal recess separates the structure from the anterior wall of the sphenoid bone (Fig. 2).

Underlying each concha/turbinate is a space, the meatus. The meatuses are named by the corresponding concha/turbinate: inferior, middle, and superior

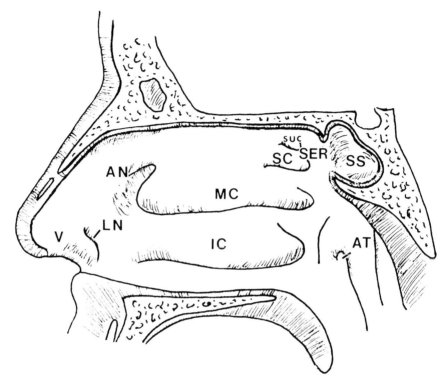

Figure 2 Schematic diagram of lateral nasal wall with conchae/turbinates intact. AN, agger nasi; AT, auditory tube; IC, inferior concha/turbinate; LN, limen nasi; MC, middle concha/turbinate; suc, supreme concha/turbinate; SC, superior concha/turbinate; SER, sphenoethmoid recess; SS, sphenoid sinus; V, vestibule.

meatuses (Figs. 3, 5). The meatuses have openings into them from a variety of sources. The opening in the inferior meatus is the nasolacrimal duct (Fig. 3). It is found in the anterior part of the meatus. In the superior meatus are openings of the posterior ethmoidal cells, and at its posterior end, within the sphenoethmoidal recess, is the sphenopalatine foramen. The latter transmits nerves and blood vessels from the pterygopalatine fossa (Fig. 3).

By far the most complicated space is the middle meatus. It lies under the concave middle concha/turbinate and receives the majority of the openings of the paranasal sinuses. Below the basal lamina is an opening or groove that has bone on each side of it, the hiatus semilunaris (Figs. 3, 5c, 6a, 7b). This opening curves anteriorly and superiorly to continue as the ethmoid infundibulum (Figs. 5a, b, 6a, 7b). The bone on the superior aspect of the groove bulges out into the

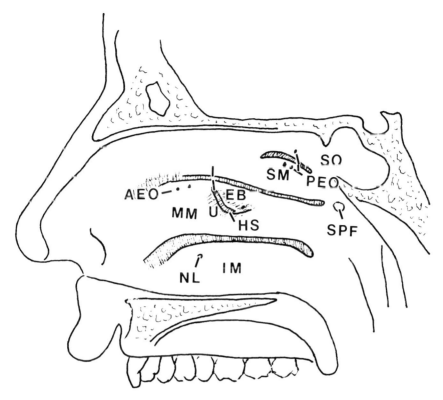

Figure 3 Schematic diagram of the lateral nasal wall with the conchae/turbinates removed. AEO, anterior ethmoidal air cell ostia; EB, ethmoid bulla; HS, hiatus semilunaris; I, infundibulum; IM, inferior meatus; MM, middle meatus; NL, nasolacrimal duct opening; PEO, posterior ethmoidal air cell ostia; SM, superior meatus; SO, Ostium of the sphenoid sinus; SPF, sphenopalatine foramen; U, uncinate process.

hiatus and is the ethmoid bulla (Figs. 3, 5b, c, 6a, 7b). On the inferior aspect of the groove is the uncinate process, a small projection of the ethmoid bone (Figs. 3, 5a–c, 7b). Openings into the hiatus semilunaris include those from the maxillary sinus, anterior ethmoidal air cells, and the frontal sinus via the infundibulum (Figs. 3, 5c, 6b).

II. PARANASAL AIR SINUSES

The paranasal sinuses include the frontal, sphenoidal, maxillary, and ethmoidal sinuses. All drain into and therefore are connected to the nasal cavity. The mucosa lining is similar to the respiratory mucosa of the nasal cavity except that it is not as thick and is less vascular and less adherent to the bone.

The following is a description of the sinuses, but it is to be remembered that the anatomy is quite variable. The sinuses vary in size from individual to individual as well as during the lifespan. Often they are extremely small at birth and expand after the teeth erupt as well as during puberty. Their growth and expansion alter the size and shape of the face during development.

III. FRONTAL SINUS

There are usually two frontal sinuses that lie between the tables of the frontal bone posterior to the supraciliary arches (Figs. 1, 5a, 7). They may be observed as separate compartments on each side of the frontal bone and be of equal size or asymmetrical. They can lie one behind the other or in some cases be connected. There are usually septa within the sinuses that subdivide it. The sinuses are small to medium in size and are usually found within the vertical or squamosal portion of the frontal bone. Occasionally they may extend into the orbital plate of the frontal bone even as far posteriorly to the lesser wing of the sphenoid bone. The frontal sinus drains into the middle meatus via the frontonasal duct and ethmoidal infundibulum (Figs. 3, 7). Important relationships of the frontal sinus are the close proximity of the anterior cranial cavity and the orbit. The bone separating these areas is quite thin. The blood supply to the sinus is the supraorbital and anterior ethmoidal arteries and veins. The nerve supply is through the supraorbital nerve. Their lymphatic drainage is to the submandibular nodes.

IV. SPHENOIDAL SINUS

The sphenoidal sinuses lie within the body of the sphenoid bone and may extend into the pterygoid processes or the greater wings of the sphenoid (Figs. 4, 7). They are separated by a septum. This septum rarely divides the sinuses equally, causing the sinuses to be asymmetrical in size. Often each sinus is further subdivided by septa. The relationship of the sinuses to surrounding structures is of utmost importance. Laterally it is related to the cavernous sinus, which contains several cranial nerves as well as the internal carotid artery (Fig. 4). The artery often causes a ridge or bulge into the sinus. The bone covering the artery may be thin or even dehiscent, causing only the sinus mucosa to separate the sinus from the artery and other cavernous sinus structures. Superiorly the sinuses are related to the hypophysis and the optic nerve in the optic canal (Fig. 4). Van Alyea noted that the optic nerve can cause a projection of bone into the sinus. When it is present there is also a projection caused by the internal cartoid artery(2). Fuji et al. noted similar results as well as a projection made by the maxillary nerve of the trigeminal nerve (3).

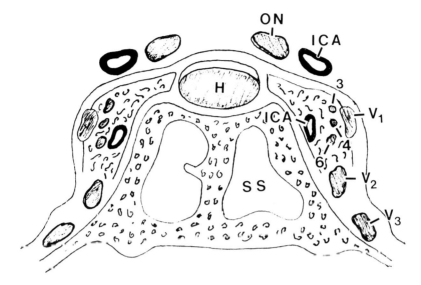

Figure 4 Schematic diagram of a coronal section through the sphenoid sinus shows its relationship to the structures surrounding it. H, hypophysis; ICA, internal carotid artery; ON, optic nerve; cranial nerves 3,4,6,V_1, V_2, V_3; SS, sphenoid sinus.

Each sinus drains into the nasal cavity by the sphenoidal ostium, which is in the anterior wall of the sinus. The drainage is into the sphenoethmoidal recess (Fig. 2). The sinus receives its blood supply from the posterior ethmoidal artery and vein and its nerve supply from the posterior ethmoidal nerve. The lymphatic drainage is to the retropharyngeal nodes.

V. MAXILLARY SINUS

The maxillary sinus, the largest of the sinuses, is pyramidal (Fig. 5). It sits within the maxilla of each side with the lateral wall of the nasal cavity as the base of the pyramid. The apex often extends into the zygomatic process of the maxilla. Superiorly the orbital plate of the maxilla separates the sinus from the orbit. There is normally a bony ridge in the roof that contains the infraorbital neurovascular bundle. Inferiorly the floor of the sinus is the alveolar ridge of the maxilla, which lies below the floor of the nasal cavity. Projections in the floor are the roots of the premolar and molar teeth. The degree of bone covering the roots is inconstant. Occasionally the vessels and nerves of the teeth are covered only by mucosa (4). Posteriorly the sinus is related to the pterygopalatine fossa. The sinus drains into the nasal cavity through its ostium, which is located usually at the anterosuperior portion of the medial wall of the sinus (Fig. 6b). It normally empties into the ethmoid infundibulum as a single ostium, but occasionally it forms a canal-like structure. The position of the ostium as it drains into the infundibulum has been described as being in one of four possible different areas (1,5). Sometimes the bony ostium is large, but it is covered by mucosa, causing the functional ostium to be quite small. Accessory ostia opening directly into the middle meatus or into the hiatus semilunaris have also been described. There may be one or more accessory ostia. They may be larger than the primary one. The sinus receives its blood supply from the facial, infraorbital, and greater palatine vessels and its nerve supply from the infraorbital and anterior, middle, and posterior alveolar nerves. The lymphatic drainage is into the submandibular nodes.

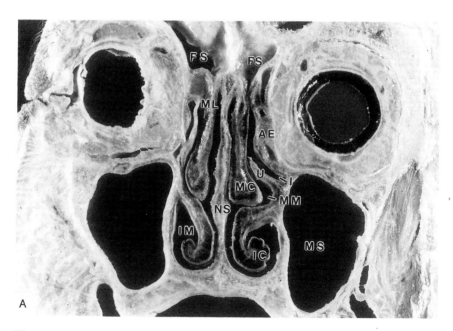

Figure 5   Series of gross coronal sections through the nasal cavities and paranasal sinuses from most anterior (A) to most posterior (E). ACC, anterior cranial cavity; AE, anterior ethmoidal air cells; EB, ethmoid bulla; CB, concha bullosa; EL, ethmoid labyrinth; FE, fovea ethmoidalis; FS, frontal sinus; I, infundibulum; IC, inferior concha/turbinate; IM, inferior meatus; LL, lateral lamella of middle concha/turbinate; MC, middle concha/turbinate; ML, medial lamella of middle concha/turbinate; MM, middle meatus; MS, maxillary sinus; NS, nasal septum; O, ostium of maxillary sinus; OE, orbital plate of ethmoid bone (lamina papyracea); PE, posterior ethmoidal air cells; SC, superior concha/turbinate; SM, superior meatus; U, uncinate process.

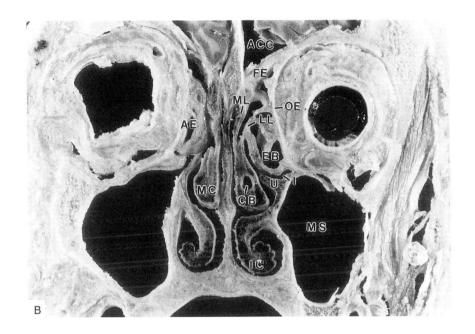

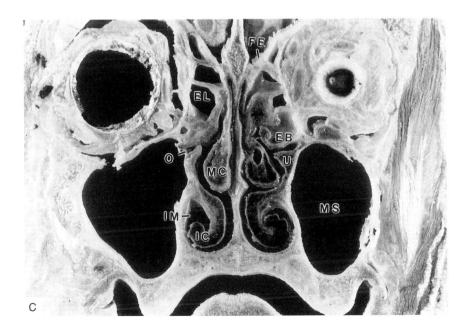

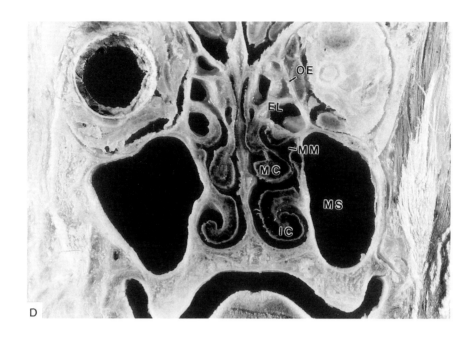

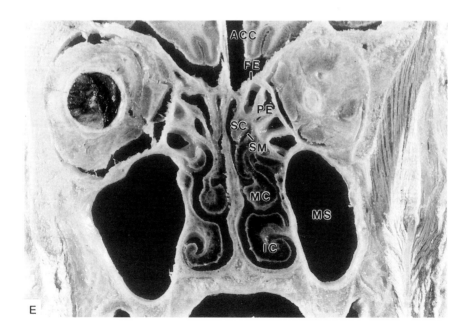

Figure 5 Continued

VI. ETHMOIDAL SINUS

The ethmoidal sinus or labyrinth of each side resembles a honeycomb with numerous air cells. Posteriorly there is a wide base of cells that abut the sphenoid sinus. The roof, which is referred to as the fovea ethmoidalis, separates the air cells from the anterior cranial cavity (Figs. 5b, c, e, 6a). The lateral wall of the labyrinth separates the air cells from the orbit. This thin plate of bone is the orbital plate of the ethmoid bone or the lamina papyracea (Fig. 5b & d). Anteriorly the air cells are in close relationship to the frontal sinus. The number of air cells varies from four to seventeen, with an average of 9 (6,7). The cells have been divided into a variety of groups, but the simplest division is into an anterior and a posterior group of air cells (Figs. 5a, b, e, 6, 7). The point of division is the attachment of the middle concha to the lateral wall of the nasal cavity, the basal lamina. The anterior cells, which are usually more numerous and smaller

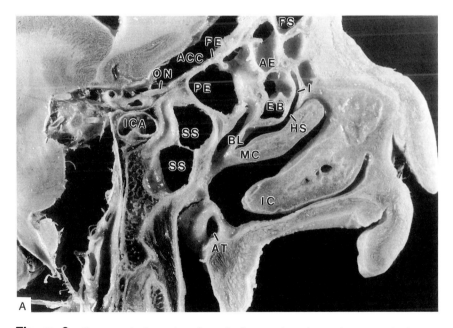

Figure 6 Gross sagittal section through the nasal cavity and paranasal sinuses. Through left nasal cavity (A) medial to (B). ACC, anterior cranial cavity; AE, anterior ethmoidal air cells; AT, auditory tube; BL, basal lamina or ground lamina of middle concha/turbinate; EB, ethmoid bulla; FE, fovea ethmoidalis; FS, frontal sinus; HS, hiatus semilunaris; I, infundibulum; ICA, internal carotid artery; IC, inferior concha/turbinate; MC, middle concha/turbinate; O, ostium of maxillary sinus; ON, optic nerve; PE, posterior ethmoidal air cells; SS, sphenoid sinus; U, uncinate process.

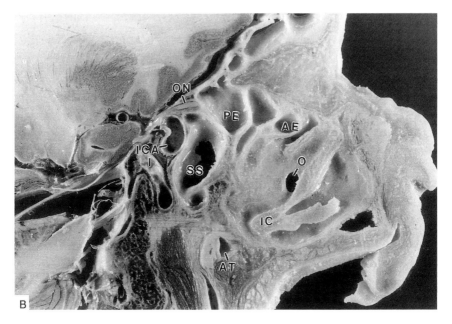

Figure 6 Continued

than the posterior cells, drain into the ethmoid infundibulum by several openings. Among the important cells of this group are the agger nasi cells, the bulla air cells, and the concha bullosa cells. The agger nasi air cells, which are deep to the agger nasi, a vestigial turbinate, lie directly anterior to the middle concha/turbinate (8). These cells are closely related to the nasolacrimal duct as it traverses the lateral nasal wall in a somewhat posteroinferior direction to drain into the inferior meatus. The duct lies lateral to the lateral nasal wall at the level of the agger nasi. The frontal sinus, agger nasi, and nasolacrimal duct lie in roughly the same frontal plane (9). Within the ethmoid bulla are the bulla air cells that can overhang the hiatus semilunaris/infundibulum (Figs. 5b, c, 6a, 7b). When the middle concha/turbinate contains air cells, they are referred to as the concha bullosa (Fig. 5b). All of these air cells can be extremely significant

Figure 7 Gross sagittal sections through opposite nasal cavity and paranasal sinuses of specimen in Figure 6. (A) is through right nasal cavity medial to (B). AE, anterior ethmoidal air cells; AT, auditory tube; EB, ethmoid bulla with air cells; FD, frontonasal duct; FS, frontal sinus; HS, hiatus semilunaris; I, infundibulum; IC, inferior concha/turbinate; ICA, internal carotid artery; MC, middle concha/turbinate; ON, optic nerve; PE, posterior ethmoidal air cells; SS, sphenoid sinus; U, uncinate process.

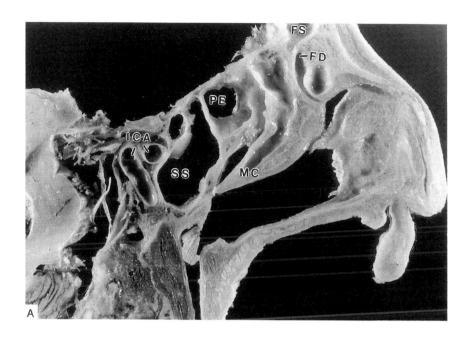

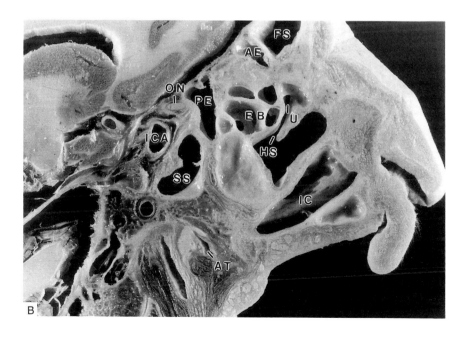

in sinus disease. The posterior ethmoidal air cells are smaller in number, but usually are larger in size. These cells may extend into the lesser wing of the sphenoid. One or more of these cells may be closely related to the optic nerve (Figs. 6b, 7b). Any of the cells related to the optic nerve is termed an Onodi cell (6). The posterior ethmoidal air cells usually drain into the superior meatus and into the supreme meatus if a supreme concha/turbinate is present (Fig. 3). They may also drain into the posterior portion of the middle meatus. Van Alyea described ethmoidal air cells as developing or encroaching on all of the other sinuses as well as passing through the nasal septum to invade structures of the opposite side or in the orbital plate of the maxilla and into pterygopalatine fossa (6).

The anterior air cells are supplied by the anterior and posterior ethmoidal arteries veins and nerves. The posterior air cells are supplied by the anterior and posterior ethmoidal artery as well as branches from the sphenopalatine artery. Therefore the ethmoid labyrinth is supplied by both the internal and external carotid artery systems. The lymphatic drainage of the anterior cells is into the submandibular nodes and from the posterior cells into the retropharyngeal nodes.

REFERENCES

1. Hollinshead WH. Anatomy for Surgeons: The Head and Neck, 3rd ed. Philadelphia: J.B. Lippincott, 1982.
2. Van Alyea OE. Sphenoid sinus. Arch Otolaryngol 1941; 34:225–53.
3. Fujii K, Chambers SM, Rhoton AL. Neurovascular relations of the sphenoid sinus. J. Neurosurg 1979;50:31–9.
4. Alberti PW. Applied surgical anatomy of the maxillary sinus. Otolaryngol Clin North Am 1976; 9:3–20.
5. Van Alyea OE. The ostium maxillare. Arch Otolaryngol 1936; 24:553–69.
6. Van Alyea OE. Ethmoid labyrinth. Arch Otolaryngol 1939; 29:881–902.
7. Rice DH, Schaeffer SD. Endoscopic Paranasal Sinus Surgery. New York: Raven Press, 1988.
8. Mattox DE, Delaney RG: Anatomy of the ethmoid sinus. Otolaryngol Clin North Am 1985; 18:3–14.
9. Wigand ME. Endoscopic Surgery of the Paranasal Sinuses and Anterior Skull Base. New York: Thieme Verlag, 1990.

3

Physiology of Sinusitis

JAMES N. BARANIUK
Georgetown University
Washington, D.C.

I. INTRODUCTION

Nasal sinuses, and specifically the ostiomeatal complex of the middle meatus, have a major design flaw. Sinuses are air-filled spaces connected to the rest of the nasal mucosa by narrow orifices. Obstruction of a sinus orifice by any of a legion of causes leads to retention of mucosal secretions within the sinus. Inoculation of micro-organisms into this luxuriant culture media leads to infection. Acute, intermittent, or chronic obstruction can lead to sinusitis (1).

Mucosal secretions are generated as a component of the normal homeostatic defense function of the upper airway. In the maxillary sinus, these secretions must be swept by mucociliary action upward, against the pull of gravity, and out of the narrow sinus meatus. Similar mucociliary mechanisms are at work in the bronchial tree, but in that location cough serves as a useful adjunct for clearance. Sinuses, which are encased in bone, do not cough. The respiratory maneuvers that can dislodge sinus secretions, and particularily mucus obstruction of sinus orifices, are limited to sneezing and snorting, which produce rapid, but limited changes in nasal cavity air pressure in the hope of developing an air pressure gradient between the sinus and nasal cavities that could "uncork" the sinus. As a result, any condition that can lead to obstruction of a sinus orifice can lead to acute, recurrent, or chronic sinusitis. Successful treatment of sinusitis is totally dependent on opening the obstructed orifice, draining the obstructed viscus, permitting mucociliary clearance of secretions, eliminating microbiological overgrowth, and addressing the underlying cause of the ostial obstruction.

I will discuss the anatomy and physiology of the respiratory mucosa with the hope of identifying mechanisms that could contribute to obstruction of the sinus ostia, and the initiation, continuation, and resolution of sinusitis.

II. EPITHELIUM

The mucosae of the nasal cavity, ostiomeatal complex, sinuses, and bronchi have both similarities and differences. The epithelium in each location is very similar, and consists of ciliated epithelial cells, nonciliated secretory cells, mucus-containing goblet cells, and basal cells. Goblet cells decrease in density from the nose to bronchi, with sinuses having an intermediate density of 9,700 cells/mm^2 (2).

Mucus, which is the product of goblet cells and submucosal glands, forms a gel phase that floats above a 5 μm thick sol phase. The cilia of ciliated cells are embedded in the gel phase and sweep it along with a coordinated stroke. The gel is pulled over the lubricating sol phase above the cells. The mucus is swept towards the ostia of sinuses, and posteriorly through the nasopharynx to the esophagus. Inhaled particles stick to the mucus and are eventually swallowed. Diffusion of allergens and other toxic substances through the mucus barrier may be limited by binding to antibodies and physicochemical interactions with glycoconjugates and other macromolecules. The viscosity of the mucus is regulated by its hydration state. Ciliary beat frequency is decreased in sinusitis, but the frequency returns to normal when infected mucus is removed from the surface of the tissue (3). Other factors, including α_2-adrenergic agonists (4), may reduce ciliary beat frequency in vivo. This reduction could lead to an inability to clear mucus and other secretions from the sinus during infection.

The basal cells rest upon a thin, continuous basement membrane. Deposition of collagen and other connective tissue components beneath the basement membrane in chronic inflammation can lead to the impression of "thickening" of the basement membrane. The mechanisms leading to this pathologic finding, and its functional significance in disease states, remain obscure.

III. VESSELS AND VASCULAR PERMEABILITY

The lamina propria is very vascular. Postcapillary venules are the sites of plasma exudation and leukocyte diapedesis. Fenestrated capillaries are present. Although it is tempting to suggest that plasma and interstitial fluid may freely exchange through the fenestrations of these highly specialized capillaries as occurs in the renal glomerulus, there is no good evidence that this can in fact occur in the nasal mucosa. Regulation of arterial blood flow to the superficial vascular plexus is thought to be a crucial regulating event in the generation of tracheal and nasal secretions (5,6). With increases in vascular hydrostatic pressure, the flux of plasma out of vessels, and the flux of interstitial fluid across the epithelium, is increased. The role of the epithelium in regulating the transepithelial flux has been the topic of much debate. Epithelial cell tight junctions, pinocytotic transport, and ion transport with passive water movement may each play significant roles (7,8). The relative importance of each mechanism may depend upon the neurohormonal environment, pathologic state, and magnitude of the hydrostatic pressure that may be driving the vascular and interstitial fluid fluxes. Increases in the volume of mucosal interstitial fluid define edema. Edema fluid can be reduced by increased flux across the epithelium (a rapid process) or lymphatic drainage (a slow process). Lymphatic drainage may be an important route for lymphocyte, antigen processing cell, and other cell traffic out of the respiratory mucosa towards draining lymphatic structures.

Increased sinus cavity hydrostatic pressures after orifice obstruction could oppose vascular hydrostatic pressures and reduce the flux of plasma. This could reduce the flow of plasma from vessels into the interstitium and across the epithelium into the sinus cavity. Under such unusual high-pressure circumstances, local blood flow may also be impaired, leading to reduced oxygen delivery that could promote the development of an anaerobic environment. Inoculation of micro-organisms into a stagnant, exudate-rich, closed space is a formula for sinus disaster.

IV. PLASMA IMMUNOGLOBULINS

Plasma exudation is the source of albumin, IgG, IgM, fibrinogen, complement, and other plasma proteins in the interstitial fluid and respiratory secretions (Table 1). These factors have important roles in antigen-specific and nonspecific antimicrobial defense and inflammation. IgG, IgM, and IgA to *Haemophilus influenzae* lipopolysaccharides are generated during active sinusitis, and are secreted into the maxillary sinuses (9). Increased convalescent antibody levels are present in plasma. Antibodies to *Streptococcus pneumoniae*, *Haemophilus influenzae*, and *Branhamella catarrhalis* have also been isolated from middle ear fluid, indicating that circulating antibodies to the most prevalent micro-organisms infecting sinuses and other upper airway structures are readily secreted by mucosal surfaces. Intravenously administered immunoglobulin (predominantly IgG) is secreted by the maxillary sinus, even in chronic sinusitis, indicating that vascular and epithelial permeability are maintained in disease states (10). It is unlikely that there is any impairment in the vascular delivery of antimicrobial agents, such as plasma proteins and drugs, to the sinus mucosa in disease states. However, limitation of diffusion of these factors into an organizing exudate may restrict their effectiveness.

Table 1 Concentrations of Proteins in Anterior Nasal Secretions Collected 10 min after Saline Challenge

Proteins	Mean (μg/ml)	(95% Confidence limits)	% Total protein
Vascular origin			
Albumin	12	(−3–27)	15
IgG	3	(1–6)	4
monomeric IgA	2	(0–4)	2
IgM	<2		<2
Serous cell origin			
Lysozyme	12	(9–14)	14
Secretory IgA	12	(4–27)	14
Lactoferrin	3	(1–8)	4
Glycoconjugate[a]	93	(55–130)	
Protein content[b]	23	(15–32)	28
Total protein	82	(38–126)	

Method used is that of Raphael et al. (19,25,29,40).
[a]Concentration compared to a standard mucin.
[b]Concentration converted to equivalent μg human serum albumin protein.

Continued infection and sinusitis must be due to other factors, such as the obstruction of a sinus orifice and inoculation with bacteria resistant to inactivation by specific antibody and nonspecific plasma and epithelial defense molecules. Subjects with selective specific antibody deficiencies, delayed acquisition of specific humoral immunity, or immunoglobulin subtype deficiency (11) may be at greater risk for bacterial overgrowth and sinusitis since they would lack specific antibodies in their sinus secretions (Table 2). In 1 series, 34 of 61 patients with recurrent sinusitis had some type of immunologic abnormality, with low IgG$_3$ concentrations and poor amnestic antibody responses to pneumococcal antigen 7 being the most prevalent (12). Prevalent, defective responses to *Haemophilus influenzae* type B capsular polysaccharide and selective IgG$_2$ deficiency have also been described (13).

Alterations of secretory IgA (sIgA) also occur in chronic sinusitis. sIgA is locally synthesized by respiratory mucosal plasma cells and is secreted via serous cells of submucosal glands. sIgA is an IgA dimer with a J-piece protein connected to secretory component. Serum IgA is generally a monomer with no secretory component, and is probably produced in gut and lymph node tissues. sIgA will be discussed along with other submucosal gland products below.

Table 2 Acute, Intermittent, and Chronic Conditions that Predispose to Ostiomeatal Obstruction

---

Anatomical: Septal and turbinate deformities
  Trauma
  Congenital/developmental
Rhinitis
  Allergic rhinitis after allergen exposure
  Nonallergic rhinitis with mucosal swelling
  Viral infection
  Occupational rhinitis [75]
  Toxic gas exposure
Nasal polyps
  Idiopathic
  Aspirin sensitivity
  Secondary to chronic inflammation
  Choanal polyps [76]
Ciliary dyskinesias: Kartagener's syndrome
Cystic fibrosis
Acute facial or head trauma
  Trauma-induced mucosal swelling
  Neurogenic mucosal swelling (?)
  Nasotracheal intubation [77]
Wegener's granulomatosis
Squamous cell carcinoma

V. VENOUS SINUSOIDS AND THE ERECTILE NATURE OF RESPIRATORY MUCOSA

Deep in the nasal mucosa lie venous sinusoids. Arterial blood flows into sinusoids through arteriovenous anastomoses (AVA). Increases in blood flow in conjunction with contraction of the draining "throttle" veins leads to filling of the sinusoids. As the sinusoids swell, they increase the thickness of the turbinate and septal mucosa. Filling of turbinate and septal venous sinusoids regulates airflow in the so-called "nasal valve" region of the anterior nasal cavity. Constriction of AVA reduces blood flow and sinusoidal filling, permits the mucosa to shrink, and increases nasal patency. Autonomic nerves coordinate the cyclical filling and contraction of sinusoids that regulate nasal airflow ("nasal cycle") (14). Cyclic changes in nasal mucosal volumes have been seen in the turbinates, nasal mucosa, and ethmoid sinus using magnetic resonance imaging (15).

However, no variation in thickness was seen in the maxillary, frontal, and sphenoid sinuses, suggesting that they do not participate in this circadian rhythm. Circadian rhythms may also regulate the amount of secretion generated from the nasal turbinates by plasma exudation and glandular secretion (16).

Sinusoidal filling and mucosal swelling can completely obstruct airflow bilaterally in pathologic conditions. The distributions of venous sinusoids and the erectile apparatus in the ostiomeatal region and sinus mucosa are poorly documented. However, dilation of vessels can rapidly thicken the mucosa. Swelling of the orifice mucosa may be a common mechanism that contributes to the obstruction of sinus passages and the impeded clearance of sinus secretions.

Constriction of blood vessels in the mucosa, however, can increase both nasal and sinus ostial patency. The α-adrenergic agonist, phenylpropanolamine (100 mg), and exercise increase maxillary ostial patency in both normal patients and those with chronic maxillary sinusitis (17,18). The effects of exercise are likely to be mediated by the sympathetic nervous system. These observations suggest that vasoconstriction reduces mucosal blood flow, reduces the filling of capacitance vessels, and, therefore, reduces the thickness of the mucosa. These vessels may contribute to the pathologic basis of sinusitis, and be targets for effective adjunctive therapy.

VI. SUBMUCOSAL GLANDS AND MUCUS

Submucosal glands are present in highest density in the turbinates (e.g., approximately 9,000 glands in the inferior turbinate alone (2)) and trachea and larger bronchi with lower densities in the smaller bronchi, and few in the sinuses. Fewer than 100 submucosal glands are present in the maxillary sinus (2). Submucosal glands at all sites are similar. They are tubuloacinar, and contain serous cells grouped as a so-called serous cap at the distal pole of the gland with more centrally located mucous cells. The acini are surrounded by contractile myoepithelial cells that squeeze exocytosed cellular products into ducts and onto the mucosal surface. Serous cell products (19) include lysozyme, lactoferrin, secretory IgA, proteases, antiproteases, fibronectin (20), and many other enzymes (Table 1), while mucous cells secrete sulfated mucins (21,22). Proteoglycans may be secreted by several populations of cells. These exocytosed macromolecules coat the surface of the mucosa and protect against inhaled micro-organisms and other damaging substances.

Stammberger (23) has postulated that glandular hyperplasia in the region of the anterior ethmoidal sinus and ostiomeatal complex is the cause of the permanent and nonreducible membrane thickening near the orifice of the maxillary sinus (see below and Fig. 1). Goblet cell hyperplasia is common in the epithelium, and ducts, with mucous cell hyperplasia in the glands. The factors that regulate mucous cell proliferation are poorly understood (24). Distention of the

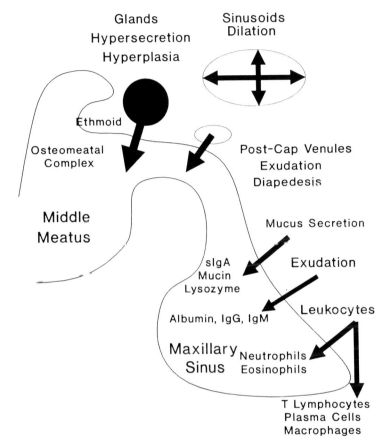

Figure 1 The ostiomeatal complex of the middle meatus contains the ethmoid sinus and maxillary sinus orifice. Submucosal gland secretion and hyperplasia, sinusoidal dilatation, edema, and plasma exudation can obstruct the ostia. Maxillary sinus secretions are derived from plasma exudation, goblet cell secretion, and some mucosal gland exocytosis. In the event of obstruction, mucociliary transport cannot remove these secretions from the sinus. If microbial inoculation occurs, plasma exudation is increased, and neutrophils, lymphocytes, and other imflammatory cells are recruited to the area. These processes contribute to the signs and symptoms of sinusitis.

glandular acini with disruption of their architecture can lead to mucus extravasation and the formation of mucoceles: mucus-generating epithelia that secrete into a closed, submucosal space and become cystic. In addition to the secretion of abundant, viscous mucus, the hypertrophic glands themselves can physically increase mucosal thickness and contribute to permanent obstruction.

Secretory IgA can be considered a serous cell product, and is particularly important for mucosal defense. sIgA is synthesized by nasal mucosal plasma cells that congregate adjacent to submucosal glands (25). The IgA is dimeric, connected by the J-chain. The locally synthesized $(IgA)_2$–J complex is bound to secretory component (SC) on the surface of serous cells, and is transported through those cells, and exocytosed into glandular lumens as a $(IgA)_2$–J–SC complex (sIgA) (26). Specific sIgA directed against the M-protein of *Streptococcus pyogenes* protects against bacterial infection by coating the microbe and preventing its adhereance to the mucosa (27). The number of bacteria that can adhere to nasal mucosal cells is greater in subjects with chronic sinusitis than in normal subjects. The presence of specific anti-M-protein sIgA reduced bacterial adherence. Subjects with chronic sinusitis have increased total IgA concentrations in nasal secretions, but reduced specific antibody reactivity against the M-protein (28). This suggests that with prolonged infection, there is a loss of specific antibody production, but an increase in nonspecific IgA production. These complex changes in IgA synthesis and secretion during chronic sinusitis require additional evaluation.

Regulation of secretion from nasal submucosal glands is altered in patients with chronic sinusitis compared to normal subjects (29). Subjects with chronic sinusitis are less responsive to methacholine on nasal provocation testing, and secrete significantly reduced amounts of sIgA and lysozyme. They may also have marginally reduced plasma exudation. Responses to histamine appear to be similar to those in normal subjects. These data, and others recorded after bradykinin nasal provocation (30), suggest that there are functional changes in mucosal secretion in chronic sinusitis, but the mechanisms remain obscure.

In contrast to the ostiomeatal region, the sinus mucosa itself appears to have a low number of submucosal glands, suggesting that there may be a relative paucity of the diverse and potent glandular antimicrobial factors in sinus secretions. Exudated plasma protein factors may be of greater antimicrobial importance in the sinus that in turbinate and tracheobronchial secretions.

VII. NEURAL REGULATION OF MUCOSAL SECRETION AND VASCULAR TONE

The nasal and sinus mucosa is innervated by sensory, parasympathetic, and sympathetic nerves (5,31).

The sensory nerves are generally of small diameter, and are mechanical and chemosensitive (5,31). These trigeminal neurons may play roles in detecting the conditions of inhaled air and in regulating the response of the mucosa to drying, cooling, or other conditions. These nerves innervate vessels, glands, and lamina propria, and extend into the epithelium. Each nerve is extensively branched. They respond to histamine, bradykinin, SO_2, H^+, K^+, capsaicin, and other nocifers by depolarizing. A wave of depolarization is conducted from the initial axon branch to the entire neuron including all the peripheral and central branches. In the periphery, the depolarization leads to the release of neuropeptides from specialized neurosecretory varicosities present near glands and vessels. This efferent function of these afferent nerves is called the "axon response." It represents a rapid recruitment mechanism that can respond to an initially limited mucosal injury and amplify the inflammatory response. Immunohistochemical studies indicate that these nerves contain and release combinations of neuropeptides including substance P (SP), neurokinin A (NKA), calcitonin gene-related peptide (CGRP), and probably other peptides (5,31). The distribution of peptide-binding sites on nasal epithelium, glands, and vessels suggests that they play an important role in the regulation of mucosal secretion after injury. The axon response may include arterial and venous dilation with increased blood flow (SP, CGRP), vascular permeability (SP), glandular secretion (SP, gastrin-releasing peptide [GRP]), and epithelial permeability and/ or secretion (SP, GRP). In pig mucosa, the magnitude of the axon response has been assessed and found to amount to a small increase in superficial blood flow (32). The potential glandular contribution has not been measured.

A much more important effect of sensory nerve stimulation appears to be the notification of central registries of nasal injury and the recruitment of systemic and parasympathetic reflexes (5,31). Nasal sensory nerve stimulation produces sensations of itch, burning pain, and "congestion" or "fullness," and "airflow" (may actually represent mucosal "cooling"). Itch and pain may be related to stimulation of specific nerve populations by histamine and bradykinin. Sensations of "congestion" may be related to increased sensory neural messages emanating from sinusoids or other capacitance vessels as they dilate, or "warm" receptors as they are stimulated by increased blood flow and an influx of 37°C blood into the 30–34°C nasal mucosa. Nasal anesthesia leads to a sensation of nasal patency or improved "airflow." Could this be due to inactivation of "warm" receptors? Nasal "cold" receptors, which may also be present in the nose to detect the temperature of inhaled air, appear to be stimulated by menthol, a popular component of proprietary nasal and sinus remedies that promote a sensation of airflow (33). Confusion about subjective sensations and pharmacologic effects of drugs on specific neural receptors has hampered our understanding of the roles of sensory nerves in the nose.

Stimulation of these populations of nociceptive sensory nerves clearly occurs in sinusitis since sensations of pain and congestion are universal complaints. The pressure symptoms and pain in sinusitis may be due to vascular engorgement with stimulation of mechanoreceptors in mucosal walls; pressure changes due to absorption of oxygen from air in obstructed sinuses that stimulate mechanoreceptors; and release of nocifers such as bradykinin, histamine, prostaglandins, and other inflammatory factors that stimulate chemosensitive nociceptive nerves.

Sensory nerves also may play roles in pathologic syndromes. Irritants, cold air, and stimulants of sensory nerves induce nasal obstruction and rhinorrhea in both normal and rhinitic subjects, but patients with vasomotor rhinitis (nonallergic perennial rhinitis, chronic cholinergic rhinitis) have exaggerated responses. Patients with vasomotor rhinitis that is characterized by profuse discharge have larger secretory responses to topical capsaicin, nicotine, and methacholine than either patients with vasomotor rhinitis with nasal obstruction and sneezing alone as their primary complaints, or normal control subjects (34). The mechanisms of the nasal sensory and cholinergic "hyperreactivity" remain unresolved.

Stimulation of the central nervous system by these trigeminal nociceptive nerves recruits central systemic reflexes including the sneeze (35). Nasobronchial and sinobronchial reflexes have been postulated to explain cough, bronchoconstriction, and bronchial hyperreactivity that coincides with sinus disease, but at present this remains a controversial topic (36). Pharyngeal pooling of rhinosinal secretions with stimulation of laryngeal nociceptive nerves or stimulation of bradykinin-sensitive pharyngeal nociceptors may play roles in this symptom complex.

Trigeminal nerve stimulation leads to recruitment of parasympathetic reflexes (5,31). These reflexes regulate glandular secretion, increase mucosal blood flow, and dilate capacitance vessels. Their effects are far greater than those of the axon response. Parasympathetic nerves contain combinations of acetylcholine, vasoactive intestinal peptide (VIP), and possibly other peptides. Acetylcholine likely acts upon M_1 and M_3 muscarinic receptor subtypes to cause vasodilation and serous and mucous cell exocytosis (37,38). VIP-binding sites are present on vessels, glands, and epithelium (39). VIP is likely a vasodilator in vivo, but also has secretagogic properties in vitro. The cholinergic component of parasympathetic nerves regulates glandular secretion after allergen challenge (19,40). In sinus mucosa, these nerves are probably more important in stimulating vasodilation given the relative paucity of submucosal glands. As such, they may cause increases in the thickness of the mucosa and hydrostatic pressure-driven plasma exudation (6) and so contribute to the pathology of sinusitis. For example, swimmer's sinusitis does not seem to be related to inhaled water, but could result from stimulation of anterior nasal sensory nerves with recruitment of bilateral, vasodilatory parasympathetic reflexes that lead to swelling of the sinus and ostiomeatal mucosa (41). Anticholinergic drugs have not been well studied in sinusitis, and so the role of cholinergic mechanisms is not established. Parasympathetic mechanisms may be overwhelmed by local inflammatory responses in infectious sinusitis, and it may not be possible to deliver therapeutic doses of these drugs to their sites of action.

The actions of sympathetic nerves have been alluded to above. Exercise, and α-adrenergic agonists, decrease the thickness of the mucosa and increase nasal and ostial patency (17,18). Sympathetic nerves innervate arterial and venous vessels including arteriovenous anastomoses, with only occasional nerves found around glands. Sympathetic nerves contain either norepinephrine, or norepinephrine plus neuropeptide Y (NPY) (42). Norepinephrine and NPY are both vasoconstrictors, but NPY is slower in onset, and very long in duration (43). NPY-binding sites are present on arterial, AVA, and venous vessels (42). The presence of both NPY-containing nerves and NPY-binding sites in AVA suggests that NPY acts as a vasoconstrictor at this key location in vivo. NPY nasal provocation leads to decreased nasal airflow resistance and reduced plasma exudation (44). NPY agonists may be excellent long-acting vasoconstrictors that may augment or replace α-adrenergic agonists. Vasoconstrictors have a place in the treatment of sinusitis since they can reduce the vasodilation that occurs during mucosal inflammation and so assist in increasing ostial patency, which will facilitate the clearance of non-impacted sinus secretions. Overuse of α-adrenergic vasoconstrictors leads to rhinitis medicamentosa and refractory and bothersome sensations of nasal congestion and decreased airflow.

Sensory and parasympathetic reflexes probably act in concert to stimulate vasodilation, vascular permeability, and glandular secretion, and other pro-inflammatory events after mucosal injury. Activity of the vasodilating parasympathetic and vasoconstricting sympathetic systems likely are coordinated at a central level, and may regulate the nasal cycle and other circadian rhythms. Disruption of sympathetic innervation of the nasal mucosa, as in Horner's syndrome, for example, can lead to intractible hypersecretion and congestion indicating the importance of both limbs of the autonomic nervous system in maintaining normal nasal function.

VIII. INFECTION

Stammberger contends that

> Most infections of the paranasal sinuses are rhinogenic, spreading from the nose into the sinuses. The common focus of infection in cases of recurring sinusitis is the stenotic areas of the anterior ethmoid, with infection recurring in the large sinuses. The anterior ethmoid, especially the infundibulum, is thus a key location for infection or cure, and maxillary as well as frontal sinuses are fully dependent on the pathophysiologic conditions there. Histological examination demonstrates that massive changes of the nasal glands are the reason for permanent mucosal thickening. Retention cysts, highly viscous mucus, mucus extravasations, and metaplastic epithelial changes add to the vicious cycle of blockage in the ostium–meatus unit (23).

Table 3 Origins of Microbes Inoculated into Obstructed Sinuses

Rhinogenic hypothesis
    Normal nasopharyngeal/oropharyngeal flora infect the partially/intermittently
      obstructed sinus by local inoculation with nasal cavity secretions
Dentogenic hypothesis
    Orosinusal fistula
    Perforation of maxillary sinus during root canal or other dental work
    Gingivitis with local bacteremia/fungemia via shared, collateral venous blood flow
      or lymphatic channels to maxillary sinus

This classic description identifies the anterior ethmoid cells of the middle meatus as the original culprit that leads to the subsequent involvement of larger sinuses.

These observations indicate that sinusitis is a two-step process that involves obstruction and infection. Recent studies in rabbits in vivo support this contention (45). Obstruction of the sinus orifice is necessary, but not sufficient by itself: infection of the obstructed sinus is also necessary. Infection of an unobstructed sinus with virulent *Streptococcus pneumoniae* alone did not result in infection.

Based upon this observation, it is conceivable that many acute and chronic causes of ostiomeatal "swelling" can lead to obstruction of a sinus orifice, the intermittent or long-term retention of sinus secretions, and the inoculation of micro-organisms from the nasal mucosa ("rhinogenic" hypothesis) into those secretions with their subsequent proliferation within the protected habitat of the viscid mucus. "Infection" leads to a mucosal response including leukocyte infiltration. Mucosal edema, vasodilation, and hypersecretion may worsen the picture by increasing the degree of ostial obstruction until total obstruction and retention of all secretions occurs. Chronic infectious sinusitis may result from recurring microbial inoculation of intermittently obstructed sinuses, or infections in sinuses that cannot drain their infected, inspissated secretions spontaneously. The crucial role of drainage is indicated by the high success rate of permanent sinus drainage systems (46). Current practice indicates that these conditions are beyond the reach of medical therapy, and require the exacting slice of the endoscopic knife (23,47).

Up to half of cases (40.6%) of chronic maxillary sinusitis, which has an incidence of 0.02% in one population, may have a dental cause ("dentogenic theory," Table 3) and require oral and sinus evaluations (48,49). Marginal periodontitis and periapical granuloma account for 83% of all dental causes. This cause of sinusitis is thought to be rare before age 30 years.

Virus infections lead to mucosal swelling and may alter local mucosal defense factors and secretion so that bacteria can more easily invade and proliferate in partially or intermittently occluded sinuses.

In acute and subacute sinusitis, the predominant organisms are commensal strains of *Streptococcus pneumoniae*, *Haemophilus influenzae*, and *Branhamella catarrhalis* (50). Chronic infections have a different spectrum of organisms. In chronic maxillary sinusitis, up to 92% of carefully collected samples can be successfully cultured, and yield anaerobic bacteria alone (56%), mixed anaerobic, facultative and aerobic bacteria (32%), or aerobic or facultative bacteria (12%) (51). The predominant anaerobes were cocci and *Bacteroides* spp., while the predominant aerobes and facultative organisms were *Streptococcus* spp. and *Staphylococcus aureus*. *Staphylococcus aureus* carriage in the upper respiratory tract can be a source for toxic shock syndrome (52). The differences in organisms between acute and chronic disease suggest that the conditions leading to the sinus obstruction, the source of the innoculum, and the presence of inflammatory responses, and the evolution of the bacterial environment can determine which organisms are selected to proliferate in the ecologic niche, and that there may be an evolutionary progression of organisms in different phases of the chronic or developing disease. Additional host factors may have an impact on the proliferating organisms. Diabetes, for example, may facilitate fungal infection, while atopic subjects may develop allergic *Aspergillus* sinusitis (see below). Fungal infection may follow partially treated bacterial infections, or inadequately drained sinusitis.

IX. LEUKOCYTES

Bacterial and fungal infections induce vigorous host responses. Neutrophil infiltration with the production of pus is a hallmark of acute infectious sinusitis. There are many chemotactic stimuli for neutrophils that are generated during sinusitis including bacterial products, complement fragments, LTB_4, and neutrophil chemotactic factor from injured or other recruited cells. Neutrophils adhere to specific adhesion molecules in postcapillary venules, and, in the presence of chemotactic stimuli, diapedese. Their role is to phagocytose and kill infecting bacteria, and they have a wide range of enzymes and oxidant-generating systems to carry out their tasks. Neutrophils in the sinus and even in circulating blood become activated and express CR1 receptors that facilitate C3b-mediated opsonization (53). Neutrophils are the primary source of lactate, a product of glycolysis, in purulent secretions (54). Anaerobic bacteria are isolated only from secretions containing high amounts of lactate. This indicates the absence of oxidative metabolism and oxygen delivery in these patients.

In chronic maxillary sinusitis, the neutrophilic infiltrate can be augmented or replaced by a mononuclear infiltrate (55) that appears along with goblet cell hyperplasia, sub-basement-membrane connective tissue deposition, submucosal gland hyperplasia, and subepithelial edema. Infiltrating lymphocytes are an important component of the mononuclear infiltrate. On immunohistochemical analysis, CD3 + cells (representing all T cells) represent about 38% of the total mononuclear cells (56). Approximately 20% of all mononuclear cells are CD8 + (marker of suppressor/cytoxic T cells), 13% are CD4 + (marker of helper T cells), and 9% are CD20 + (B lymphocyte marker). The B cells are predominantly plasma cells. This distribution of markers is consistent in three histopathologic types of chronic maxillary sinusitis: edematous, cellular infiltrative, and mixed patterns. However, if the histologic examination demonstrates a fibrous pattern, an increase in the frequency of CD3 + cells (74% of mononuclear cells), CD8 + cells (63%), no change in CD4 + cells (13%), and a decrease in CD20 + cells (3%) were seen. Unfortunately, the total numbers of each cell population per unit area in the mucosa, and studies in control, noninfected tissues, were not available for comparison. These observations suggest that CD8 + cells may be associated with a fibrotic histologic appearance.

Abnormalities of T-cell function have been described in chronic sinusitis including reduced migration inhibition factor (cytokine) generation, reduced delayed-type hypersensitivity skin test reactivity to candidin and/or streptokinase-streptodornase (extracts of commensual upper respiratory tract organisms), and skin test reactivity to hemolytic *Streptococcus* (Table 3) (57–59). Some of these generalized defects have been reversed by treatment with the thymic hormone preparation thymostimulin (60).

These observations indicate that a relatively high percentage of sinusitis cases are associated with immunoglobulin subclass abnormalities, sIgA defects, lacunar deficits in antibody repetoires, and that modulation of cellular and humoral immunity can occur (Table 4). While each defect could play important

Table 4   Immunologic Abnormalities that May Permit Infectious Sinusitis

---

Selective IgA deficiency
Common variable hypogammaglobulinemia
IgG subclass deficiencies
Lacunar defects in immunoglobulin repertoire with selective, specific antibody
  deficiency
Developmental delay in specific immunoglobulin responses (e.g., *Haemophilus
  influenzae*)
Acquired or congenital selective cellular immune response deficiency to commensal
  bacteria and fungi

---

permissive roles in sinusitis, some of the findings could be merely epiphenomena of chronic infection. Additional, carefully controlled studies are required to determine the pathophysiological significance of these observations. In addition, the role of delayed-type hypersensitivity in chronic sinusitis remains undecided. Future studies may reveal the subtypes of T_{H1} helper T cells (associated with delayed type hypersensitivity) and T_{H2} helper T cells (associated with atopic diseases) in normal and diseased sinus mucosa.

X. ATOPY

Mast cells may play a role in sinusitis. Although only about 15–25% of cases of sinusitis are associated with allergic diseases, sinusitis can clearly be a complication of allergic rhinitis (61). Mast cell degranulation releases histamine, PGD_2, leukotrienes, and generates bradykinin, which causes vascular dilation and permeability and stimulate sensory nerves. Neural reflex mechanisms could play a role in allergen-induced sinus symptoms. Mast cell degranulation in the anterior turbinate after pollen exposure, could lead to sensory nerve stimulation and recruitment of parasympathetic reflexes that could affect the nasal mucosa in the region of the ostiomeatal complex and the sinuses and lead to further vasodilation, plasma exudation, and glandular secretion. These secretory processes could acutely increase mucosal thickness and reduce ostial patency while increasing sinus, turbinate, and other mucosal secretion. Retention of mucoid sinus secretions and intermittent ostial obstruction could result. Nasal application of allergen leads to maxillary sinus pressure symptoms, acute headache, and otalgia, indicating stimulation of sensory nerves, as well as radiologic evidence of increased maxillary sinus mucosal thickening and sinus opacification (62). This suggests that neural mechanisms can greatly amplify the inflammatory response to allergen, and that the sinuses can be affected as a result of either direct allergen-induced degranulation with mediator release in the middle meatus or sinus or neural reflex mechanisms. The frequency of sinus mucosal thickening detectable by magnetic resonance imaging has been reported to be greatest in July, August, September, and December (63). It is tempting to speculate that exposure to grass pollen, ragweed pollen, or mold, or seasonal viral epidemics during these months could have been associated with the sinus mucosal thickening.

Dust mites may also be a factor. As many as 68% of patients with chronic sinusitis have immediate skin test reactivity to mite allergen, indicating the presence of specific IgE (64). Mite-specific IgG was found in 72% of patients. The IgG titers were higher in subjects with rhinosinusitis than in a control group with asthma alone. The mite-specific IgE titers were higher in the asthma group. While bacterial-specific IgG would have a beneficial role in infectious sinusitis (e.g., complement fixation) (65), the role of allergen-specific IgG is not known.

Allergen-specific IgG in nasal secretions may be protective since it could bind to inhaled allergens and facilitate their elimination. Increased allergen-specific IgG may be one beneficial result of allergy injection therapy (61,66).

Eosinophils are recruited to the sites of mast cell degranulation and release their cytotoxic contents. Major basic protein (MBP) has been identified by immunohistochemistry in chronic sinusitis tissues (67) and has been shown to be toxic to human sinus mucosa in vitro (68,69). MBP can reduce ciliary beat frequency and disrupt epithelial integrity.

Eosinophils are also associated with allergic *Aspergillus* sinusitis. Histopathologic examination of sinus mucosa from these patients reveals eosinophils and Charcot-Leyden crystals interspersed with fungal hyphae (70). These patients have increased serum total IgE and cutaneous hyperreactivity to mold extracts. A chronic allergic reaction in the secreted mucus and mucosa leads to chronic inflammation, mucosal thickening, and retained sinus secretions that harbor the noninvasive fungus.

XI. NASAL POLYPS

Nasal polyps are found in about 17% of cases of chronic maxillary sinusitis, including 13% with dental origin and 23% with rhinogenic origin (48). Their cause is obscure, and is likely to be multifactorial. They are most commonly found in nonatopic asthmatic subjects over the age of 40 years (71). Up to 36% of subjects with aspirin intolerance may have polyps. Aspirin intolerance may be related to increased production or effect of leukotrienes since LTD_4 antagonists reduce symptoms in subjects with allergic rhinitis and asthma (72). Nasal polyps may be an indicator of as yet poorly characterized mucosal processes that lead to thickening of the mucosa and the production of masses (polyps) that can obstruct ostia. Increased nasal airflow through the middle meatus may also play a role since an "aerodynamic" theory has been proposed that suggests that the negative pressure of inspiration may lead to polypoid changes (74). Both nasal polyps and aspirin sensitivity are reviewed in greater detail elsewhere in this volume.

XII. APPROACH AND TREATMENT BASED ON THE PATHOPHYSIOLOGY OF SINUSITIS

The acute, subacute, or chronic course of the sinusitis must be established. Rhinologic causes must be sought including preceding viral infections, allergic rhinitis, polyps with or without aspirin sensitivity, septal and ostiomeatal deformities. Dental causes should be investigated. Patients with recurring sinusitis not associated with the above causes may have specific immunologic defects such as immunoglobulin deficiency states, Kartagener's syndrome, or cystic fibrosis.

The key to effective therapy is drainage of the affected sinuses. This can be approached acutely by topical application of vasocontrictors and anti-inflammatory glucocorticoids. These will reduce vascular congestion and inflammatory responses in the nasal mucosa and promote ostial patency. Antihistamines are of assistance in mast cell-related diseases such as allergic rhinitis. Endoscopic surgical debridement of the ostiomeatal complex of the middle meatus is often necessary in cases of recurring sinusitis to remove permanently thickened mucosa and facilitate drainage. More extensive surgery can now be relegated to cases of very severe disease, or disease related to dental causes that require other surgical approaches.

The other pillar of treatment is effective antibiotic therapy. Acute and chronic infection should be treated with a sufficiently long course of appropriate antibiotics aimed at eradicating the likely community or iatrogenically acquired bacteria or fungi. Culture is necessary in cases that do not respond to conventional therapy.

Each of these treatment issues will be discussed from a clinical perspective elsewhere in this volume. Understanding the differential diagnosis and pathophysiology of sinusitis makes therapeutic approaches more rational. By recognizing that "sinusitis" is not one disease but rather a series of syndromes that result from sinus orifice obstruction by any of a myriad of possible causes, with the inability to clear retained sinus secretions, and subsequent inoculation of nasophayngeal or oropharyngeal microbes into the partially or totally occluded viscus, it is possible to develop new insights into the pathogenesis of sinus inflammation and infection, and their treatment. Despite great progress, many mysteries about the underlying mucosal and immunological abnormalities that constitute the sinusitis diathesis remain to be investigated.

ACKNOWLEDGMENT

Dr. Baraniuk has been granted the Edward Livingston Trudeau Scholar Award by the American Lung Association.

REFERENCES

1. Wald ER. Sinusitis in children. N Engl J Med 1992; 326:319–23.
2. Tos M. Distribution of mucus producing elements in the respiratory tract: differences between upper and lower airways. Eur J Respir Dis Suppl 1982; 128:269–79.
3. Saano V, Nuutinen J, Virta P, Joki S, Karttunen P, Silvastin M. The effect of ATP on the ciliary activity of normal and pathological human respiratory mucosa in vitro. Acta Otolaryngol (Stockh) 1991; 111:130–4.
4. Cervin A, Bende M, Lindberg S, Mercke U, Olsson P. Relations between blood flow and mucociliary activity in the rabbit maxillary sinus. Acta Otolaryngol (Stockh) 1988; 105:350–6.

5. Baraniuk JN. Neural control of human nasal secretion. Pulm Pharmacol 1991; 4:20–31.

6. Persson CGA, Erjefalt I, Alkner U, Baumgarten C, Greiff L, Gustafsson B, Luts A, Pipkorn U, Sundler F, Svensson C, Wollmer P. Plasma exudation as a first line respiratory mucosal defence. Clin Exp Allergy 1991; 21:17–24.

7. Tackeuchi K, Suzumura E, Hirata K, Majima Y, Sakakura Y. Role of transepithelial ion transport as a determinant of mucus viscoelasticity in chronic inflammation of the maxillary sinus. Acta Otolaryngol (Stockh) 1991; 111:1133–8.

8. Peterson BT. Permeability: theory vs. practice in lung research. Am J Physiol (Lung Cell. Mol. Physiol) 1992; 262(6):L243–L56.

9. Harada T, Sakukare Y. Immunologic responses against lipopolysaccharide of *Haemophilus influenzae* in patients with acute sinusitis. Ann Otol Rhinol Laryngol 1988; 97:207–10.

10. Williams P, White A, Wilson JA, Yap PL. Penetration of administered IgG into the maxillary sinus and long-term clinical effects of intravenous immunoglobulin replacement therapy on sinusitis in primary hypogammaglobulinemia. Acta Otolaryngol (Stockh) 1991; 111:550–5.

11. Shapiro GG. Sinusitis in children. J Allergy Clin Immunol 1988; 81:1025–7.

12. Shapiro GG, Virant FS, Furukawa CT, Pierson WE, Bierman CW. Immunological defects in patients with refractory sinusitis. Pediatrics 1991; 87:311–6.

13. Umetsu DT, Ambrosino DM, Quinti I, Sibar GR, Geha RS. Recurrent sinopulmonary infection and impaired antibody responses to bacterial capsular polysaccharide antigen in children with selective IgG-subclass deficiency. N Engl J Med 1985; 313:1247–51.

14. Eccles R. The domestic pig as an experimental animal for studies of the nasal cycle. Acta Otolaryngol (Stockh) 1978; 85:431–6.

15. Zinreich SJ, Kennedy DW, Kumar AJ, Rosenbaum AE, Arrington JA. MR imaging of normal nasal cycle: comparison with sinus pathology. J Comput Assist Tomogr 1988, 12:1014–9.

16. Passali D, Bellussi L. Circadian changes in the secretary activity of nasal mucosa. Acta Otolaryngol (Stockh) 1988, 106:281–5.

17. Melen I, Andreasson L, Ivarsson A, Jannert M, Johansson CJ. Effects of phenylpropanolamine on ostial and nasal airway resistance in healthy individuals. Acta Otolaryngol (Stockh) 1986, 102:99–105.

18. Melen I, Friberg B, Andreasson L, Ivarsson A, Jannert M, Johansson CJ. Effects of phenylpropanolamine on ostial and nasal patency in patients treated for chronic maxillary sinusitis. Acta Otolaryngol (Stockh) 1986, 101:494–500.

19. Raphael GR, Baraniuk JN, Kaliner MA. How and why the nose runs. J Allergy Clin Immunol 1991, 87:457–67.

20. Ito O, Suzaki H, Nomura Y. Immunohistochemical distribution of fibronectin in the mucosa with chronic sinusitis. Acta Otolarygnol (Stockh) 1991; 111:144–8.

21. Patow CA, Shelhamer J, Marom Z, Logun C, Kaliner MA. Analysis of human nasal mucous glucoproteins. Am J Otolaryngol 1984, 5:334–43.

22. Lundgren JD, Shelhamer JH. Pathogenesis of airway mucus hypersecretion. J Allergy Clin Immunol 1990, 85:399–417.

23. Stammberger H. Endoscopic endonasal surgery—concepts in treatment of recurring rhinosinusitis. Part I. Anatomic and pathophysiological considerations. Otolaryngol Head Neck Surg 1986, 94:143–7.
24. Lundgren JD, Baraniuk JN. Mucus secretion in inflammation. Pulm Pharmacol, 1992.
25. Raphael GD, Meredith SD, Baraniuk JN, Druce HM, Banks SM, Kaliner MA. The pathophysiology of rhinitis. II. Assessment of the sources of protein in histamine-induced nasal secretions. Am Rev Respir Dis 1989; 139:791–800.
26. Brandzaeg P. Immune functions in human nasal mucosa and tonsils in health and disease. In: Bienenstock J, ed. Immunology of the Lung. New York: McGraw Hill, 1984:28–95.
27. Kurono Y, Fujiyoshi T, Mogi G. Secretory IgA and bacterial adherence to nasal mucosal cells. Ann Otol Rhinol Laryngol 1989; 98:273–7.
28. Kurono Y, Mogi G. Secretory IgA and serum type IgA in nasal secretion and antibody activity against the M-protein Ann Otol Rhinol Laryngol 1987; 96:419–24.
29. Jeney EMV, Raphael GD, Meredith SD, Kaliner MA. Abnormal nasal glandular secretion in recurrent sinusitis. J Allergy Clin Immunol 1990; 86:10–8.
30. Baraniuk JN, Brayton P, Kaliner MA, Barnes PJ. Perennial rhinitis subjects have altered vascular, glandular, and neural nasal responses to bradykinin. Am Rev Respir Dis 1991; 143:A617.
31. Baraniuk JN, Kaliner MA. Neuropeptides and nasal secretions. Am J Physiol (Lung Cell Mol Physiol 5) 1991; 261:L223–35.
32. Stjarne P, Lacroix JS, Anggard A, Lundberg JM. Compartment analysis of vascular effects of neuropeptides and capsaicin in the pig nasal mucosa. Acta Physiol Scand 1991; 141:335–42.
33. Eccles R, Morris S, Tolley NS. The effects of nasal anesthesia upon nasal stimulation of airflow. Acta Otolaryngol (Stockh) 1988; 106:152–5.
34. Stjarne P, Lundblad L, Lundberg JM, Anggard A. Capsaicin and nicotine sensitive afferent neurones and nasal secretion in healthy human volunteers and in patients with vasomotor rhinitis. Br J Pharmacol 1989; 96:693–701.
35. Raphael GD, Meredith SD, Baraniuk JN, Kaliner M. Nasal reflexes. Am J Rhinology 1988; 2:8–12.
36. Sacha RF, Tremblay NF, Jacobs RL. Chronic cough, sinusitis, and hyperreactive airways in children: an ofter overlooked association. Ann Allergy 1985; 54:195–8.
37. Okayama M, Baraniuk JN, Merida M, Kalier M. Autoradiographic localization of muscarinic receptor subtypes in human nasal mucosa. Am J Respir Cell Mol Biol 1992. submitted.
38. Baraniuk JN, Kaliner MA, Barnes PJ. Muscarinic m3 receptor mRNA in situ hybridization in human nasal mucosa. Am J Rhinol 1992. in press.
39. Baraniuk JN, Okayama M, Lundgren JD, Mullol M, Merida M, Shelhamer JH, Kaliner MA. Vasoactive intestinal peptide (VIP) in human nasal mucosa. J Clin Invest 1990; 86:825–31.
40. Raphael GD, Igarashi Y, White MV, Kaliner MA. The pathophysiology of rhinitis. V. Sources of protein in allergen-induced nasal secretions. J Allergy Clin Immunol 1991; 88:33–43.

41. Deitmer T, Scheffler R. Nasal physiology in swimmers and swimmer's sinusitis. Acta Otolaryngol (Stockh) 1990; 110:286–91.
42. Baraniuk JN, Castellino S, Goff J, Lundgren JD, Mullol J, Merida M, Shelhamer JH, Kaliner MA. Neuropeptide Y (NPY) in human nasal mucosa. Am J Respir Cell Mol Biol 1990, 3:165–73.
43. Potter EK. Neuropeptide Y as an autonomic neurotransmitter. Pharmacol Ther 1988, 37:251–73.
44. Baraniuk JN, Silver PB, Kaliner MA, Barnes PJ. Neuropeptide Y (NPY) is a vasoconstrictor in human nasal mucosa. J Appl Physiol 1991. submitted.
45. Johansson P, Kumlien J, Carlsoo B, Drettner B, Nord CE. Experimental acute sinusitis in rabbits. Acta Otolaryngol (Stockh) 1988; 105:357–66.
46. Berg O, Lejdeborn L. Experience of a permanent ventilation and drainage system in the management of purulent maxillary sinusitis. Ann Otol Rhiniol Laryngol 1990; 99:92–6.
47. Kennedy DW. First-line management of sinusitis: a national problem? Overview. Otolaryngol Head Neck Surg 1990; 103:847–54.
48. Melen I, Lindahl L, Andreasson L, Rundcranz H. Chronic maxillary sinusitis. Definition, diagnosis and relation to dental infections and nasal polyposis. Acta Otolaryngol (Stockh) 1986; 101:320–7.
49. DeFoer C, Fossion E, Vaillant JM. Sinus aspergillosis. J Craniomaxillofac Surg 1990; 18:33–40.
50. Wald ER, Byers C, Guerra N, Casselbrant N, Beste D. Subacute sinusitis in children. J Pediatr 1989; 115:28–32.
51. Brook I. Bacteriology of chronic maxillary sinusitis in adults. Ann Otol Rhinol Larygnol 1989; 98:426–8.
52. Gittelman PD, Jacobs JB, Lebowitz AS, Tierno PM Jr. Staphylococcus aureus nasal carriage in patients with rhinosinusitis. Laryngoscope 1991; 101:733–7.
53. Berg O, Carenfeld C, Hallden G, Hed J. CR1-expression and C3b-mediated phagocytosis of granulocytes in purulent maxillary secretion and peripheral blood from patients with sinusitis. Acta Otolaryngol (Stockh) 1989; 107:130–5.
54. Stierna P, Soderlund K, Hultman E. Chronic maxillary sinusitis. Energy metabolism in sinus mucosa and secretion. Acta Otolaryngol (Stockh) 1991; 111:135–43.
55. Stierna P, Carlsoo B. Histopathological observations in chronic maxillary sinusitis. Acta Otolaryngol (Stockh) 1990; 110:450–8.
56. Nishimoto K, Kotaro U, Teruhiko H, Shun JC, Sakakura Y. Lymphocyte subsets in maxillary mucosa in chronic inflammation. Acta Otolaryngol (Stockh) 1988; 106:291–8.
57. van de Plassche-Boers EM, Drexhage HA, Kokje-Kleingeld M, Leezeenberg HA. Parameters of T cell mediated immunity to commensal micro-organisms in patients wioth chronic purulent rhinosinusitis: a comparison between delayed type hypersensitivity skin test, lymphyocyte transformation test and macrophage migration inhibition factor assay. Clin Exp Immunol 1986; 66:516–24.
58. van de Plassche-Boers EM, Tas M, de Haan-Meulman M, Kleingeld M, Drexhage HA. Abnormal monocyte chemotaxis in patients with chronic purulent rhinosinusitis: an effect of retroviral p15E-related factors in serum. Clin Exp Immunol 1988; 73:348–54, 1988.

59. Toppozada H. Haemolytic streptococcus infection of chronic maxillary sinusitis. An immunological study using the skin window test. J Laryngol Otol 1988; 102:890–3.

60. Tas M, Leezenberg JA, Drexhage HA. Beneficial effects of the thymic hormone preparation thymostimulin in patients with defects in cell-mediated immunity and chronic purulent rhinosinusitis. A double-blind cross-over trial on improvements in monocyte polarization and clinical effects. Clin Exp Immunol 1990; 80:304–13.

61. Naclerio RM. Allergic rhinitis. N Engl J Med 1991; 325:860–9.

62. Pelikan Z, Pelikan-Felipek M. Role of nasal allergy in chronic naxillary sinusitis—diagnostic value of nasal challenge with allergen. J Allergy Clin Immunol 1990; 86:484–91.

63. Conner BL, Roach ES, Laster W, Georgitis JW. Magnetic resonance imaging of the paranasal sinuses: frequency and type of abnormalities. Ann Allergy 1989; 62:457–60.

64. Freudenberger T, Grizzanti JN, Rosenstreich DL. Natural immunity to dust mites in patients with chronic rhinosinusitis. J Allergy Clin Immunol 1988; 82:855–62.

65. Chapman AJ, Jr, Musher DM, Jonsson S, Clarridge JE, Wallace RJ Jr. Development of bactericidal antibody during *Branhamella catarrhalis* infection. J Infect Dis 1985; 151:878–82.

66. Platts-Mills TAE, von Maur RK, Ishizaka K, Normal PS, Lichtenstein LM. IgA and IgG anti-ragweed antibodies in nasal secretions: quantitative measurements of antibodies and correlation with inhibition of histamine release. J Clin Invest 1976; 57:1041–50.

67. Fujisawa T, Kephart GM, Gray BH, Gleich GJ. The neutrophil and chronic allergic inflammation. Immunohistochemical localization of neutrophil elastase. Am Rev Respir Dis 1990; 141:689–97.

68. Hisamtasu K, Ganbo T, Nakazawa T, Murakami Y, Gleich GJ, Makiyama K, Koyama H. Cytotoxicity of human eosinophilic major basic protein to human sinus mucosa in vitro. J Allergy Clin Immunol 1990; 86:52–63.

69. Harlin SL, Ansel DG, Lane SR, Myers J, Kephart GM, Gleich GJ. A clinical and pathological study by chronic sinusitis: the role of the eosinophil. J Allergy Clin Immunol 1988, 81:867–75.

70. Allphin AL, Strauss M, Abdul-Karim FW. Allergic fungal sinusitis: problems in diagnosis and treatment. Laryngoscope 1991; 101:815–20.

71. Settipane GA. Nasal polyps: epidemiology, pathology, immunology, and treatment. Am J Rhinol 1987; 1:119–26.

72. Stechschulte DJ. Leukotrienes in asthma and allergic rhinitis. N Engl J Med 1990; 323:1769–70.

74. Ogawa H. A possible role of aerodynamic factors in nasal polyp formation. Acta Otolaryngol (Suppl) (Stockh) 1986; 430:18–20.

75. Fukuda F, Shibata A. A case-control study of past history of nasal diseases and maxillary sinus cancer in Hokkaido, Japan. Cancer Res 1988; 48:1651–2.

76. Berg O, Carenfelt C, Silversward C, Sobin A. Origin of the choanal polyp. Arch Otolaryngol Head Neck Surg 1988; 114:1270–1.

77. Salord F, Gaussorgues, P, Marti-Flich J, Sirodot N, Allimant C, Lyonnet D, Robert D. Nosocomial maxillary sinusitis during mechanical ventilation: a prospective comparison of orotracheal versus the nasotracheal route for intubation. Intensive Care Med 1990; 16:390–3.

4

Microbiology of Sinusitis

JACK M. GWALTNEY, JR.
University of Virginia Health Sciences Center
Charlottesville, Virginia

I. INTRODUCTION

The paranasal sinuses are sterile under normal conditions (1–4), although intermittent, transient microbial contamination, by way of the sinus ostia, is believed to occur. When conditions are normal, micro-organisms entering the sinuses are thought to be promptly removed by mucociliary clearance. Therefore, for the purpose of understanding the microbiology of sinusitis, it is possible to consider the sinus cavity as a closed space. In the setting of clinical sinus disease, the recovery of a micro-organism from the sinus cavity usually implies some causative importance.

Collection of samples from the sinus cavity for microbial culture and other diagnostic tests requires sinus puncture to avoid contamination of the specimen with the indigenous nasal flora. The rationale for this is discussed below in the section on bacteriology. The results of sample collection by sinus endoscopy, a technically appealing procedure, have not been rigorously compared to the result with sinus puncture. Therefore, the endoscopic method of specimen collection cannot be currently relied upon to provide accurate sinus culture results. In the microbial studies reviewed in this chapter, cultures were performed mainly on specimens obtained by sinus puncture. In many of the studies, quantitative bacterial cultures were also performed to help avoid misinterpretation of culture results due to low-level contamination of the specimens.

The variety of micro-organisms that has now been firmly implicated in acute infection of the sinus cavity is large and includes the viruses, bacteria, and fungi. Evidence implicating other groups, such as the *Chlamydia*, is also being collected. Because of the large number of possible pathogens and the similar illness they produce, the microbial causes of sinusitis cannot be determined by clinical evaluation of the patient. Therefore, the physician must know the usual causes of the infection and plan treatment accordingly or, when indicated, obtain a sinus aspirate for culture. Also, the infectious causes of sinusitis differ in the community and hospital as well as in the impaired host, and these will be considered separately.

The condition often known as chronic sinusitis will be referred to as chronic sinus disease in this chapter. The latter terminology has been selected because chronic sinus disease is best viewed as a condition in which anatomical abnormalities of the nasal passage or other medical conditions have altered the host's resistance so that infection is no longer the primary focus of treatment, although infection may have been important in the initial pathologic process and may still be an active part of the problem.

II. GENERAL PRINCIPLES

Certain microbial organisms are found normally in the nasal cavity and nasopharynx, and those of interest in sinusitis are primarily in the bacterial and fungal families. *Staphylococcus aureus* resides primarily in the nasal vestibule; streptococcal species, including *S. pneumoniae* and *S. pyogenes* and *Haemophilus influenzae* are found in the posterior nasal passages and nasopharynx (Table 1) (5). The latter is also the probable site of colonization for *Moraxella catarrhalis*. The location of the indigenous fungi in the nose has not been as well defined as for the bacteria.

In contrast to the bacteria, the viruses of importance in sinusitis are not part of the normal nasal microbial flora but appear in the upper airway during acute self-limited infections. These infections, which are clinically recognized as common colds and influenzal illnesses, are of primary importance in the pathogenesis of acute community-acquired sinusitis. The role of viruses in the pathogenesis of sinusitis is supported by the clinical observation that acute sinusitis is most often preceded by a common cold and by the recovery of viruses from the sinus cavity of patients with sinusitis (3,6). Also, changes indicative of early sinus disease have been observed in magnetic resonance imaging (MRI) scans of volunteers with experimental rhinovirus infection (7).

Although direct evidence is not available, the current view is that viral infection of the nasal passage and/or sinus leads to and promotes secondary bacterial infection of the sinus cavity. The harmful effects of viral infection on the normal protective mechanisms of the upper airway could be by both promoting

Table 1 Indigenous Bacterial Flora of the Nose

	Frequency of recovery (%)	
	Infants/Children	Adults
Nasal vestibule		
Staphylococcus epidermidis and Micrococcus	35–60	40–100
Staphylococcus aureus	30–85	25–40
Diphtheroids (lipophilic)	15–40	90–100
Gram-negative bacteria	2	1
Posterior nasopharynx		
Streptococcus pneumoniae	45–90	15–25
Haemophilus influenzae	15–70	6–40
Streptococcus pyogenes	3–50	6
Staphylococcus aureus	35–45	12
Diphtheroids	35–50	
Gram-negative bacteria	6	13
Neisseria meningitidis	3–8	4–27

inflammatory changes in the ostiomeatal complex of the nasal cavity and by damaging the epithelial lining of the sinus cavity. These conditions can result in impaired sinus drainage through subosteal or osteal obstruction and impaired mucociliary clearance in the sinus cavity itself.

III. ACUTE COMMUNITY-ACQUIRED SINUSITIS

A. Virologic Characteristics

Several families of viruses have been implicated as causes of the common cold and presumably play a role in the pathogenesis of acute sinusitis (Table 2). Rhinovirus, parainfluenza virus, and influenza virus have been recovered from sinus aspirates of patients with acute community-acquired sinusitis (3,6). The difficulty of growing coronavirus and, to a lesser extent, respiratory syncytial virus has made investigation of these agents more difficult.

The various virus families appear to have different mechanism of pathogenesis. Rhinovirus infection is associated with minimal detectable damage to the epithelial lining of the upper airway (9) and appears to exert its clinical affects primarily through triggering the release of inflammatory mediators. After rhinovirus is deposited in the nasal cavity, it is apparently promptly transported to the adenoid area of the nasopharynx where infection begins. Within 16 hr of viral challenge in volunteers, kinin (10) and interleukin-1 (11) concentrations

Table 2   Viruses Associated with the Common Cold and Influenzal Illnesses

	Primary clinical illness	Recovery from sinus cavity
Rhinovirus	Common cold	Yes
Coronavirus	Common cold	No
Influenza virus	Common cold, influenza, pneumonia	Yes
Parainfluenza virus	Common cold, croup, pneumonia	Yes
Respiratory syncytial virus	Common cold, bronchiolitis, pneumonia	No
Adenovirus	Pharyngoconjunctival fever, adult respiratory distress syndrome	No[a]

[a]The importance of the recovery of an adenovirus from the sinus tissue of a patient with chronic sinus disease (8) is uncertain and may represent a coincidental finding.

are elevated in nasal secretions, which is also at the time when symptoms are beginning. In addition, other mediators and neurogenic reflexes have been implicated in the inflammatory events of rhinovirus colds, including the parasympathetic and adrenergic nervous systems, prostaglandins, and, to a lesser extent, histamine (12). During the second and third day of infection, there appears to be an anterior progression of the infection to involve sites in the nasal passages (9). In most uncomplicated rhinovirus colds, symptoms subside rapidly during the fourth and fifth day of infection and have ended by a week. In adults, viral shedding in nasal secretions continues for an average duration of 3 weeks although the clinical illness has subsided.

In one-quarter of natural rhinovirus colds that persist into the second week (13), the sinuses may have become involved in the pathologic process. Infection and/or inflammation in the anterior ethmoid air cells, poorly visualized on standard sinus radiographs (14), is now recognized as being important in the development of acute sinusitis. In one small study, one-third of volunteers with experimental rhinovirus colds developed MRI scan changes of mucosal thickening or fluid accumulation in the sinuses during the course of their illness (7). Of particular interest was the finding that nasal mucus secretion weights were fourfold higher in the volunteers with sinus MRI abnormality than in those without. Such studies are helping to define the role of respiratory virus in the pathogenesis of sinusitis.

The clinical observation has been made repeatedly that influenza epidemics are frequently associated with an increase in the incidence of cases of community-acquired sinusitis. Also, next to rhinovirus, influenza virus has been most often recovered from sinus aspirates of patients with acute sinusitis (6). Influenza virus causes a destructive infection of respiratory epithelium (15), which probably explains its importance in precipitating secondary bacterial infection of the sinuses.

B. Bacteriologic Characteristics

Sinus puncture was used by Urdal (16) in 1949 to study the bacterial causes of acute community-acquired sinusitis. His work was followed by similar studies by other Scandinavian investigators (2,17–19) and more recently by workers in the United States (3,20,21) and Finland (22). In the puncture studies, specimen collection has been limited to the maxillary sinus with but a few exceptions. That the findings of these studies can be extrapolated to the cause of infection in the other sinuses is not certain but is probably justified. In this regard, antimicrobial selection, based on the antral puncture results, has been successful in treating patients with involvement of the other sinuses.

Nasal bacterial cultures have been correlated with simultaneous cultures of aspirates obtained by sinus puncture (3,19,20,23). The predictive value obtained from nasal culture is not sufficient to be useful in determining cause or selecting antimicrobial treatment for sinusitis. Although a comparison of nasal and sinus aspirate results showed a good predictive value for *S. pyogenes*, it was not good for *H. influenzae* and *S. pneumoniae* and was poor for *M. catarrhalis* (23). Also, the results between nasal and sinus aspirate cultures for *S. aureus* are notoriously poor, with nasal cultures yielding a falsely high incidence of staphylococcal infection (3,19,23). Further complicating the problem of using nasal cultures to diagnosis the bacterial cause of sinusitis is the fact that some patients with acute community-acquired sinusitis have more than one bacterial pathogen recovered from the same sinus cavity and others have bilateral sinus involvement due to different bacterial species (3,20,23).

Sinus puncture, when performed by an experienced physician, is a technically easy and safe procedure (Table 3). The findings of the puncture studies have been in good agreement except for minor differences in the relative importance of the different bacterial species. The relative importance of the different species has not changed over several decades, although there have been changes in the antimicrobial susceptibilities of some species.

S. pneumoniae and *H. influenzae* are the major bacterial causes of acute community-acquired sinusitis, accounting for up to three-quarters of cases (Table 4) (2,3,16–22). Also, they are the most frequent cause of dual infections in the same sinus. All other bacterial species are relatively infrequent causes of infection compared to these two bacteria. Infections due to anaerobic bacteria and *M. catarrhalis* are next in frequency. The mixed anaerobic infections have been observed mainly in adults. They often contain multiple species including anaerobic streptococci, facultative gram-positive cocci, *Bacteroides* species, and *Fusobacteria*, reflecting their endodontic origin (24). *M. catarrhalis* appears to be of special importance in children, accounting for 19% of cases in one study (20). A limited amount of information based on sinus puncture cultures indicates that the bacteriologic cause of acute and subacute sinusitis in children is similar to that of adults (20,25–27).

Table 3 Sinus Puncture Technique for Obtaining Specimens for Microbial Culture and Other Diagnostic Tests of Sinus Contents

Anterior nares and area below the inferior turbinate cleansed with an antiseptic
 solution
Puncture site below the inferior turbinate anesthetized
Medial wall of antrum punctured with 12 gauge needle[a]
Sinus contents aspirated with a syringe or 1 ml normal saline instilled and
 aspirated[b]
Capped syringe transported promptly to the laboratory for processing

[a]Insertion of a plastic catheter through the needle runs the risk of shearing off the end of the catheter in the sinus cavity when the catheter is removed.
[b]Positioning of the head by flexion of the neck in different directions improves the specimen yield. The normal saline should not contain antibacterial preservatives.

Table 4 Bacterial Causes of Acute Community-Acquired Sinusitis Determined by Puncture of the Maxillary Antrum

Bacteria	Percentage of cases (range)	
	Adults	Children
Streptococcus pneumoniae	20–41	36
Haemophilus influenzae	6–50	23
S. pneumoniae and H. influenzae	1–9	—
Anaerobic bacteria	0–10	—
Moraxella catarrhalis	2–4	19
Streptococcus pyogenes	1–8	2
Other streptococcal species	2	—
Staphylococcus aureus	0–8	—
Gram-negative bacteria[a]	0–24	2

[a]One study showed a 24% isolation of gram-negative bacteria, but in other studies the recovery rate was not over 5%. Gram-negative bacteria recovered included P. aeruginosa, K. pneumoniae, and E. coli.

S. aureus, S. pyogenes, and other streptococcal species, such as Streptococcus intermedius, also account for a small proportion of cases. The importance of the enterobacteria and other gram-negative bacteria that were reported in some studies is not certain. Although some of these isolates may represent true pathogens, others may be contaminants that were inadvertently encountered in the collection of the specimens. Most of the community studies have reported a very low percentage of gram-negative bacteria.

In one study that focused on infection of the sphenoid sinus, specimens were collected by puncture or from sinus tissue obtained from the operative site (28). Streptococcal species accounted for 41%; *S. aureus*, 29%; and *S. pneumoniae* for 17% of the cases. Again, the possibility of specimen contamination, especially of the surgical tissues, must be considered in interpreting these results.

It is important to recognize that approximately one-quarter to one-half of patients with the clinical diagnosis of acute community-acquired sinusitis will not have bacterial growth from specimens collected by antral sinus puncture (21,22). The reasons for this are unclear. Some of these patients may be having an uncomplicated cold with clinical features suggestive of sinusitis. Another possibility is that antral infection is not the cause of the patient's complaints and that infection of other sinuses, especially of the ethmoids, is present. Some cases of sinusitis may be the result of a pure viral infection, as suggested in some puncture studies, or of infections with hard to grow, newly recognized, or as yet undiscovered organisms.

Leading the list of the new agents that may have a role in acute community-acquired sinusitis is *Chlamydia pneumoniae* (strain TWAR). The importance of this agent as a respiratory pathogen is receiving increasing recognition, including evidence of its role in sinus infection. The clinical diagnosis of sinusitis was present in 16% of 19 older children and adults with *C. pneumoniae* infection (29). As a possible cause of sinusitis, *C. pneumoniae* is of special interest because it does not respond to currently recommended antimicrobial treatment for acute sinusitis (21). Also, the chronic nature of *C. pneumoniae* infection in some patients (30) and its reported association with prolonged cough, bronchospasm, and adult-onset asthma make this infection of particular importance (29). There have been no reports of *C. pneumoniae* recovery from sinus aspirates, and more information is needed to determine its role in sinus infection, but it should be considered in the causative diagnosis of the disease.

C. Mycologic Characteristics

Fungi are well established as a cause of sinusitis in the community setting, where these infections are being recognized with increasing frequency (31,32). It is not clear whether the incidence of fungal sinusitis is increasing or that recognition of the infection has improved. Marijuana smoking has been proposed as a possible risk factor in some patients (33,34).

Community-acquired fungal sinusitis tends to be more insidious in onset than its bacterial counterpart and typically presents with pressure rather than inflammatory symptoms. Bony destruction may occur and characteristic dark or "peanut butter-like" exudates are present in the sinus cavity of some patients. Also, a syndrome of allergic fungal sinusitis has been recognized in patients with

Table 5 Fungal Infections Associated with Disease of the Paranasal Sinuses

Fungal infections and agents	Community acquired	Impaired host	Allergic syndrome
Aspergillosis	Yes	Yes	Yes
(*A. fumigatis*, *A. flavus*, *A. niger*, *A. oryzae*,			
A. nidulans)			
Cryptococcosis		Yes	
(*C. neoformans*)			
Pseudallescheriasis	Yes	Yes	
(*P. boydii*)			
Sporothrichosis	Yes		
(*S. schenkii*)			
Homobasidiomycosis	Yes	Yes	
(*Schizophyllum commune*)			
Hyalohyphomycosis	Yes		
(*Penicillium melini*)			
Phaeohyphomycosis	Yes	Yes	Yes
(*Bipolaris hawaiiensis*, *B. spicifera*, *Exserohilum*			
rostratum, *E. mcginnisii*, *Alternaria alternata*,			
Curvularia lunata)			
Zygomycosis	Yes	Yes	
(*Mucor* spp. *Rhizophus* spp. *Cunninghamella*			
bertholletiae)			

normal immunocompetence (35,36). This condition is characterized by persistent sinusitis with nasal polyps, asthma, and peripheral eosinophilia. Various immunologic parameters of reaction to fungal antigens are used in making the diagnosis. "Allergic mucin," a pale eosinophilic or basophilic material containing eosinophils and crystals, is also characteristic of the condition.

Several fungal groups including *Aspergillus* (37–39), *Homobasidiomyces* (40), *Hyalohyphomyces* (3,41), *Phaeohyphomyces* (32,42–45), *Pseudallescheria* (46), *Sporothrix* (46), and zygomycoses (37) have been implicated in community-acquired sinusitis (Table 5). Most papers have described individual cases or small series of cases. Fungal infections still are responsible for only a small proportion of sinusitis acquired in the community setting. The role of fungi in sinus infection in the immunocompromised host is discussed below.

IV. NOSOCOMIAL SINUSITIS

Sinusitis developing in the hospitalized patient is due primarily to the bacterial species associated with other nosocomial infections. Bacteria recovered by antral sinus puncture have included *S. aureus*, some methicillin-resistant, and a variety of gram-negative bacteria (47–51). Among the latter are *Pseudomonas aeruginosa*, *Enterobacter* species, *Klebsiella pneumoniae*, *Proteus mirabilis*, and *Escherichia coli*. *Bacteroides fragilis* and *B. melaniogenecus* strains as well as occasional β-hemolytic streptococci (group A and non-group A), *S. pneumoniae*, and *Haemophilus* species were also encountered. Nasal intubation of different kinds as well as nasal packing, cranial and facial fractures, and mechanical ventilation are risk factors in these infections. Sinus puncture is usually required to determine the infecting organism and its antimicrobial susceptibilities in order to plan effective therapy.

V. SINUSITIS IN THE IMPAIRED HOST

The diseases that adversely affect immunity and resistance and are associated with sinus infection include diabetes mellitus, leukemia and lymphomas, cystic fibrosis, and other diseases affecting cilial function, and, more recently, acquired immunodeficiency syndrome (AIDS). Also, patients receiving organ transplants and chemotherapy are at risk for developing sinus infection. In addition to the usual pathogens associated with community- and hospital-acquired infection discussed above, a variety of other micro-organisms have been implicated in sinusitis in immunocompromised patients.

Fungal infections are particularly important (Table 5). Mucormycosis was originally recognized as a fulminant infection in patients with diabetes mellitus, usually during episodes of ketoacidosis (52–54). Other predisposing conditions for this infection include neutropenia, burns, leukemias and lymphomas, uremia, and prolonged immunosuppressive therapy. Diagnosis is made by fungal stains of specimens obtained by biopsy of involved sites.

Sinus infection with *Aspergillus* species also occurs in patients with a variety of immune problems including blood dyscrasias, diabetes mellitus, and renal and bone marrow transplants (39,46). *A. fumigatus* is the most common causative agent in this setting, with other *Aspergillus* species being seen less frequently. Other fungal infections of the sinus reported in immunocompromised patients include cryptococcosis (55), pseudallescheriasis (56), homobasidiomycosis (40,57), and phaeohyphomycosis (42).

Other classes of organisms associated with sinus infection in the impaired host include *Legionella pneumophilia* which was recovered from the sinus of a patient with AIDS (58) and *Mycobacterium chelonei*, which has been reported as the cause of sinusitis in a patient with diabetes mellitus (59).

Persistent bacterial infection is the major problem when resistance is impaired by abnormal mucociliary clearance in the sinus cavity (60). A sinus puncture study in patients with cystic fibrosis found that *P. aeruginosa* was the most important cause of infection (61). Other bacteria implicated in patients with cystic fibrosis were *H. influenzae*, β-hemolytic streptococci, *E. coli*, *S. aureus*, *Peptostreptococcus* species, and *Bacteroides* species.

VI. CHRONIC SINUS DISEASE

The diagnosis of chronic sinus disease (chronic sinusitis) is usually made in the patient with persistent upper respiratory tract symptoms associated with irreversible changes on sinus x-ray or other imaging studies. The duration of illness may be months or years. Although the detailed events in the pathogenesis of this condition are not well understood, it usually follows an acute infection or series of infections of the sinuses. To this extent, the condition clearly has an infectious component, although by the time it is well established other factors, such as ostiomeatal obstruction and allergy or problems with immunity, are usually implicated in the process. Also, as discussed above, noninfectious diseases such as cystic fibrosis, Kartagener's syndrome, and other ciliary dismotility syndromes predispose to the development of sinus disease. Once chronic sinus disease has developed, it is difficult to evaluate the causative importance of micro-organisms recovered from the upper airway, even from sinus aspirate specimens.

Attempts to assign a microbial "cause" for chronic sinus disease have not been illuminating. Most of the micro-organisms recovered from the sinus cavity of patients with chronic disease are of the type that would be expected to colonize a site such as a functionally impaired sinus. With the human upper airway normally populated with anaerobic bacteria in concentrations of up to 10^{11} organisms per ml of fluid or gram of tissue (62), it is not surprising that these bacteria would be found in a sinus cavity with functional impairment of clearance. Therefore, the recovery of anaerobic bacteria from the sinus cavity of patients with chronic sinus disease (63,64) does not necessarily establish them as the primary cause of the condition.

However, it is possible that micro-organisms, because of the severity or chronicity of the infection that they produce, are the direct cause of chronic sinus disease. One attractive but unproven candidate for this role is *C. pneumoniae*, which is discussed above. What is clinically well established is that intensive and prolonged antimicrobial treatment is usually not sufficient to "cure" patients of their disease.

Some recent success in treating and reversing chronic sinus disease has been achieved with surgical procedures directed at relieving osteal and substeal obstruction of the sinus and thus re-establishing or improving drainage of the sinus cavity. Also, treatment of immune deficiencies and allergic conditions may be helpful in some patients. The favorable results obtained with ostiomeatal surgery, immunotherapy, and treatment of allergy indicate that causal factors other than infection alone play a role in the pathogenesis of chronic sinus disease. Further study is needed to determine the relative importance of various risk factors in this disease.

VII. MICROBIAL CONSIDERATIONS IN THERAPY

A. Antimicrobial Susceptibility and Resistance

Not all of the bacterial causes of community-acquired sinusitis were sensitive to penicillin or the other early-generation antibiotics. Thus, when antibiotics became available, it was not possible to treat all potential sinusitis pathogens with one drug. The resistance of *H. influenzae* to penicillin was the primary problem. When the ampicillins became available, they were recognized as meeting the need for an effective broad-spectrum treatment for acute sinusitis. However, even the ampicillins did not provide complete coverage since they were not effective for the small proportion of sinus infections due to penicillin-resistant *S. aureus*.

More recently, beta-lactamase production by strains of *H. influenzae* and *M. catarrhalis* and the development of methicillin resistance by *S. aureus* have further complicated the problem of antimicrobial treatment for acute community-acquired sinusitis. In recent years, 54% of strains of *H. influenzae* and 74% of *M. catarrhalis* recovered from sinus aspirates have been ampicillin-resistant (21). Methicillin resistance in *S. aureus*, although not reported in cases of community-acquired sinusitis, is nonetheless a potential problem that also must be recognized in selecting treatment, especially for serious cases of sinusitis and those with known or suspected intracranial complications.

The availability of the second-generation cephalosporins, like cefuroxime axetil and of the amoxicillin/clavulanate and trimethroprim–sulfamethoxazole combinations, has provided excellent antimicrobial coverage for the initial treatment of acute community-acquired sinusitis. These drugs, which have been proven effective in sinus puncture studies (21), remain useful to the present time, although treatment for known or suspected *S. aureus* sinus infections still requires special consideration.

A recent event affecting bacterial susceptibility in acute sinusitis is the emerging resistance of *S. pneumoniae* to penicillin. Also, if *C. pneumoniae* is established as an important cause of sinusitis, its antimicrobial susceptibilities will have to be considered in selecting therapy.

B. Drug Concentrations in the Sinus Cavity and Duration of Treatment

Limited attempts have been made to measure antimicrobial concentrations in sinus cavity secretions of patients with acute sinusitis. In two studies (65,66), the drug being given was detected in some, but not all, sinus aspirates, and the correlation between measured drug concentrations in the sinus and the presence of bacterial growth was inexact. In another study, drug was detected in only 1 of 21 sinus aspirates although the bacteriologic cure rate was 91% (67). In this study, measurements in serum simultaneously showed the presence of drug although concentrations were low, probably reflecting the prolonged interval between drug ingestion and sample collection. Also, the sinus aspirate measurements were made on the tenth day of treatment, at a time when inflammation in the sinus had subsided.

The effectiveness of antimicrobial treatment for sinusitis has been most accurately determined by studies employing pre- and posttreatment quantitative bacterial cultures (21). Until reliable methods are developed for measuring antimicrobial concentrations in sinus cavity secretions and tissues and until these results can be correlated with antimicrobial dosage and bacteriologic cure rates, pre- and post-therapy sinus puncture will remain the gold standard for determining treatment efficacy with new drugs. Because of ethical and practical considerations, paired pre- and post-treatment sinus punctures are more difficult to obtain in children (27).

Two examples have shown the value of paired pre- and post-treatment sinus punctures in determining microbial cure rates in sinusitis. In a limited trial of clindamycin, microbial failures were demonstrated with *H. influenzae* infection, although some patients reported clinical improvement, suggesting that they were receiving effective treatment (3). Acute sinusitis is usually a self-limited disease, and patients with sinusitis experience clinical improvement despite ineffective treatment as proven by sinus punctures showing persistent exudate and high bacterial concentrations in the sinus cavity. For this reason, objective measures of efficacy are necessary when new treatments are being evaluated. Sinus imaging techniques have value in this regard, but because of the slow resolution of imaging abnormalities are not as useful as puncture.

Another example of the value of paired sinus punctures was the repeated observation of failure of bacteriologic cure after treatment with inadequate dosages of cefaclor. In one study, the daily dosage of cefaclor was raised from 1 g to 2 g (68) before evidence of acceptable bacteriologic response was obtained. In another, a daily dosage of 1 g compared unfavorably to the bacteriologic cure rate obtained with a comparison drug (21). Clinical observation alone would have been unlikely to have detected the therapeutic failures disclosed by the paired bacterial cultures.

An important unresolved question relating to the antimicrobial treatment of acute sinusitis is duration of treatment. In the Charlottesville studies, in which pre- and post-therapy sinus aspirations were performed, 10 days of treatment with an appropriate drug gave cure rates of 90% or better (21). However, it is possible that the diagnostic sinus aspirations was of sufficient therapeutic benefit in itself to augment the effect of the antibiotic treatment and give the favorable results observed after 10 days of treatment. Sinus aspiration alone, however, did not produce bacteriologic cure when the infecting bacteria were insensitive to the drug given.

REFERENCES

1. Bjuggren G, Kraepelien S, Lind J. Sinusitis in children at home and in day-nurseries. Ann Paediatr 1949; 173:205–21.
2. Björkwall T. Bacteriological examination in maxillary sinusitis: bacterial flora of the maxillary antrum. Acta Otolaryngol [Suppl] (Stockh) 1964; 188:390–9.
3. Evans FO Jr, Sydnor JB, Moore WEC, Moore GR, Manwaring JL, Brill AH, Jackson RT, Hanna S, Skaar JS, Holdeman LV, Fitz-Hugh GS, Sande MA, Gwaltney JM Jr. Sinusitis of the maxillary antrum. N Engl Med 1975; 293:735–9.
4. Shapiero ED, Wald ER, Doyle WJ, Rohm DD. Bacteriology of maxillary sinuses of the rhesus monkey. Ann Otol Rhinol Laryngol 1982; 91:150–1.
5. Gwaltney JM Jr, Hayden FG. The nose and infection. *In*: Proctor DF, Andersen IB, eds. The Nose. Upper Airway Physiology and the Atmospheric Environment. New York: Elsevier Biomedical Press, 1982:399–422.
6. Hamory BH, Sande MA, Sydnor A Jr, Seale DL, Gwaltney JM Jr. Etiology and antimicrobial therapy of acute maxillary sinusitis. J Infect Dis 1979; 139:197–202.
7. Turner BW, Cail WS, Hendley JO, Hayden FG, Doyle WJ, Sorrentino JV, Gwaltney JM Jr. Physiologic abnormalities in the paranasal sinuses during experimental rhinovirus colds. J Allergy Clin Immunol 1992; 90:474–8.
8. Spector SL, English GM, McIntosh K, Farr RS. Adenovirus in the sinuses of an asthmatic patient with apparent selective antibody deficiencies. Am J Med 1973; 55:227–31.
9. Winther B, Gwaltney JM Jr, Mygind N, Turner RD, Hendley JO. Sites of recovery after point inoculation of the upper airway. JAMA 1986; 256:1763–7.
10. Naclerio RM, Proud D, Kagey-Sobotka A, Lichtenstein LM, Hendley JO, Gwaltney JM Jr. Kinins are generated during experimental rhinovirus colds. J Infect Dis 1988; 157:133–42.
11. Proud D. Personal communication.
12. Gwaltney JM Jr. Combined antiviral and antimediator treatment of rhinovirus colds. J Infect Dis. 1992; 166:776–82.
13. Gwaltney JM Jr., Hendley JO, Simon G, Jordan WS Jr. Rhinovirus infections in an industrial population. II. Characteristics of illness and antibody response. JAMA 1967; 202:494–500.
14. Som PM, Lawson W, Biller HF, and Lanzieri CF. Ethmoid sinus disease: CT evaluation in 400 cases. Part I. Nonsurgical patients. Radiology 1986; 159:591–7.
15. Mulder J, Hers JF. Influenza. Groningen, The Netherlands: Wolters-Noordhoff, 1972: 1–272.
16. Urdal K, Berdal P. The microbial flora in 81 cases of maxillary sinusitis. Acta Oto-Laryngol 1949; 37:20–5.
17. Lystad A, Berdal P, Lund-Iversen L. The bacterial flora of sinusitis with an in vitro study of the bacterial resistance to antibiotics. Acta Otolaryngol [Suppl] (Stockh) 1964; 188:390–9.
18. Rantanen T, Arvilommi H. Double-blind trial of doxicycline in acute maxillary sinusitis: a clinical and bacteriological study. Acta Otolaryngol(Stockh) 1973; 76:58–62.
19. Axelsson A, Brorson JE. The correlation between bacteriological findings in the nose and maxillary sinus in acute maxillary sinusitis. Laryngoscope 1973; 83:2003–11.

20. Wald ER, Milmoe GJ, Bowen A, Ledesma-Medina J, Salamon N, Bluestone CD. Acute maxillary sinusitis in children. N Engl J Med 1981; 304:749–54.
21. Gwaltney JM Jr, Scheld WM, Sande MA, and Sydnor A. The microbial etiology and antimicrobial therapy of adults with acute community acquired sinusitis: a 15-year experience at the University of Virginia and review of other selected studies. J Allergy Clin Immunol. 1992; 90:457–62.
22. Jousimies-Somer HR, Savolainen S, Ylikoski JS. Bacteriological findings of acute maxillary sinusitis in young adults. J Clin Microbiol 1988; 26:1919–25.
23. Jousimies-Somer HR, Savolainen S, Ylikoski JS. Comparison of the nasal bacterial floras in two groups of healthy subjects in patients with acute maxillary sinusitis. J Clin Microbiol 1989; 27:2736–43.
24. Williams BL, McCann GF, Schoenknecht FD. Bacteriology of dental abscesses of endodontic origin. J Clin Microbiol 1983; 18:770–4.
25. Wald ER, Byers C, Guerra N, Casselbrant ML, Beste D. Subacute sinusitis in children. J Pediatr 1989; 115:28–32.
26. Wald ER. Sinusitis in children. N Engl J Med 1992; 326:319–23.
27. Giebink GS. Criteria for evaluation of antimicrobial agents and current therapies for acute sinusitis in children. Clin Infect Dis 1992; 14(Suppl 2):S212–5.
28. Lew D, Southwick FS, Montgomery WW, Weber AL, Baker AS. Sphenoid sinusitis. N Engl J Med 1983; 309:1149–54.
29. Hahn DL, Dodge RW, Golubjatnikov R. Association of *Chlamydia pneumoniae* (strain TWAR) infection with wheezing, asthmatic bronchitis, and adult-onset asthma. JAMA 1991; 266:225–30.
30. Hammerschlag MR., Chirgwin K, Roblin PM, Gelling M, Dumornay W, Mandel L, Smith P, Schachter J. Persistent infection with *Chlamydia pneumoniae* following acute respiratory illness. Clin Infect Dis 1992; 14:178–82.
31. Washburn RG, Kennedy DW, Begley MG, Henderson DK, Bennett JE. Chronic fungal sinusitis in apparently normal hosts. Medicine 1988; 67:231–47.
32. Zieske LA, Kipke RD, Hamill R. Dematiaceous fungal sinusitis. Otolaryngol Head Neck Surg 1991; 105:567–77.
33. Kagen SL. *Aspergillus*: an inhalable contaminant of marijuana. N Engl J Med 1981; 304:483–4.
34. Schwartz IS. Marijuana and fungal infection. Am J Clin Pathol 1985; 84:256.
35. Hartwick RW, Batsakis JG. Sinus *Aspergillosis* and allergic fungal sinusitis. Ann Otol Rhinol Laryngol 1991; 100:427–30.
36. Corey JP. Allergic fungal sinusitis. Otolaryngol Clin North Am 1992; 25:225–30.
37. Stevens MH. Primary fungal infections of the paranasal sinuses. Am J Otolaryngol 1981; 2:348–57.
38. Romett J, Newman R. Aspergillosis of the nose and paranasal sinuses. Laryngoscope 1982; 92:764–6.
39. Rinaldi MG. Invasive aspergillosis. Rev Infect Dis 1983; 5:1061–77.
40. Kern ME, Uecker FA. Maxillary sinus infection caused by the homobasidiomycetous fungus *Schizophyllum commune*. J Clin Microbiol 1986; 23:1001–5.

41. Morriss FH Jr., Spock A. Intracranial aneurysm secondary to mycotic orbital and sinus infection. Report of a case implicating penicillium as an opportunistic fungus. Am J Dis Child 1970; 119:357–62.
42. Padhye AA, Ajello L, Wieden MA, Steinbronn KK. Phaeohyphomycosis of the nasal sinuses caused by a new species of *Exserohilum*. J Clin Microbiol 1986; 24:245–9.
43. MacMillan RH III, Cooper PH, Body BA, Mills AS. Allergic fungal sinusitis due to *Curvularia lunata*. Hum Pathol 1987; 18:960–4.
44. Killingsworth SM, Wetmore SJ. *Curvularia/Drechslera* sinusitis. Laryngoscope 1990; 100:932–7.
45. Aviv J, Lawson W, Bottone E, Sachdev V, Som P, Biller H. Multiple intracranial mucoceles associated with phaeohyphomycosis of the paranasal sinuses. Arch Otoloryngol Head Neck Surg 1990; 116:1210–3.
46. Morgan MA, Wilson WR, Neel B III, Roberts GD. Fungal sinusitis in healthy and immunocompromised individuals. Am J Clin Pathol 1984; 82:597–601.
47. Pope TL, Stelling CB, Leitner YB. Maxillary sinusitis after nasotracheal intubation. South Med J 1981; 74:610–2.
48. Via-Reque E, Rattenborg CC. Prolonged oro- or nasotracheal intubation. Crit Care Med 1981; 9:637–9.
49. Caplan ES, Hoyt NJ. Nosocomial sinusitis. JAMA 1982; 247:639–41.
50. Deutschman CS, Wilton PB, Sinow J, et al. Paranasal sinusitis: a common complication of nasotracheal intubation in neurosurgical patients. Neurosurgery 1985; 17:296–9.
51. Linden BE, Aguilar EA, Allen SJ. Sinusitis in the nasotracheally intubated patient. Arch Otolaryngol Head Neck Surg 1988; 114:860–1.
52. Pillsbury H. Rhinocerebral mucormycosis. Arch Otolaryngol 1977; 103:600–4.
53. McNulty J. Rhinocerebral mucormycosis: predisposing factors. Laryngoscope 1982; 92:1140–3.
54. Parfrey NA. Improved diagnosis and prognosis of mucormycosis. Medicine 1986; 65:113–23.
55. Choi SS, Lawson W, Bottone EJ, Biller. Cryptococcal sinusitis: a case report and review of literature. Otolaryngol Head Neck Surg 1988; 99:414–8.
56. Gluckman SJ, Ries K, Abrutyn. *Allescheria (Petriellidium) boydii* sinusitis in a compromised host. J Clin Microbiol 1977; 5:481–4.
57. Rosenthal J, Katz R, DuBois DB, Morrissey A, Machicao A. Chronic maxillary sinusitis associated with the mushroom *Schizophyllum commune* in a patient with AIDS. Clin Infect Dis 1992; 14:46–8.
58. Schanger G, Lutwick LI, Kurzman M, Hoch B. Sinusitis caused by *Legionella pneumophila* in a patient with the acquired immune deficiency syndrome. Am J Med 1984; 77:957–60.
59. Eron LJ, Huckins C, Park CH, Poretz DM, Gelman HK, Ball MF. *Mycobacterium chelonei* infects the maxillary sinus: a rare case. VA Med 1981; 108:335–8.
60. Corkey CWB, Levison H, Turner JAP. The immotile cilia syndrome. Am Rev Respir Dis 1981; 544–8.

61. Shapiro ED, Milmoe GJ, Wald ER, Rodnan JB, Bowen A. Bacteriology of the maxillary sinuses in patients with cystic fibrosis. J Infect Dis 1982; 146:589–93.
62. Busch DF. Anaerobes in infections of the head and neck and ear, nose, and throat. Rev Infect Dis (Suppl) 1984; 6:S115–22.
63. Frederick J, Braude AI. Anaerobic infection of the paranasal sinuses. N Engl J Med 1974;290:135–7.
64. Brook I. Bacteriologic features of chronic sinusitis in children. JAMA 1981; 246:967–9.
65. Gullers K. Penicillin in paranasal sinus secretions. Chemotherapy 1969; 14:303–7.
66. Carenfelt C, Eneroth C-M, Lundberg C, Wretlind B. Evaluation of the antibiotic effect of treatment of maxillary sinusitis. Scand J Infect Dis 1975; 7:259–64.
67. Scheld WM, Sydnor A Jr, Farr B, Gratz JC, Gwaltney JM Jr. Comparison of cyclacillin and amoxicillin for therapy of acute maxillary sinusitis. Antimicrobial Agents Chemother 1986; 30:350–3.
68. Gwaltney JM Jr, Sydnor A Jr, Sande MA. Etiology and antimicrobial treatment of acute sinusitis. Ann Otol Rhinol Laryngol 1981; 90:68–71.

5

Radiologic Diagnosis of the Nasal Cavity and Paranasal Sinuses

S. JAMES ZINREICH
Johns Hopkins Medical Institutions
Baltimore, Maryland

Of the 31 million people affected by sinusitis each year, roughly half will seek the help of a physician. Yet sinusitis, especially as it relates to allergies, is one of the most frequently overlooked and misunderstood diseases in clinical practice. It is often misdiagnosed and treated inappropriately.

With a better understanding of the pathophysiology of sinus disease, advances in diagnostic techniques, and the advent of endoscopic surgery, the evaluation and treatment of sinusitis are undergoing a major evolution.

Coupled with these new developments, the role of allergies as they relate to sinusitis has commanded greater attention. A recent study found that nasal allergy is present in a very high frequency in patients with sinusitis (1). We will examine the relationship of allergy to sinusitis and explore the radiographic appearance and anatomical characteristics that must be considered in the diagnosis and treatment of sinusitis.

I. OSTIOMEATAL COMPLEX AND MUCOCILIARY CLEARANCE

Until recently, the diagnosis and therapy of sinusitis predominantly addressed problems of the maxillary and frontal sinuses. In the past, standard roentgenograms were used to best display these sinuses. This led to the belief that the primary site of mucosal inflammation was the maxillary sinus. Not surprising, then, was the fact that the majority of surgical procedures aimed at helping patients with chronic sinusitis were focused on the maxillary sinuses (Caldwell-Luc and nasal antrostomy; 2,3). Several noted otolaryngologists, including Messerklinger, Proctor, and Hilding, however, pointed out that the ethmoid sinus is the most common site of inflammatory disease, and infection here is probably the precursor of disease in the frontal and maxillary sinuses (4–7).

Later, Messerklinger and Drettner demonstrated that obstruction of the ostia is the usual precursor of sinusitis (7,8). They showed that apposition of contiguous mucociliary surfaces within the paranasal sinuses results in a disruption of sinonasal drainage, with retention of secretions, which in turn leads to inflammation and infection. Messerklinger also showed that the infundibulum and the middle meatus are the channels most frequently affected by anatomical variations. These variations may also result in juxtaposition of the mucosal surfaces in the narrow ostiomeatal channels and in turn facilitate mucosal inflammation (4). Aust and Drettner discovered a high frequency of ostial dysfunction in subjects with a history of recurrent maxillary sinusitis, and reported that maxillary ostial patency is almost always reduced in patients with chronic sinusitis (9).

Other evidence further supports the concept that the anterior and middle ethmoid sinuses are the primary sites of pathologic involvement in this area. The mucosa covering these structures bears the brunt of inspiratory airflow. Inspired air moves with high velocity through the nasal valve and particulate impaction occurs as it changes direction of flow. Walsdorf et al. showed that inhaled tagged water aerosol was primarily deposited in this area. It is also the primary site for the development of adenocarcinoma in woodworkers, and squamous cell carcinoma in workers exposed to nickel fumes (10–12).

The importance of the middle meatus–anterior ethmoid complex in the pathogenesis of frontal and maxillary sinus disease led Neumann to describe the area as the ostiomeatal unit (13).

The ostiomeatal complex is composed of narrow channels and is subject to wide normal anatomical variation (Fig. 1). It contains the ostia not only for the drainage of the anterior ethmoid sinuses but also for the frontal and maxillary sinuses. These sinuses are therefore dependent upon the integrity of the ostiomeatal complex for ventilation and mucociliary clearance. Local inflammation or anatomical obstruction within the ostiomeatal complex may result in secondary disease within the maxillary and frontal sinuses. It is evident that if surgery is contemplated, primary consideration should be given to establishing the patency of the narrow passages of the ethmoid sinuses rather than focusing only on removal of disease from the maxillary sinuses (2,4,5)

In the case of a nasal allergic reaction, a recent study found that decreased mucociliary clearance is a contributory factor in decreased ventilation of the sinuses (1).

Understanding the pattern of mucociliary clearance is important for both the radiologist and the surgeon. The thin layer of mucus covering the inner surface

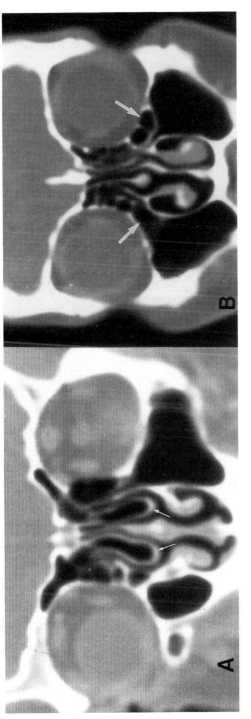

Figure 1 Anatomical variations. Coronal CT images through the anterior ethmoid sinuses reveal (A) bilateral conchae bullosa (fine arrows) and (B) bilateral Haller cells (large arrows).

of sinuses receives the largest deposits of inhaled particulate matter. The cilia and the thin mucous layer here are in constant motion in predetermined pathways toward the various sinus ostia. If mucosal transport of bacteria, mucus, and debris is obstructed, the sinus is susceptible to infection.

Mucociliary clearance in the frontal sinuses advances along the septal wall to the sinus roof, then moves laterally along the roof and medially along the floor toward the ostium. Backflow, resulting from recirculation in the frontal recess, may be a cause of initial infection (7).

In the maxillary sinus, mucociliary movement is toward the ostium. It starts at the sinus floor and radiates along the wall of the sinus superiorly. Even in the presence of nasal antral windows after inferior meatotomy, intended to clear mucus from the maxillary sinus, mucociliary movement persists in its upward movement toward the sinus ostium.

Unobstructed flow through the ostiomeatal complex and its narrow communicating passages within the sinus ostia is integral to mucociliary clearance and ventilation. It is of particular importance that the anterior and posterior ethmoid sinus channels be patent because the primary sites for mucociliary drainage include the anterior middle meatus and the posterior sphenoethmoid recess. With anatomical distortion or even minor swelling, two mucosal layers may become opposed and lead to stenosis or obstruction in the ostiomeatal complex. Reduced aeration or accumulated secretions in the major maxillary and frontal sinuses then appear to predispose again to infection.

On the basis of these observations, the guiding principle of management is to reverse the sinusitis cycle involving the ostiomeatal complex. Understanding how to do this has yielded research exploring new techniques that have dramatically changed standards in the care of patients with sinusitis.

II. RADIOGRAPHIC EVALUATION

The primary aims of the radiologic evaluation of the nose and paranasal sinuses are to provide an accurate and perceptible display of regional anatomy and to establish the extent of disease. Proper display of the anatomy will reveal regional airway obstructions that may block ventilation and mucociliary clearance and, thus, explain the cause of recurrent bouts of infection. Establishing the extent of bone erosion in the presence of neoplasia allows presurgical perception of possible sites of intracranial and/or intraorbital invasion. This information subsequently facilitates safe surgery with a well-defined "road map" (Fig. 2).

A. Standard Roentgenograms

Standard radiographs are still the most frequently used radiographic modality when evaluating sinus disease. The anterior-posterior (A-P) and Waters views best demonstrate the frontal and maxillary sinuses. The lateral view best dis-

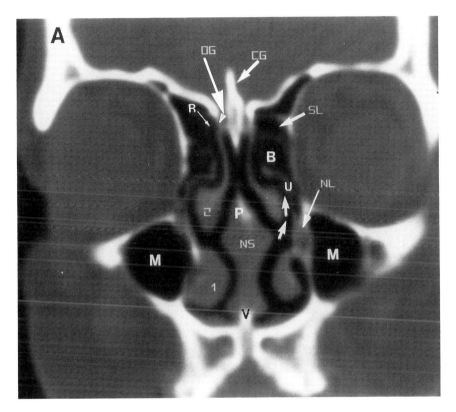

Figure 2 Anterior ostiomeatal channels. Coronal CT images through the anterior ethmoid sinuses reveal the frontal sinus (F); maxillary sinus (M); ethmoid beulla (B); uncinate process (U); sinus lateralis (SL); frontal recess (R); middle meatus (arrows); nasolacrima duct (NL); nasal septum (NS); perpendicular plate (P); vamer (V); crista galli (CG); olfactory groove (OG); inferior turbinate (1); middle turbinate (2).

plays the sphenoid sinus. The fine bony anatomy of the ethmoid sinuses, however, is poorly displayed on all views because of the problem of structural superimposition. Even though of limited value in evaluating the patient with chronic inflammatory disease, standard radiographic views may be of value in assessing the patient with acute inflammatory disease or aggressive pathologic involvement (14).

B. Tomography

Polytomography addresses the roentgenographic limitation of structural superimposition and significantly improves the display of bony detail within the ethmoid sinuses. However, soft tissue-like densities ("phantom artifacts")

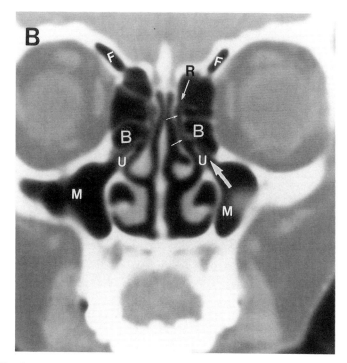

Figure 2 Continued

commonly attributed to this modality) may be mistaken for inflammatory disease. Thus, although bony detail is viewed more clearly, the associated artifacts preclude accurate interpretation of the extent of soft tissue inflammatory disease (3,15).

C. Computed Tomography

Computed tomography (CT) is currently the modality of choice in the evaluation of the nose and paranasal sinuses (Fig. 3). Its ability to display bone, soft tissue, and air optimally facilitates accurate definition of regional anatomy and extent of disease.

The cross-sectional plane that most closely correlates with the surgical approach and best shows both the ostiomeatal channels and the relationship of brain to fovea ethmoidalis to ethmoid sinus is the coronal plane. The following are the parameters we use when performing this evaluation:

Patient position: prone with chin hyperextended.
Gantry angulation: perpendicular to bony palate.
Extent of examination: from anterior frontal sinus through sphenoid sinus.

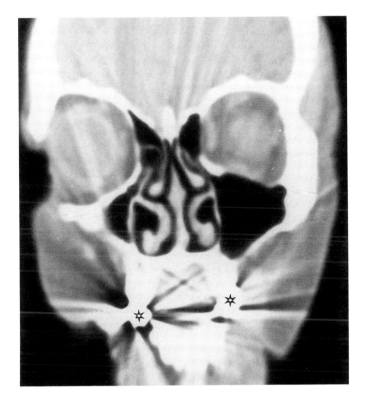

Figure 3 Metallic artifacts on coronal CT images. ''Spray'' artifacts emitted by dental amalgam (stars) do not obscure display of the ostiomeatal anatomy.

Slice thickness: 3 mm (using GE-9800 scanner).

Table incrementation: 3mm (with thicker slices should overlap scans for optimal MPR).

Field of view: adjusted to include only the nasal cavity and paranasal sinuses.

Windowing: for soft tissue and air passages, start with window width of +2000 and a center of −200. Adjust potentiometers for best display of uncinate process and bulla ethmoidalis. Record images at this setting for entire examination. For bone structures, window width of +1500 and a center of +300.

D. Magnetic Resonance Imaging

Magnetic resonance imaging (MRI) provides better imaging of soft tissue than CT, but it is less suited to imaging the anatomy of this region. Because bone and

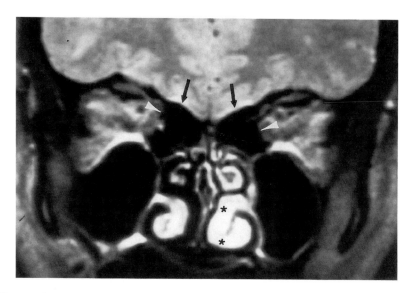

Figure 4 MRI of nasal cavity and paranasal sinuses. Due to the absence of signal the forea ethmoidalis (arrows) and lamina papyracea (arrowheads) are not displayed. The normal nasal mucosa (asterisk) has a signal intensity similar to bacterial and viral inflammation.

air yield similar signal intensities on MRI, precise definition of the ostiomeatal air passages and their bony perimeter is difficult (Fig. 4). Furthermore, in the patient with extensive inflammatory disease, the signal intensity of this pathologic process is indistinguishable from the appearance of the normal mucosa in the edematous phase of the nasal cycle (14,16–18) [Fig. 4]. These factors limit the MRI evaluation of underlying anatomy in a patient with chronic inflammatory disease, especially since the mucosa in the ethmoid sinus "cycles" with the mucosa in the nasal cavity.

Although MRI has significant limitations in the definition of anatomy, it is extremely sensitive in evaluating paranasal sinus mucosa disease in the frontal, maxillary, and sphenoid sinuses, because the mucosa in these sinuses does not undergo the cyclic edema described above. The causes of certain disease processes may be differentiated by MRI. Bacterial and viral inflammation have a high signal intensity on T2-weighted images, whereas neoplastic processes (90% are squamous cell carcinoma) assume an intermediate bright signal on T2-weighted images (19). Fungal concretions have a very low signal intensity on T2-weighted images (similar to air) (20) (Fig. 5:T_1 & T_2).

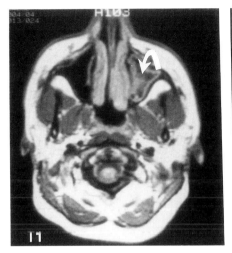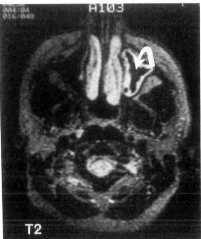

Figure 5   MRI of aspergilloma. Axial T_1- and T_2-weighted images reveal the low signal intensity of an aspergilloma on the T_2-weighted scan.

E. Radiographic Anatomy

The radiographic evaluation of the nasal cavity and paranasal sinuses should stress the display of the ostiomeatal channels. These aerated channels provide airflow to mucociliary clearance from the frontal, maxillary, ethmoid, and sphenoid sinuses. The anterior ostiomeatal channels consist of the air passages between the frontal recess, the middle meatus, and the infundibulum, and therefore provide communication between the anterior ethmoid sinus and the frontal and maxillary sinuses. Mucus from the posterior ethmoid and sphenoid sinuses is deflected toward the sphenoethmoid recess and supreme meatus.

At the CT evaluation, the first images display the outline of the frontal sinus. The frontal recess is an hourglass-like narrowing between the frontal sinus and the anterior middle meatus. It is the point of communication between these airspaces. It is not a tubular structure as the name nasofrontal duct might imply, and therefore the term recess is preferred. Anterior, lateral, and inferior to the frontal recess is the agger nasi cell, an aerated cavity representing a remnant ethmoturbinal. It usually borders the primary ostium/floor of the frontal sinus, and thus its size may directly influence the patency of the frontal recess and the anterior middle meatus. These air passages are the narrowest air channels anteriorly and are frequently the site of inflammation, subsequently blocking ventilation and mucociliary clearance of the frontal sinus. The uncinate process is a superior extension of the lateral nasal wall (medial wall of the maxillary sinus).

Anteriorly, the uncinate process fuses with the medial wall of the agger nasi cell and the posteromedial wall of the nasolacrimal duct. The uncinate process has a ''free'' (unattached) superoposterior edge. Laterally this free edge delimits the infundibulum and posterior to it is the ethmoid bulla, usually the largest of the anterior ethmoid cells. The ethmoid bulla is enclosed laterally by the lamina papyracea. The gap between the ethmoid bulla and the ''free'' edge of the uncinate process defines the hiatus semilunaris. Medially the hiatus semilunaris communicates with the middle meatus, and the airspace lateral to the middle turbinate. Laterally and inferiorly, the hiatus semilunaris communicates with the infundibulum, the air channel between the uncinate process, and the inferomedial border of the orbit. The infundibulum in turn communicates with the primary ostium of the maxillary sinus and the maxillary sinus proper.

The structure medial to the ethmoid bulla and the uncinate process is the middle turbinate. Anteriorly it attaches to the medial wall of the agger nasi cell and superior edge of the uncinate process. Superiorly, it adheres to the cribriform plate. As the middle turbinate extends posteriorly it emits a laterally coursing bony structure that fuses with the lamina papyracea just posterior to the ethmoid bullae: the basal or ground lamella. In most patients, the posterior wall of the ethmoid bulla is intact and an airspace is usually found between the ground lamella and the ethmoid bulla. This airspace may extend superior to the ethmoid bullae and communicate with the frontal recess, and is the sinus lateralis. A dehiscence or total absence of the posterior wall of the ethmoid bulla is not uncommon and may provide communication between these two usually separated airspaces. The posterior ethmoid sinus consists of air cells between the basal lamellae and the sphenoid sinus. The number, shape, and size of these air cells varies significantly from person to person.

The sphenoid sinus is the most posterior sinus. It is usually imbedded into the clivus, and bordered superoposteriorly by the sella turcica. Its ostium is usually located anteriorly superior to the nasal septum, optimally demonstrated with a paramedian sagittal reconstruction.

The relationship between the aerated portion of the sphenoid sinus and the posterior ethmoid sinus needs to be accurately perceived by the surgeon so as to avoid complications during surgery. This morphology is best displayed in the axial plane and with three-dimensional imaging. In most patients the posterior ethmoid sinus aeration is wider and somewhat higher than that of the sphenoid sinus. Usually in the paramedian sagittal plane, the sphenoid sinus is the most superior and posterior airspace. More laterally (1.5–2.0 cm from the nasal septum) the sphenoid sinus is situated more inferiorly and the most posterior–superior airspace is the posterior and ethmoid sinus. Thus, when in this lateral plane the surgeon must be cautious with the posterior advancement of the endoscopic instruments to avoid inadvertent penetration into the optic canal.

One should be equally aware of the relationship between the sphenoid sinus and the carotid artery, optic canal and nerve course, foramen rotundum, and vidian canal. The number and position of septations within the sphenoid sinus are subject to anatomical variation. Some of these septations may adhere to the bony wall covering the carotid artery that, not infrequently, penetrates into the sphenoid sinus. This relationship should be clearly understood, especially in the presence of concomitant inflammatory disease. An infracture of the communication between a sphenoid sinus septum and the carotid canal should clearly be avoided to preclude the risk of traumatizing the carotid artery.

F. Anatomical Variations

Even though the nasal anatomy varies significantly from patient to patient, certain anatomical variations have been documented in the general population and appear even more frequently in patients with chronic inflammatory disease. The significance of such an anatomical variation is determined by the degree of compromise of the major ethmoidal and nasal cavity air passages. In patients with chronic inflammation, recurrence of chronic sinusitis can be attributed to these variations that narrow or obstruct the airways. In our experience, the most common variations in order of decreasing frequency are as follows.

Concha bullosa (36%) prevails when an aerated middle turbinate enlarges to obstruct the middle meatus and even the infundibulum. This variation may be unilateral or bilateral. As an airspace the conchae bullosa has its own mucociliary flow, directed to the frontal recess in most patients. However, not infrequently, it can follow the basal lamella to the sinus lateralis. Inflammatory disease that obstructs the frontal recess and sinus lateralis could therefore block the concha bulla ostium and produce a mucocele.

Nasal septal deformity (21%) is an asymmetrical bowing of the nasal septum that may compress the middle turbinate laterally, narrowing the middle meatus. Excessive bony spurring associated with this variation may further contribute to the narrowing of the nasal air passages including the middle meatus.

Paradoxical middle turbinate (15%) occurs when the greater curvature of the middle turbinate is concave to the nasal septum and may contribute to the narrowing of the middle meatus and even the infundibulum.

Haller cells (10%) are ethmoid cells that extend along the medial roof of the maxillary sinus. These air chambers lateral to the uncinate process often contribute to the narrowing of the infundibulum, especially when affected by an inflammatory process.

Prominent ethmoid bulla (8%): Even though the ethmoid bulla is one of the largest "air cells" within the ethmoid sinus, it may excessively enlarge to narrow or obstruct the middle meatus and infundibulum.

Deviation of the uncinate process (3%) occurs when the superior edge of the uncinate process deviates laterally to obstruct the infundibulum, or deviates medially to obstruct the middle meatus.

A less frequent variation is the uncinate process bulla (0.4%). This is an air chamber adherent to the superior edge of the uncinate process, blocking the middle meatus and infundibulum. This anatomical variation also may be unilateral or bilateral. Various shapes and sizes of the inferior middle meatus are encountered, some of which can obstruct the middle meatus and nasal passage.

Sixty-two percent of our patient population with chronic sinusitis had at least one anatomical variation. These variations were only present in 11% of a normal control group.

G. Use of CT During Functional Endoscopic Sinus Surgery

Decisions regarding surgical intervention should never be based on CT findings alone, because CT may demonstrate asymptomatic mucosal disease (24–39% of asymptomatic population) (21). Surgery is reserved for patients whose condition fails to respond to medical management. A decision to operate is based on the combination of history, CT findings, and endoscopic findings. The functional endoscopic approach provides the greatest reduction in morbidity over conventional techniques, and hence is of the greatest benefit, when careful diagnosis reveals a limited underlying cause for widespread sinus disease. The most frequent indications for surgical intervention are chronic and recurrent acute sinusitis, diffuse nasal polyposis, and mucoceles.

The surgery itself is typically performed under local anesthesia with sedation. The extent of surgery is individualized depending on the pathologic involvement. It may vary from an infundibulotomy to a total sphenoethmoidectomy with middle meatal antrostomy and removal of maxillary sinus disease. Important landmarks, such as the frontal recess, the ethmoid bulla, the medial orbital wall, and the skull base, need to be identified before surgery. During this identification process the information available on the CT examination becomes critical (Fig. 6). The extent of disease in the maxillary sinuses is assessed and a decision is made about the need for a direct maxillary sinuscopy. The degree of mucoperiosteal disease in the frontal sinuses will determine whether the frontal recess needs to be enlarged. The size of the agger nasi cells and the presence of mucoperiosteal disease within the middle meatal boundaries (findings easily established on CT) are critical to the surgeon. Because this area is hidden from the endoscopist's direct view, its position and distance from the anterior nasal spine can be determined with a sagittal reconstruction performed through the middle of the ethmoid sinus.

During functional endoscopic surgery the uncinate process is usually partially resected to widen the infundibulum. Care must be taken not to infringe on

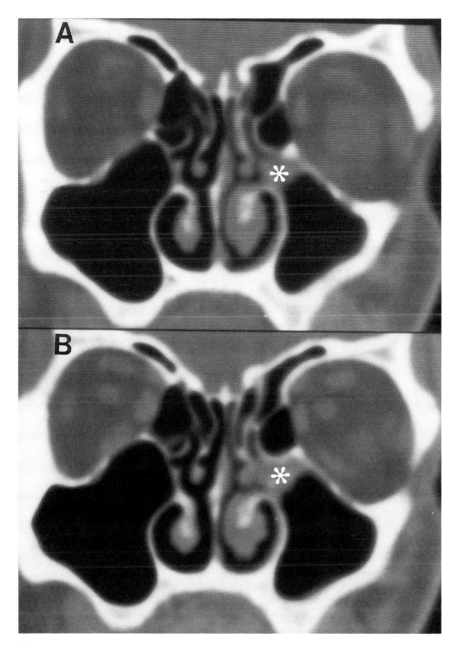

Figure 6 Inflammatory disease obstructing the infundibulum (asterisk) and primary aostium of the maxillary sinus.

the patency of the nasolacrimal duct, which borders the uncinate process ventrally. The position of this tubular structure can be defined on sagittal and axial reconstructions.

Coronal images provide an excellent display of the fovea ethmoidalis (the ethmoidal roof). The roof of the ethmoid may vary in angulation from almost horizontal to almost vertical. Thus the cribriform plate lies 4–7 mm below the roof of the ethmoid in 70% of patients. In 18% of patients, the cribriform plate lies 12–16 mm below the ethmoidal roof. The integrity and position of the roof are especially critical in patients who have had multiple previous surgical procedures and widespread removal of anatomical landmarks. The bone in the vicinity of the ethmoidal sulcus is up to 10 times thinner than the adjacent fovea ethmoidalis and coronal images are invaluable in demonstrating this as well as the many anatomical variations in this area.

The primary sites for intracranial complications are the ethmoid roof just posterior to the ethmoidal dome and the lateral posterior ethmoid just above the sphenoid sinus. The anterior ethmoid artery runs below the ethmoid roof posterior to the dome. In a sagittal reconstruction the artery can usually be located at the mid level of the crista galli. If bleeding occurs during surgery in the dome, one can assume that the skull base has been reached and care should be taken not to invade the intracranial compartment. The sagittal reconstruction can be invaluable to show these relationships and provide distance and angulation measures that would show the surgeon the permissible path and advancement of instrumentation into the depth of the sinuses.

III. CONCLUSION

Once the clinician has gained an understanding of the pathophysiology of sinusitis and the possible contribution of a nasal allergic reaction, diagnosis and treatment of this entity are greatly facilitated. A thorough radiographic evaluation as well as nasal endoscopy are valuable tools in the diagnosis and treatment of sinusitis.

REFERENCES

1. Holmström M, Lund VJ, Scadding G. Nasal ciliary beat frequency after nasal allergen challenge. Am J Rhinology 1992;6(3):101–5.
2. Kennedy DW, Zinreich SJ, Rosenbaum AE, et al. Functional endoscopic surgery: theory and diagnosis. Arch Otolaryngol 1985;111:576–82.
3. Zinreich SJ, Kennedy DW, Rosenbaum AE, et al. Paranasal sinuses: CT imaging requirements for endoscopic surgery. Radiology 1987;163:769–73.
4. Messerklinger W. Endoscopy of the Nose. Urban and Schwartzenberg, 1978.
5. Proctor DF. The nose, paranasal sinuses and pharynx. In: Walters W, ed. Lewis-Walters Practice of Surgery. Hagerstown, MD: W. F. Prior Co., 1986: 1–37.

6. Hilding AC. Physiologic basis of nasal operations. Calif Med J 1950; 94:147–56.
7. Messerklinger W. On the drainage of the normal frontal sinus of man. Acta Otolaryngol 1967;643:176–81.
8. Drettner B. The obstructed maxillary ostium. Rhinology 1967;5:100.
9. Aust R, Drettner B. Oxygen tension in the human maxillary sinus under normal and pathological conditions. Acta Otolaryngol (Stockh) 1974;78:264–9.
10. Wolfstorf J, Swift DL, Avery ME. Mist therapy reconsidered: an evaluation of the respiratory deposition of labelled water aerosols produced by jet and ultrasonic nebulizers. Pediatrics 1969;43:799–808.
11. Hadfield EH: A study of adenocarcinoma of the paranasal sinuses in woodworkers in the furniture industry. Ann R Coll Surg Engl 1970;46:301–19.
12. Torjussen W, Solberg L, Hogetveit A. Histopathologic changes of nasal mucosa in nickel workers. Cancer 1979;44:963–74.
13. Naumann H. Pathologische Anatoie der chronischen rhinitis and sinusitis. In Proceedings VIII International Congress of Oto-rhinolaryngology. Amsterdam: Excerpta Medica, 1965.80.
14. Eccles R, Eccles KSJ. Asymmetry in the autonomic nervous system with reference to the nasal cycle, migraine, anisocoria and Meniere's syndrome. Rhinology 1981;19:121–5.
15. Dolan K. Radiology of nasal cavity and paranasal sinuses. In: Cummings C, Krouse CJ, eds. Otolaryngology, Head and Neck Surgery, Chicago: Mosby Year Book, 1989: 853–62.
16. Zinreich SJ, Kennedy DW, Kumar AJ, Rosenbaum AE, Arrington JA, Johns ME. MR imaging of normal nasal cycle: comparison with sinus pathology. J Comput Assist Tomog 1988;12:1014–9.
17. Eccles R. The central rhythm of the nasal cycle. Acta Otolaryngol (Stockh) 1978;86:464–8.
18. Eccles R, Elwell D, Lee RL. Nasal vasoconstriction induced by electrical stimulation of the cat hypothalamus. J Physiol (Lond) 1979;193:48.
19. Som PM, Shapiro MD, Biller HF, et al. Sinonasal tumors and inflammatory tissues: differentiation with MR imaging. Radiology 1988;167:803–8.
20. Zinreich SJ, Kennedy DW, Malat J, Curtin HD, Epstein JI, Huff LC, Kumar AJ, Johns ME, Rosenbaum AE. Fungal sinusitis: diagnosis with CT and MR imaging. Radiology 1988;169:439–44.
21. Havas TE, Motbey JA, Gullane PJ. Prevalence of incidental abnormalities on computerized tomographic scans of the paranasal sinuses. Arch Otol Head Neck Surg 1988;114:856–9.

6

Medical Management of Sinusitis in the Adult

HOWARD M. DRUCE
Hoffmann-La Roche Inc.
Nutley, New Jersey
and University of Medicine and Dentistry
of New Jersey—New Jersey Medical School
Newark, New Jersey

I. PATHOPHYSIOLOGY

It has been suggested that chronic sinusitis results from incomplete resolution of an initial episode of acute sinusitis. Acute sinusitis is a secondary bacterial infection following a viral upper respiratory infection (1). The initial episode may well go unrecognized and be perceived as a severe head cold. The paranasal sinuses are generally considered to be microbiologically sterile in the absence of active infection. For infectious organisms to reach the sinuses during a head cold, there must be either a failure of the mucociliary clearance system, which conducts surface fluid out of the sinuses into the nasal cavity, or direct cell-to-cell infection. In either case, pus-producing organisms enter the sinus cavities. Pus in the antrum may not completely resorb and its presence generates secondary inflammation (2). This leads to swelling and possibly hypertrophy of the sinus mucosa with resulting occlusion of the sinus ostia. Accumulation of secretions leads to stasis and impaired mucociliary clearance. There is also histologic evidence of formation of new glands in chronic sinusitis and hyperactivity of the normal seromucous glands (3). A decrease in ciliary beat frequency may also be observed (4). These processes have been termed collectively the "sinusitis cycle" and predispose an individual to further infection. It is difficult to assess the relative contributions of infection, inflammation, and anatomical destruction in most cases of chronic sinusitis. If fever and visible pus

73

persist, they are indicative of an active infectious process. However, chronic symptoms of postnasal drainage, headaches, and pressure may persist once all infection is eradicated. For this reason, therapy is directed at all aspects of pathophysiology.

II. MEDICAL MANAGEMENT

Management of acute sinusitis usually includes an oral antibiotic. However, it has been estimated that about 45% of cases will resolve without the use of antibiotics. In one study of 50 patients with chronic anterior or posterior purulent nasal discharge, 20 patients were treated with topical dexamethasone and decongestant sprays, 20 patients with the above medications and topical neomycin, and 10 with matched placebo sprays or propellants alone. Significantly more patients receiving the active treatments demonstrated improvement in symptoms than those receiving placebo. The authors concluded that improved sinus draining permitted host mechanisms to recover and that topical antibiotics added no additional benefit. However, systemic antibiotics were not used (5). In another study of 80 allergic children with asthma, 4–14 years of age, sinus abnormalities were detected on x-ray in 55 patients. The findings of mucosal thickening >2 mm, opacification, or air-fluid level were defined as abnormal radiographs. Those children with purulent postnasal drip (n = 13) were treated with ampicillin, phenylephrine, and triprolidine. In 42 children without purulent drainage, the ampicillin was replaced by intranasal beclomethasone spray for 1 month, together with phenylephrine and triprolidine. In both treatment groups, sinus radiographs improved with a decrease in severity of the asthma. However, the presence of bacterial sinusitis was not adequately documented and all children received topical decongestant, so the role of the intranasal beclomethasone could not be adequately assessed (6).

Both these studies suggest that systemic antibiotics are not required. However, the serious complications of sinusitis, such as intracranial extension of infection, have decreased in frequency since the advent of antibiotics; consequently, antibiotics are now generally prescribed as primary therapy.

Although treatment of sinusitis is associated with resolution of radiographic abnormalities, and improves symptoms of asthma, scarce data exist on the efficacy of treatment for chronic sinusitis. Because of the pathophysiology of chronic sinusitis, medical management should be designed to treat infection in the sinuses effectively, reduce tissue swelling in the region of the sinus ostia that may block egress of secretions, facilitate drainage of retained secretions, promote ciliary function, and maintain ostial patency, both during and after therapy.

I use treatment protocols such as the example detailed in Table 1. The rationale for this is based on clinical experience rather than formal trials.

Table 1 A Sample Regimen to Treat Chronic Sinus-Related Symptoms in the Absence of Concomitant Allergic Disease

Amoxicillin 500 mg three times daily or trimethoprim–sulfamethoxazole DS twice daily for 21 days
Beclomethasone aqueous nasal spray, 2 sprays twice daily for 30 days
Guaifenesin 600 mg/pseudoephedrine 120 mg combination tablets twice daily for 30 days
Steam inhalations twice daily for 30 days
Nasal saline sprays or irrigation

A. Antibiotic Choice

Many patients have previously taken multiple courses of 7–10 day antibiotic therapy at dosages appropriate for acute upper respiratory infections. This leads to a partial and temporary improvement in symptoms. Many practitioners (7) have found that prescription of larger dosages, as described in Table 2, for a minimum of 21 days, has a more salutary effect. The contents of maxillary antral cavities may be sterilized in 7–10 days, but the dosage and duration required to penetrate the ethmoid sinuses and ostiomeatal complex tissues has not been demonstrated. In most adults who yield mixed flora on maxillary sinus aspiration, broad-spectrum antibiotics such as amoxicillin or sulfamethoxazole–trimethoprim generally suffice if given at adequate dosages (8–10). In children, and resistant cases in adults in whom *M. catarrhalis* is the predominant pathogen, amoxicillin/clavulanate is currently the antibiotic of choice (11). The temptation to treat recurrent episodes with successive short courses of increasingly potent and expensive agents alone should be vigorously resisted. Persistence of frank pus or air-fluid levels should prompt the physician to obtain aerobic, anaerobic, and fungal cultures. The prevalence of chronic fungal sinusitis in immunocompetent hosts is uncertain (12).

B. Other Antibiotics in Sinusitis

1. Cephalosporins
Comparative studies of cephalosporins suggest that cefuroxime axetil (250 mg twice daily) is more effective than cefaclor in the treatment of acute maxillary sinusitis (13). Cefuroxime had similar efficacy to amoxicillin (14).

2. Macrolide Antibiotics
Although erythromycin is not recommended for acute sinusitis, recent studies have evaluated the modified macrolide molecules azithromycin and clarithromycin. The data suggest efficacy comparable to amoxicillin for acute maxillary sinusitis of both these molecules (15–18).

Table 2 Efficacy of Selected Antimicrobial Agents for the Common Pathogens in Acute Sinusitis

Antimicrobial agents	Recommended dosage: adult	Streptococcus pneumoniae (30)	Haemophilus influenzae (20)	Moraxella catarrhalis (20)	Streptococcus pyogenes (<5)	Staphylococcus aureus (<5)*
Ampicillin	500 mg every 6 hr	+	±	±	+	±
Amoxicillin	500 mg every 8 hr	+	±	±	+	±
Amoxicillin-clavulanate potassium (500/125)	1 tablet every 8 hr	+	+	+	+	+
Cefaclor	500 mg every 6 hr	+	+	±	+	+
Cefuroxime axetil	250 mg every 12 hr					
Trimethoprim-sulfamethoxazole (160/800)	1 DS tablet every 12 hr	+	+	+	−	+

*values in parentheses = percentage of cases of acute sinusitis caused by this pathogen.

Source: Adapted from Stafford CT. The clinician's view of sinusitis. Otolaryngol Head Neck Surg 1990; 103:870–5.

3. Ciprofloxacin

This drug has also been tested in sinusitis, and was found to be superior to pen-icillin V (19).

4. Investigational Agents

Third-generation cephalosporins have been used in sinusitis with good results (20). A variety of agents, such as cefprozil and cefpodoxime, are under study (21). Various other antibiotics have been used in clinical studies (22).

Antibiotics not recommended in sinusitis include tetracycline, because of resistant pneumococci, and penicillin, erythromycin, and cefalexin, because of resistant *H. influenzae* (23).

I use various adjunctive agents together with antibiotics to fulfill treatment goals as outlined above.

C. Pharmacologic Adjuncts

1. Decongestants

Oral decongestants are alpha-adrenergic agonists that produce a reduction in na-sal blood flow (24). They increase sinus ostial patency, which is narrowed in chronic sinusitis (25–26). There has been concern that α-sympathomimetics may cause ciliary stasis that might counteract any beneficial effect. However, the presence of pus in active infection inhibits ciliary activity, so the clinical effects of this are not apparent. Oral preparations are safe for long-term administration. Topical nasal formulations should not be used for more than 3–5 consecutive days because of development of tolerance and rhinitis medicamentosa. The ef-ficacy of topical preparations may diminish after several days of therapy, but this does not occur with oral formulations. The reasons for this are unclear, but may be related to downregulation of alpha-adrenoceptors at the high topical dosages (27). However, these agents are not always well tolerated. Side effects of hy-peractivity, insomnia, and inhibition of micturition are not uncommon. There is some controversy as to the safety of using these drugs in the presence of hyper-tension (28–29). The former two symptoms may be mitigated by prescribing a lower dosage or using a combined decongestant–antihistamine preparation.

2. Topical Corticosteroids

Topical corticosteroids (beclomethasone, dexamethasone, triamcinolone, fluni-solide, or budesonide) may theoretically increase sinus ostial diameter by reduc-ing inflammation in the area of the sinus ostia. No evidence has been presented to suggest that they induce superinfection or encourage development of resistant organisms. Data showing their clinical efficacy as adjunctive therapy has re-cently appeared (30). The use of nasal steroids has been restricted by some practitioners to those patients with overt nasal obstruction, coexisting nasal polyposis, or allergic rhinitis. The rationale for using them more widely is to suppress inflammation of the nasal mucosa at the sinus ostia (31). There is evidence that topical corticosteroids do reach the affected area by ciliary transport, and have the capability to suppress inflammation. In patients with severe nasal obstruction, it is not feasible to use topical nasal steroid preparations initially. In that case I prescribe a topical nasal decongestant, such as oxymetazoline 0.05%, for the first 3 days of treatment. The patient takes the topical steroid preparation after decongestion is obtained. The steroid also mitigates the development of rhinitis medicamentosa. For those patients who cannot tolerate any nasal medication, a short course (7–10 days) of prednisone is a possible alternative. The use of a combined topical corticosteroid and decongestant preparation was found to produce symptomatic relief in patients with chronic mucopurulent rhinosinusitis in a British trial (5).

Long-term safety of topical nasal steroids has been demonstrated, provided the patient develops no overt symptoms attributable to the drug, such as epistaxis. There is no good reason to restrict use of these drugs to a short course, if the patient is continuing to obtain benefit. There have been isolated reports of nasal septal perforation occurring in patients receiving chronic nasal steroid therapy. These have not been specific to any one steroid molecule or formulation. However, the perforations have usually been preceded by crusting and ulcer formation. I therefore examine the nasal septum carefully before initiating topical steroid treatment. I do not prescribe more than 6 month's supply without an office visit to check the septum. I instruct patients on correct usage of the spray devices and on how to recognize adverse effects. Topical nasal steroids should not be prescribed for patients who have recently undergone nasal septum surgery.

3. Mucoevacuants

a. Guaifenesin.   Guaifenesin (glyceryl guaicolate) is a water- and alcohol-soluble substance that has been used as an expectorant (32). This use was based on its pharmacologic property of increasing respiratory tract fluid, and hence reducing the viscosity of tenacious secretions. It has been used in the symptomatic management of coughs associated with the common cold, bronchitis, laryngitis, pharyngitis, influenza, and measles, as well as sinusitis. There is clinical evidence that guaifenesin is an effective expectorant in that it increases expectorated sputum volume over the first 4–6 days of a productive cough, decreases sputum viscosity and difficulty in expectoration, and improves associated symptoms. There is currently insufficient evidence to support efficacy of the drug as an antitussive or an adjunct in sinusitis (32). High-dosage guaifenesin (1200 mg twice daily) has been used empirically for its ability to thin tenacious respiratory secretions, based on data derived from its effects on sputum. No clinical trials have been reported to demonstrate its efficacy.

Iodine-containing compounds such as potassium iodide or iodinated glycerol might be expected to have similar empiric effects. They have not proved as popular in clinical use. This may be because of the potential adverse effects of iodine hypersensitivity or chronic iodine ingestion.

  b. Bromhexine.   Nebulizations with bromhexine, a mucolytic agent, were symptomatically beneficial, but not superior to saline in one study (33).

4. Antihistamines

Antihistamines and other "allergy" medications are generally withheld unless the patient has a history of concomitant allergic disease, supported by appropriate positive laboratory tests. Antihistamines are only of value in treating conditions associated with histamine liberation. There are two instances in which antihistamines are of value in sinusitis therapy.

  The first is when a patient has symptoms of allergy in conjunction with acute sinusitis in the allergy season, for example, in the ragweed season from mid-August until the first frost. This is the patient who manifests a typical clinical picture of thin, watery nasal discharge, sneezing, and itchy nose, together with nasal obstruction, head pain, and congestion. A sinus radiograph, if taken, would be abnormal. This may indicate sinusitis related to an allergic reaction. In such a situation, it is impossible to say whether the problem is allergic rhinitis or an allergic reaction occurring within the sinus cavities. Nevertheless, it is evident the patient needs therapy with either a topical corticosteroid or an antihistamine or both to reduce mucosal swelling and keep the ostia open. This strategy helps prevent escalation of an allergic reaction into the infectious process of acute sinusitis as a result of obstruction of the ostiomeatal complex.

  The second instance is when during allergy season the patient has signs of infection: fever and purulent rather than thin discharge. First-line treatment of infection using antibiotics and decongestants is indicated. Once the infection is resolved, antihistamines help prevent recurrence. It would also be sensible to put the patient on antiallergy therapy (e.g., topical corticosteroids) before the start of each allergy season. This would help prevent obstruction of the sinus ostia and progression into the sinusitis cycle, and also inhibit the mast cell-mediated late-phase reaction.

  The association of allergy and sinusitis is important. European investigators have studied allergy in association with sinusitis with interesting results. In Finland, Savolainen (34), in a study of 224 young adults with verified acute maxillary sinusitis, found allergy in 25% and probable allergy in another 7%. This is compared with corresponding percentages of 16.5% and 3% in a control group of 103 healthy young adults of comparable age. In Belgium, De Cleyn et al. (35) studied 270 patients with asthma or rhinitis or both for sinus pathology involvement and found that asthma was significantly more often associated with sinus x-ray film abnormalities (65%) than with rhinitis or chronic cough or both (44%).

Whether allergy or sinusitis is the primary event in these cases is unknown. However, it is clear that the treatment of sinusitis is an important aspect of the therapy of asthma. It has been suggested that children with chronic allergic asthma may be predisposed to sinusitis (36,37). Many children with asthma fail to respond to appropriate therapy for that disease until their sinusitis is diagnosed and treated (38).

5. Analgesics

Analgesics may be beneficial in the short-term relief of pain. I often recommend an over-the-counter sinus preparation that contains a decongestant as well as acetaminophen or ibuprofen, provided there are no contraindications to the decongestants. I avoid the use of aspirin because of the risks of Reye's syndrome in children and of gastrointestinal bleeding in adults.

Sensitivity to aspirin or the nonsteroidal anti-inflammatory drugs or both occurs in about 10% of patients who have both asthma and sinusitis, particularly in patients who have asthma and nasal polyps (39). So, although many patients may find pain relief from these drugs, a few patients may compound their symptoms by taking them. Only rarely should a patient with acute sinusitis require an analgesic containing a controlled substance.

D. Nonpharmacologic Adjuncts

Many nonpharmacologic measures are advocated for symptomatic relief of acute sinusitis (Table 3). Because scientific data their on efficacy are lacking, research-oriented physicians may dismiss some of these measures as folk medicine. For many patients, however, one of more of these treatments may provide effective relief of distressing symptoms while the infection is resolving. Most of these measures are short-lived in effectiveness, and they must be repeated as symptoms recur.

Table 3 Adjunctive Therapies for Acute Bacterial Sinusitis

Nonpharmacologic measures	Pharmacologic measures
Steam inhalation	Decongestants, topical (for 3 days)
Astringents (pine oil, menthol)	Decongestants, oral (>3 days)
Spicy foods (garlic, horseradish)	Corticosteroids, topical
Saline sprays	Mucoevacuants/decongestants
	(guaifenesin, iodinated compounds)
Hot, dry air	Analgesics

Source: Adapted from Druce HM. Adjuncts to medical management of sinusitis. Otolaryngol Head Neck Surg 1990; 103:880–3.

1. Steam and Saline

Steam and saline prevent crusting of secretions in the nasal cavity and especially in the region of the ostiomeatal complex. By liquefying secretions, they also help mucociliary clearance. Repetitive saline applications also act as a mild vasoconstrictor of nasal blood flow (24). The combination of steam and saline instillation has a beneficial effect on pressure symptoms and prevents nasal crusting. Apart from their action in liquefying secretions, there is some evidence that saline has a mild decongestant effect by reducing nasal blood flow (24). Saline nebulizations were demonstrated to be beneficial in one study in children (33).

The traditional method of steam inhalation is to instruct the patient to do the following:

1. Pour boiling water into a pan or basin set on a low table.
2. Sit at the table with a towel draped over the head to make a tent over the pan of water.
3. Hold the face a few inches above the water and breathe through the nose for approximately 10 min.

This procedure liquefies and softens crusts while moisturizing the dry, inflamed mucosa. Many patients find that two such treatments a day, with or without additives discussed below, provide effective symptomatic relief.

If a patient is unable to perform this simple procedure, using a vaporizer or a facial sauna or taking long, hot showers may be beneficial, but none of these is a good substitute for the steam and tent method. The ritual of boiling the kettle, preparing the tent, and relaxing over the steamy brew probably has a good psychological effect, enhancing the therapeutic benefit. Some patients, however, may need to be reminded not to breathe steam directly from a boiling kettle.

Astringents. Adding pine oil, mentholated preparations such as Vicks VapoRub, oil of eucalyptus, or similar aromatics may add to the beneficial effect of the steam treatment. Such additions may help relieve stuffiness, or at least give a subjective sensation of increased air flow. Again, there are no scientific data to support this view, but patients say they work.

2. Spicy Foods

Garlic has an active ingredient (n-allylthiosulphinate) that provides short-lived decongestant effects. Eating foods highly seasoned with garlic has been considered therapeutic. Ziment (40) included a recipe for his wife's garlic-and-chicken soup in his textbook on treatment of respiratory ailments. This was not, however, tested by his peers. Encapsulated garlic powder is sometimes recommended by patients who do not like the flavor of the garlic in their food.

Chewing horseradish root, which is available from many food markets, is another home remedy reported effective in "clearing the sinuses" by some patients. Because horseradish is extremely pungent, and just a generous nibble can produce an intense burning sensation in the oral mucosa, this is probably a remedy best left to self-discovery by patients not known to be spicy food enthusiasts. Again, no scientific data support its reported benefits.

3. Saline

Nasal instillation of saline spray two or three times a day, between steam treatments, provides a mild decongestant action. Saline spray also helps to liquefy nasal secretions and moisturize the nasal and sinus mucosa. Irrigation with saline, or antral lavage, is a familiar procedure, but one best left to otolaryngologic surgeons after purulent matter is aspirated from the sinuses of severely congested patients.

4. Hot, Dry Air

Some patients report benefit from breathing hot, dry air. This dries secretions and also generates or enhances a feeling of well-being. Air at 41°C has been reported to be viricidal in vitro (41), and some commercially available devices provide heated air. However, maxillary sinusitis is usually bacterial, not viral, and, to my knowledge, only anecdotal evidence supports the premise that hot, dry air is viricidal in vivo.

There is no clear evidence that the use of these adjunctive agents prolongs the symptom-free period or reduces the eventual need for surgery. After patients have obtained relief of symptoms, it is important to maintain ostial patency to prevent recurrence of infection. I maintain nasal steroids and saline sprays as tolerated, and oral decongestants if the patient continues to derive benefit from them. I do not routinely obtain follow-up imaging tests to asses progress, but do so if the pattern of symptoms change or new ones develop. Surgical referral is indicated if there is any suspicion of malignancy, such as appearance of unilateral nasal polyposis, unilateral symptoms, deep pain behind the eyes, bleeding, or visual disturbance. Medical management is less likely to be effective if anatomical blocks to sinus drainage coexist, if hypertension or glaucoma prevents use of decongestants, if nasal ulcers or perforation precludes administration of topical agents, or if there is significant untreated allergy or intolerance to multiple antibiotics. Patients may simply not accept the inconvenience of multidrug therapy. In chronic cases with anatomical reasons to prevent sinus drainage, surgery is the ultimate mode of therapy.

There is a need for further research in the management of sinusitis. Most recent studies have addressed the choice of antibiotic, and generally consist of small comparative study populations with acute maxillary sinusitis. Other studies are now appearing that evaluate the site of adjunctive agents. These studies are difficult to design. Because patients present with a variety of symptoms, it is hard to conceive of a scientifically valid study based on objective parameters. A "sham" surgical procedure to ensure blinding would be unethical. Since the use of adjunctive agents has become the accepted "standard of care," it is hard to withhold them.

III. CONCLUSION

Appropriate therapy of acute sinusitis today includes measures designed to prevent recurrence of acute disease or development of chronic sinusitis, or both. Although there is a paucity of scientific data to support the addition of pharmacologic and nonpharmacologic adjuncts to appropriate antibiotic therapy, there are still compelling theoretic and practical reasons for doing so. These reasons are backed by clear clinical impressions of favorable effects, not only of the pharmaceuticals but also of the popular remedies such as steam inhalation, irrigations, and breathing hot, dry air. To determine the precise role of pharmacologic adjuncts (topical and oral decongestants, topical corticosteroids, and mucoevacuants), scientifically validated, double-blind, placebo-controlled clinical studies are indicated.

REFERENCES

1. Weinstein L. Acute sinusitis. In: Petersdorf RG, Adams RD, Braunwald E, et al, eds. Harrison's Principles of Internal Medicine, 10th ed. New York: McGraw-Hill, 1983: 1570.
2. Ohashi Y, Nakai Y. Functional and morphological pathology of chronic sinusitis mucous membrane. Acta Otolaryngol Suppl 1983; 397: 11–48.
3. Tos M, Mogensen C. Mucus production in chronic maxillary sinusitis: a quantitative histopathological study. Acta Otolaryngol 1984;97:151–9.
4. Ohashi Y, Nakai Y. Reduction of ciliary action in chronic sinusitis. Acta Otolaryngol Suppl 1983;397:3–9.
5. Sykes DA, Wilson R, Chan KL, Mackay IS, Cole PJ. Relative importance of antibiotic and improved clearance in topical treatment of chronic mucopurulent rhinosinusitis. A controlled study. Lancet 1986;2:359–60.
6. Businco L, Fiore L, Frediani T, Artuso A, Di Fazio A, Bellioni P. Clinical and therapeutic aspects of sinusitis in children with bronchial asthma. Int J Pediatr Otorhinol 1981;3:287–94.
7. Druce HM, Heiberg E, Rutledge J. Imaging in chronic sinusitis: disparity between radiographic and ultrasound interpretation. Am J Rhinol 1988;2:61–4.
8. Hamory BH, Sande MA, Sydnor A Jr, Seale DL, Gwaltney JM Jr. Etiology and antibiological therapy of acute maxillary sinusitis. J Infect Dis 1979;139:197–202.
9. Slavin RG. Nasal polyps and sinusitis. In: Middleton E, Adkinson NF Jr, Busse WW, Ellis EG, Reed CD, Yunginger JW, eds. Allergy: Principles and Practice, 4th ed. St. Louis: Mosby-Year Book. 1993

10. Evans FO, Sydnor JB, Moore WEC, et al. Sinusitis of the maxillary antrum. N Engl J Med 1975;293:735–9.

11. Gwaltney JM. Microbiology of sinusitis. In: Druce HM, ed. Sinusitis—Pathophysiology and Treatment. New York: Marcel Dekker, 1993.

12. Washburn RG, Kennedy DW, Begley MG, Henderson DK, Bennett JE. Chronic fungal sinusitis in apparently normal hosts. Medicine 1988;67:231–47.

13. Sydnor A Jr, Gwaltney JM Jr, Cocchetto DM, Scheld WM. Comparative evaluation of cefuroxine axetil and cefaclor for treatment of acute bacterial maxillary sinusitis. Arch Otolaryngol Head Neck Surg 1989;115:140–3.

14. Brodie DP, Knight S, Cunningham K. Comparative study of cefuroxime axetil and amoxycillin in the treatment of acute sinusitis in general practice. J Int Med Res 1989;17:547–51.

15. Felstead SU, Daniel R. Short-course treatment of sinusitis and other upper respiratory tract infections with azithromycin: a comparison with erythromycin and amoxycillin. J Int Med Res 1991;19:363–72.

16. Casiano RR. Azithromycin and amoxicillin in the treatment of acute maxillary sinusitis. Am J Med 1991;91:275–305.

17. Karma P, Pukander J, Penttila M, Yeikoski J, Savolainen S, Olen L, Melen I, Loth S. The comparative efficacy and safety of clarithromycin and amoxicillin in the breathrough of outpatients with acute maxillary sinusitis. J Antimicrob Agents Chemother 1991;27:Suppl A:83–90.

18. Marchi E. Comparative efficacy and tolerability of clarithromycin and amoxycillin in the treatment of outpatients with acute maxillary sinusitis. Curr Med Res Opin 1990;12:19–24.

19. Falser N, Mittermayer H, Weuta H. Antibacterial treatment of otitis and sinusitis with ciprofloxacin and penicillin V—a comparison. Infection 1988;16:Suppl 1:S51–4.

20. Gauger U, Inoka P, Gesmano G, Kissling M. Cefetamet in the treatment of acute sinusitis in adult patients. J Int Med Res 1990;18:228–34.

21. Gehanno P, Depondt J, Barry B, Simonet M, Dewever H. Comparison of cefpodoxime proxetil with cefaclor in the treatment of sinusitis. J Antimicrob Chemother 1990;26:Suppl E:87–91.

22. Boezeman AJ, Kayser AM, Siemelink RJ. Comparison of spiramycin and doxycycline in the empirical treatment of acute sinusitis: preliminary results. J Antimicrob Chemother 1988;22:Suppl B:165–70.

23. Winther B, Gwaltney JM Jr. Therapeutic approach to sinusitis: anti-infectious therapy as the baseline of management. Otolaryngol Head Neck Surg 1990;103;876–9.

24. Druce HM, Bonner RF, Patow C, et al. Response of nasal blood flow to neurohormones as measured by laser-Doppler velocimetry. J Appl Physiol 57(4): 1984; 1276–83.

25. Melen I, Friberg B, Andreasson L, et al. Effects of phenylpropanolamine on ostial and nasal patency in patients treated for chronic maxillary sinusitis. Acta Otolaryngol 101:1986;494–500.

26. Melen I, Friberg B, Andreasson L, Ivarsson A, Jannert M, Lindahl L. Ostial and nasal patency in chronic maxillary sinusitis. Acta Otolaryngol 1986;102:500–8.

27. Mygind N. Pharmacotherapy of nasal disease. N Engl Reg Allergy Proc 1985; 6:245–8.
28. Pentel P. Toxicity of over-the-counter stimulants. JAMA 1984;252:1898–903.
29. Radack K, Deck CC: Are oral decongestants safe in hypertension? An evaluation of the evidence and a framework for assessing clinical trials. Ann Allergy 1986; 56:396–401.
30. Meltzer EO, Busse WW, Druce HM, et al. Assessment of flunisolide nasal spray vs placebo as an adjunct to antibiotic treatment of sinusitis. J Allergy Clin Immunol 1992; 89:301 (abstr).
31. Patow CA, Kaliner M. Corticosteroid treatment of rhinologic diseases. Ear Nose Throat J 1983;62:14–27.
32. McEvoy GK, ed. AFHS Drug Information. Bethesda, MD: American Society of Hospital Pharmacies. 1992:1600–1.
33. Van Beuer HPS, Bosmans J, Stevens WI. Nebulization treatment with saline compared to bromhexine in treating chronic sinusitis in asthmatic children. Allergy 1987;42:33–6.
34. Savolainen S. Allergy in patients with acute maxillary sinusitis. Allergy 1989; 44:116–22.
35. De Cleyn KM, Kersschot EA, De Clerck LS, et al. Paranasal sinus pathology in allergic and nonallergic respiratory tract diseases. Allergy 1986;41:3131–8.
36. Rachelsfsky GS, Shapiro GG. Diseases of paranasal sinuses in children. In: Bierman CD, Pearlman DS, eds. Allergic Diseases of Infancy, Childhood and Adolescence. Philadelphia: WB Saunders, 1980;526–35.
37. Rachelefsky GS, Goldberg M, Katz RM, et al. Sinus disease in children with respiratory allergy. J Allergy Clin Immunol 1978;61:310–4.
38. Shapiro GG. Role of allergy in sinusitis. Pediatr Infect Dis 1985:4(suppl):55–8.
39. Slavin RG, Friedman WH. Nasal allergy: medical and surgical treatment. Adv Otolaryngol Head Neck Surg 1987;91–108.
40. Ziment I. Respiratory Pharmacology and Therapeutics, 1st ed. Philadelphia: WB Saunders, 1978.
41. Yerushalmi A, Karman S, Lwoff A. Treatment of perennial allergic rhinitis by local hyperthermia. Proc Natl Acad Sci 1982;79:4766–9.

7

Medical Management in Children

FRANK S. VIRANT and GAIL G. SHAPIRO
University of Washington
Seattle, Washington

I. ANATOMY

The paranasal sinuses are a series of paired mucosa-lined cavities that surround the nose and are adjacent to the orbit. As early as 10 weeks of gestation, the maxillary sinuses begin to develop as a small ridge superior to the inferior turbinates, projecting medially into the middle meatus. Subsequently, during the third to fifth month of fetal life, the frontal, sphenoid, and ethmoid sinuses begin to develop as well. Pneumatization of all of the sinuses continues throughout the childhood years until early adulthood. The mucosal lining of the sinuses, or mucoperiostium, contains cilia and mucus glands quite similar (although less dense) than those found in the nasal mucosa. Normally this mucosa is covered with a small amount of mucus that is naturally propelled by the cilia toward the ostia of the sinuses (1).

It is important to realize that the maxillary antra and ethmoids are sufficiently pneumatized early in infancy to be a site for active, acute or chronic disease. When evaluating children with recurrent middle ear disease, it is also important to realize that the sinus ostia are located only slightly anterior and superior to the orifice for the eustachian tube. Infected sinuses may therefore serve as a source for chronic purulent middle ear disease and middle ear disease may affect the sinuses.

Table 1   Sources of Sinus Ostial Obstruction

Mucosal swelling	Mechanical factors
Viral upper respiratory infection	Choanal atresia
Allergic rhinitis	Septal deviation
Asthma	Polyps
Cystic fibrosis	Foreign bodies
Immunodeficiency	Tumor
Immotile cilia syndrome	
Down's syndrome	
Trauma, barotrauma	
Dental infections	
Cigarette smoke (?)	
Pollution (?)	

II. PATHOPHYSIOLOGIC BASIS

The focal points for sinus disease are the sinus openings, or ostia. The ostia of the maxillary sinuses are round or oval, approximately 2.5–4 mm in diameter, and lie in the middle meatus between the inferior and middle turbinate bones. Within the sinus itself, the ostia are located immediately below the orbital floor at the highest point of the antrum, a position not conducive to gravity-dependent drainage while the patient is upright. The ostia of the individual ethmoid air cells are even smaller, with a typical diameter of only 1 or 2 mm. This renders the ethmoid sinuses particularly susceptible to occlusion from mucosal edema or granulation tissue. Although the ostia of the frontal and sphenoid sinuses in the superior meatus are also quite small, their position is more ideal in that gravity can enhance the normal ciliary clearance of mucus (2).

The many factors that predispose to ostial obstruction, and hence increased risk of sinus disease, can be divided into those that principally cause swelling of the mucosa and secondary obstruction and those that cause direct, primary mechanical obstruction (see Table 1) (3). Swelling of the mucosa, often on an inflammatory basis, may occur as a consequence of a systemic disease, for example cystic fibrosis, Down's syndrome, or immunodeficiency, or may be a consequence of localized tissue insult, for example, diving or cigarette smoking. From a clinician's perspective, viral and allergic rhinitis are the most commonly encountered causes of sinus ostia obstruction.

Persistent obstruction of the sinus ostia promotes the development of sinusitis by creating a milieu of negative intranasal pressure and congestion (4). In this setting the patient responds by sniffing and blowing the nose, which increases the likelihood of introduction of bacteria into the sinus cavities. This is particularly enhanced when the ostia open transiently and the secretions are exposed to relatively higher atmospheric pressures. Simultaneously, with less nasal breathing due to congestion the sinus cavities become a relatively anaerobic area that favors the multiplication of many bacterial pathogens.

In addition to sinus ostia obstruction, disorders of the mucociliary apparatus are another important factor in the development of sinus disease. This system includes the cilia, which are thin, hairlike projections on the surface of the columnar epithelia and the mucus layer itself. Normal ciliary structure includes a ring of nine doublet microtubules surrounding two central microtubules. In rare cases there can be a congenital defect in the construction of the cilia that does not permit normal beating activity and hence reduces the ability of the cilia to clear secretions. More commonly, external factors will impair the normal mucociliary transport, such as cold or dry air, viral infections (5), or altered mucus such as in the context of purulent sinus secretions.

III. INCIDENCE

The precise incidence of sinus disease in children is not available, primarily because the gold standard for the diagnosis of sinusitis (i.e., radiographic imaging), is inappropriate for the routine surveying of a pediatric population. Studies would suggest that as many as 5% of upper respiratory tract infections can be complicated by acute sinusitis in children (6). Based on the assumption that prolonged upper respiratory tract infections symptoms might equate with sinusitis, other research would suggest that up to 6–13% of children in various child care situations may experience sinusitis in the first 3 years of life (7). This particular study is notable in that the incidence of prolonged upper respiratory symptoms was twice as common in children in day care than in home care settings. Considering that children typically average many more upper respiratory tract infections than adults (particularly in the first few years of life), it is reasonable to expect that chronic sinus disease would be a more frequent occurrence in clinical pediatrics (8).

Chronic sinus disease is very often overlooked as a clinical diagnosis because the symptoms can be subtle and often mimic other conditions such as allergic rhinitis, viral upper respiratory tract infections, or mild asthma (9). These other conditions frequently coexist in the patient with sinus disease, and can be important pathophysiological factors. Several studies suggest that the incidence of atopy in children with sinus disease is much higher than that observed in the general population, and that aggressive treatment of underlying allergic rhinitis can reduce the likelihood of sinusitis (10,11). The work of Hisamatsu and co-workers suggests that the eosinophil may play a major pathophysiological role in the association of atopy and sinusitis (12). Major basic protein, a significant component of the eosinophil granules, alters the mucosal surface of the allergic airway and inhibits ciliary function, more so in atopic than nonatopic individuals. Further indirect evidence of a link between atopy and the development of sinus disease is suggested by the work of Pelikan et al. (13). In this study of allergic patients with chronic maxillary sinusitis, nasal provocation tests with relevant inhalant allergens yielded an 80% incidence of increased mucosal edema or opacification based on sinus radiographs before and after challenge.

In summary, allergy and viral illness are the two most common causes for sinus disease in children. There is evidence that both of these underlying disorders can damage the mucosa, impair ciliary function, and lead to ostial obstruction. It is not difficult to imagine that the combination of allergic rhinitis and prolonged viral upper respiratory infection would provide an ideal environment for the development of sinus disease.

IV. HISTORY

Although the clinical presentation of a child with sinus disease is somewhat variable, the typical history is that of persistence of the signs and symptoms of an upper respiratory tract infection beyond the typical 7–10 day course. The most common presenting symptoms are cough and rhinorrhea (14). The cough can be either "dry" or productive, and particularly in the younger child may be associated with vomiting as the child attempts to clear secretions from the airway. Although the cough is often present during the day, it is typically worse at night. Rhinorrhea is usually purulent, although in some cases with severe congestion it may be minimal or absent. Less frequent complaints include malodorous breath, sore throat, irritability, fatigue, periorbital edema, and pallor. Fever, headache, and facial pain are fairly uncommon symptoms and are very rarely mentioned as primary complaints (15,16).

From a clinician's perspective, it is important to remember that parents may not perceive that their child has developed a new problem, but complain that the prior treatments for allergy or asthma no longer seem to be efficacious. Although such children may indeed develop more problems with atopy, chronic sinus disease invariably is present with such a history.

V. PHYSICAL EXAMINATION

The examination of the child with sinus disease should focus on the airway, but begin with general appearance. Frequently, facial pallor will be evident, along with dark periorbital circles and edema, particularly if the child is being seen early in the morning. These signs are typically a consequence of upper airway congestion impinging on normal venous and lymphatic drainage. This appearance may be intensified if paroxysms of coughing and extreme congestion have interrupted normal sleep patterns. The nasal examination typically shows evidence for inflammation with mucosal edema and erythema, and scattered purulent secretions. Frequently, thick purulent secretions will also be evident on the floor of the nasopharynx. In this regard, it is important to note that the presence of sinus disease will obscure the findings of typical uncomplicated allergic rhinitis (i.e., pale, boggy nasal mucosa and clear, watery secretions). Accordingly, the clinician must rely on other features such as past history and nasal cytologic results to assess the likelihood of underlying atopy.

The middle ear should also be carefully examined in the child with sinusitis because up to 50% of the time there will be clinical evidence for eustachian tube dysfunction based on physical examination or tympanogram (17). This is an important variable to evaluate over time, since the abnormalities may not resolve totally with resolution of the sinusitis, particularly if the child has underlying allergy.

Chronic sinus disease may enhance bronchial hyperresponsiveness. Since cough is a very common presenting feature in children with sinusitis, it is important to listen carefully to the chest for any signs of wheezing. Although a significant component of cough is often due to pharyngeal irritation and the need to clear secretions, an asthmatic component is often apparent only with careful examination or, occasionally, only evident with pulmonary function testing.

VI. DIAGNOSTIC AIDS

A. Nasal Cytologic Study

Although not infallible, examination of nasal secretions can often provide a useful clue to the cause of chronic respiratory complaints in children (see Table 2). With sinusitis, the nasal cytologic study shows a predominance of neutrophils, often with intracellular bacteria. On the other hand, neutrophilic rhinitis can also be seen with upper respiratory infections and after exposure to irritants such as cigarette or wood smoke. In this regard, it is important to view the nasal cytologic results in the context of the clinical history. The presence of more than 10% eosinophils in the nasal secretions correlates well with the presence of atopy, particularly in children, in whom nonallergic eosinophilic rhinitis is quite rare. The absence of nasal eosinophilia, especially in a child with severe, chronic sinusitis, does not exclude the possibility of underlying allergy.

In essence, nasal cytologic results can aid the clinician in confirming a suspicion of sinusitis. This may preclude the need for further evaluation. The findings may also direct the clinician to obtain more information, from imaging studies or allergy evaluation.

B. Transillumination

In general, transillumination of the paranasal sinuses is not reliable. Since many patients have congenital asymmetry in the development of their sinuses, transillumination is only useful in the setting of complete unilateral opacification

Table 2 Differential Diagnosis of Rhinitis

	Eosinophilic allergic	Eosinophilic nonallergic	Neutrophilic	Vasomotor
Age at onset	Typically during childhood	Adulthood, often young	Any age	Adulthood, rare in childhood
Symptoms	Sneezing, nasal pruritius, clear rhinorrhea	Severe obstruction; anosmia, polyps common	Purulent secretions, sinus tenderness, nocturnal cough	Congestion, minimal rhinorrhea
Frequency	Episodic or perennial	Perennial symptoms	Appearance most common during fall and winter	Variable presentation
Associated findings	Triggers are often obvious (e.g., dust mites, animals, pollens)	Often aspirin-sensitive; frequent asthma and sinus disease	Infection typical; can be caused by irritation (e.g., cigarette or wood smoke)	Can be hormonal (e.g., thyroid disease, pregnancy)
Nasal cytologic findings	Eosinophils ± Basophils ± Neutrophils	Eosinophils ± Basophils ± Neutrophils	Neutrophils often with intracellular bacteria	Unremarkable generally

(18). This is a relatively uncommon clinical occurrence, with most patients having either varying degrees of bilateral mucosal thickening or more severe symmetrical involvement, which is difficult to discern with transillumination (compared with normal anatomical variants).

C. Fiberoptic Rhinoscopy

Although direct visualization of mucopurulent secretions exuding from the sinus ostia confirms the diagnosis of sinusitis, it is not a practical test for most of the pediatric population because complete patient cooperation is required.

D. Ultrasound

Sinus ultrasonography is also not particularly useful since complete patient cooperation is required and it is typically diagnostic only in the setting of complete opacification of the maxillary sinuses (14,19). In fact, compared to radiography, the sensitivity and specificity of ultrasound are only 50–60% (20).

E. Radiography

For years routine plain film radiographs have been the mainstay of diagnosing sinus disease in children. Waters (occiputomental) and Caldwell (angled posterior/anterior) views provide information about the maxillary, frontal, and posterior ethmoid sinuses. In the past, the maxillary sinus was the primary focus of attention and, in fact, a single Waters view was recommended to "rule out sinusitis." It is now evident that the absence of maxillary sinus abnormalities does not exclude the possibility of significant sinus disease, particularly in the anterior ethmoids. Accordingly, the use of plain sinus radiographs should be highly individualized. Since most pediatric sinus disease will include a maxillary component visible on Waters view, this film may yield readily available, relatively inexpensive clinical information on both diagnosis and follow-up of sinusitis.

When children are refractory to optimal medical treatment for sinusitis, a coronal computed tomogram (CT) should be performed. Such a study offers an excellent view of the ostiomeatal complex, an area now believed to be the critical region involved in the pathophysiology of recurrent pediatric sinusitis (21). The value of such a study is enhanced if the child has already been treated with maximal antibiotic and decongestant therapy so that underlying obstructing lesions of the ostiomeatal complex can be differentiated from surrounding mucosal edema and fluid (22).

Many centers now offer limited coronal CT evaluations for evaluating sinus disease (23). Although these studies limit radiation, they do not provide adequate information for the surgeon should surgical intervention be necessary.

Since it is usually performed for complicated situations that may require surgery, the role of limited CT studies is controversial.

Children who present with potential orbital complications of sinusitis, such as periorbital swelling or proptosis, should also be examined with axial CT (24). If combined axial and coronal CT studies suggest intracranial involvement, a magnetic resonance imaging (MRI) evaluation will provide the best soft tissue examination. Otherwise, MRI has several limitations including high cost, prolonged imaging times nearly always requiring sedation, and the inability to display bony landmarks directly.

F. Allergy Assessment

The possibility of underlying allergic rhinitis as a predisposing factor should be considered in all children with recurrent sinusitis. Suspicion should be heightened in the presence of a positive family history of atopy and significant nasal eosinophilia. If allergy seems likely, the environmental history should be carefully reviewed, with particular emphasis on the heating system and the patient's bedroom. This review should elicit possible exposures to important perennial allergens, for example, dust mites, animals, and mold spores.

Appropriate allergy evaluation includes prick puncture testing for relevant inhalant allergens. In the younger child, testing should focus on exposures that can be significantly influenced by environmental control. Skin testing in older children should also include pollens, and intradermal tests should be considered in an effort to increase sensitivity. This becomes important if comprehensive immunotherapy is ultimately required in a child refractory to environmental control and pharmacotherapy.

The routine performance of skin testing for foods is to be discouraged. In the absence of a history suggesting a temporal relationship between the ingestion of a particular food and the development of respiratory symptoms, such evaluation is unlikely to be rewarding. Negative skin test results can be useful in excluding the diagnosis when the possibility of sensitivity to a particular food, for example, milk, has been raised by the parents. On the other hand, the predictive value of a positive skin test is poor: only about 40–50%.

G. Immunologic Assessment

The possibility of immunodeficiency should be considered in any child with recurrent sinus disease. This should be a particular concern in children needing surgical treatment for their sinusitis since immunodeficient patients rarely experience long-term benefits from such procedures (25).

Before embarking on an immunodeficiency evaluation, the clinician should remember that the majority of sinusitis-prone children are much more likely to be allergic than immunodeficient (26). If appropriate allergic studies have been performed or if efforts to control the effect of respiratory allergens adequately have been unhelpful, the possibility of immunodeficiency should be studied further.

The types of immunodeficiency associated with recurrent sinusitis all involve defects of antibody production (27). An appropriate evaluation for possible immunodeficiency should therefore include a measurement of serum IgG, IgM, IgA, IgE, and IgG subclasses. In the child older than 2 years, qualitative studies of antibody response to antigen, such as pneumococcal polysaccharide or unconjugated *H. influenzae* type B, may also detect immunodeficiency (28,29).

Many patients with sinusitis associated with immunoglobulin deficiency have transient disease. The use of prophylactic antibiotics may be adequate for them. In other cases, the detection of bona fide immunodeficiency provides the clinician with a rationale for instituting intravenous immunoglobulin infusions on a regular basis (30,31). This is important to document because such treatment is expensive and not without significant risk of side effects.

VII. BACTERIOLOGIC FINDINGS

Although sinus disease is clinically important in children, there have been relatively few adequate studies of the microbiological basis of sinus infections. The primary reason for this is that appropriate studies involve direct aspiration of sinus contents, a procedure that requires anesthesia and is generally poorly tolerated.

Wald and co-workers recently performed maxillary sinus aspiration on children with acute sinusitis documented by abnormal radiographs (with sinus opacification, air-fluid level, or mucosal thickening > 4 mm). From the sinus aspirates bacteria in high density ($> 10^4$ colony-forming units/ml) were recovered 70% of the time (32). Although a variety of bacterial isolates were observed (see Table 3), the most common were *S. pneumoniae*, *M. catarrhalis*, and *H. influenzae*. *Moraxella* and *Haemophilus* species were frequently beta-lactamase-producing and, hence, amoxicillin resistant. The *H. influenzae* found were typically nontypable organisms, rather than *H. influenzae* type B. Notably, anaerobes were only isolated once and staphylococci were never recovered.

Another study of sinus aspirates in children with acute disease revealed positive cultures in half of the subjects. Again, *S. pneumoniae* and *H. influenzae* species were quite common, with *N. subflava* being more apparent than *M. catarrhalis* (33). In general, studies of children with chronic sinus disease reveal similar pathogens to those observed in acute disease (34–36). *M. catarrhalis*, in particular, seems quite common and frequently is resistant to amoxicillin. In

Table 3 Bacterial Isolates in Acute Sinusitis

Bacterial isolate	Single isolates	Multiple isolates	Total
Streptococcus pneumoniae	14	8	22
Moraxella catarrhalis	13	2	15
Haemophilus influenzae	10	5	15
Eikinella corrodens	1	0	1
Group A *Streptococcus*	1	0	1
Group C *Streptococcus*	0	1	1
Alpha *Streptococcus*	1	1	2
Pepto *Streptococcus*	0	1	1
Moraxella species	1	0	1

addition to *H. influenzae* species and *S. pneumoniae*, other streptococci and *S. aureus* were noted. Studies in children with cystic fibrosis frequently revealed *P. aeruginosa* and occasional anaerobes (37). Brook's research into children with protracted and severe sinusitis showed a somewhat different pattern, with the isolation of anaerobes from 37 of 40 patients (38). Studies on cultures from the ethmoid bullae of patients with chronic disease have shown a preponderance of staphyloccoci (39).

In summary, children with acute or chronic bacterial sinusitis generally will demonstrate sinus aspirates containing *S. pneumoniae*, *H. influenzae*, or *M. catarrhalis*. Children with protracted or severe symptoms tend to show increasing isolates of anaerobes and staphylococci (and occasionally other alpha-hemolytic streptococci).

VIII. MEDICAL THERAPY

A. Antimicrobials

The primary form of medical treatment for acute and chronic sinusitis is antimicrobial agents (see Table 4). The choice of antimicrobials should be based on an appreciation of bacteria generally responsible for infection. In acute and most cases of chronic sinusitis, the most common bacteria are *S. pneumoniae*, *M. catarrhalis*, and *H. influenzae*. In most areas 75–100% of *M. catarrhalis* and 20–30% of *H. influenzae* is beta-lactamase positive (32). Given the relative prevalence of the various bacteria, about 20–30% of sinus pathogens will be resistant to amoxicillin. As chronic sinus disease becomes protracted or severe, anaerobic bacteria become increasingly important pathogens.

Amoxicillin remains the drug of choice in patients who have uncomplicated sinus disease. It has the advantages of being effective in most patients, relatively inexpensive, and showing a good safety record. Probably the only major disad-

Table 4 Antimicrobials for Sinusitis in Children

Antimicrobial	Daily dosage (mg/kg)	Administration (times/day)
Amoxicillin	40	3
Amoxicillin/potassium clavulanate	40/10	3
Erythromycin/sulfisoxazole	50/150	4
Sulfamethoxazole/trimethoprim	40/8	2
Cefaclor	40	3
Cefadroxil monohydrate	30	2
Cefuroxime axetil	250 -500 mg	2
Cefixime	8	1

vantage of amoxicillin is that it is susceptible to the beta-lactamase of several *H. influenzae* and *M. catarrhalis* species. This problem can be overcome by combining amoxicillin with potassium clavulanate, a beta-lactam salt that can inhibit beta-lactamase enzymes. The combination of amoxicillin/potassium clavulanate, marketed as Augmentin, enhances the spectrum of amoxicillin to include beta-lactamase-producing *H. influenzae*, *M. catarrhalis*, *S. aureus*, and many anaerobes (40). However, Augmentin frequently causes gastrointestinal symptoms including abdominal cramping and diarrhea. Most of the diarrhea is relatively mild and tolerable; if it is not, this side effect reverses quickly when use of the agent is stopped.

Erythromycin–sulfisoxazole is another combination of drugs that can be used for sinusitis in pediatric patients. Erythromycin alone is not a good choice because it is effective only against gram-positive cocci, and therefore, does not provide coverage for *H. influenzae*. Disadvantages of the erythromycin–sulfisoxazole combination include the need for four times daily administration and not infrequent gastrointestinal symptoms. Occasionally, some children will also be hypersensitive to the sulfa component.

Sulfamethoxazole–trimethoprim (SMX-TMP) is another potential alternative treatment for sinusitis. Although hypersensitivity to sulfa is again a potential problem, SMX-TMP has a broad spectrum of antimicrobial action and has the advantages of being inexpensive and only given twice daily. Occasionally, resistance to group A *Streptococcus* and *S. pneumoniae* can also be a problem.

Cephalosporins represent another major group of antimicrobials that can be used for treating both acute and chronic sinusitis in children (41). First-generation cephalosporins do not provide adequate *H. influenzae* coverage and, hence, are not a reasonable choice for sinusitis. Cefaclor, a second-generation cephalosporin, provides better coverage than first-generation analogs but still is resisted by some strains of *H. influenzae* and *M. catarrhalis*. Although cefaclor allegedly can be given twice daily, efficacy studies would suggest that three times daily administration is preferable (42). Like sulfa drugs, cefaclor also can occasionally be associated with severe serum sickness-like reactions.

Attractive newer cephalosporins are cefadroxil monohydrate and cefuroxime axetil. These agents have the advantage of resistance to the action of the beta-lactamases produced by *H. influenzae*, *M. catarrhalis*, and *S. aureus* (43). Both cefadroxil monohydrate and cefuroxime also have the advantage of twice daily administration. Cefadroxil monohydrate, in particular, is very useful for young children, with its availability as a 125 mg/5 ml, 250 mg/5ml, and 500 mg/5ml preparations. Cefuroxime axetil is more useful in older children and adolescents, available as a 125 mg, 250 mg, or 500 mg tablet. In general, both agents are well tolerated, although cefuroxime axetil is very bitter and is occasionally associated with gastrointestinal side effects.

Cefixime is a third-generation cephalosporin that can be given orally once daily. Although cefixime has not been studied in sinus disease, it has been evaluated for the treatment of pediatric acute otitis media (44). From these studies it is apparent that cefixime is effective against beta-lactamase-producing bacteria but that it has somewhat reduced activity against *S. pneumoniae*. Accordingly, it should probably only be used in a child in whom treatment with an antibiotic that has adequate coverage for *S. pneumoniae* has failed, for example, amoxicillin.

Newer agents with broad-spectrum coverage include cefprozil, azithromycin, and clarithromycin. Further studies need to be performed to assess the value of these antimicrobials in treating pediatric sinusitis.

In addition to bacterial infection with *S. pneumoniae*, *M. catarrhalis*, and *H. influenzae*, anaerobes should be considered as a pathogen, particularly in severe protracted cases. Most of these anaerobic organisms are penicillin-sensitive and others, for example, *Bacteroides* species, should respond to amoxicillin/potassium clavulanate combination treatment. As an alternative, other antibiotics such as clindamycin and metronidazole can be used if an anaerobe is a clear pathogen. In refractory cases of sinusitis particularly in the absence of a sinus aspirate, the clinician should consider combination therapy with a beta-lactamase-resistant antimicrobial and clindamycin. The anecdotal success of this approach may relate to the observation that 25% of cultures from children with subacute sinusitis yield multiple isolates (36). Although the major drawback of clindamycin therapy is the potential for severe pseudomembranous enterocolitis, this adverse effect can be encountered with other potent antimicrobials used for sinusitis and is not unique to clindamycin.

The duration of antimicrobial treatment for children with sinusitis has not been adequately studied. Generally, a 10–14 day course of antimicrobials is adequate for children with acute sinus disease. In fact, patients' conditions should be markedly improved in the first 2–3 days of treatment, with diminution of cough, rhinorrhea, and fever. If the expected improvement has not occurred, an alternative antimicrobial should be considered after 72 hr of therapy.

Subacute or chronic sinusitis frequently requires much more prolonged treatment. Not infrequently, some children will require 3, 4, or even 6 weeks of treatment with antimicrobial agents. In fact, it seems reasonable to prolong the course of antimicrobial therapy for at least 7–10 days beyond the time when symptoms have resolved.

As suggested earlier, children with recurrent sinus disease should be carefully scrutinized for possible allergic rhinitis, immunodeficiency, or anatomical abnormalities. When appropriate treatment for allergies fails to alter the pattern of recurrent sinusitis, or when there is an evident selective antibody deficiency, antibiotic prophylaxis should be considered. Although this approach has not yet been well studied, the potential value of prophylaxis for acute otitis media would suggest that this approach might also be useful for sinusitis. In the presence of more broadly based immunodeficiency, a 6–12 month trial of intravenous gammaglobulin, 200–400 mg/kg per month, should be contemplated.

B. Ancillary Treatment

A variety of ancillary treatments aimed at improving nasal and sinus ostial patency, for example, antihistamines, decongestants, cromolyn, corticosteroids, and nasal irrigation, might be helpful in both the treatment and prevention of sinusitis.

Although allergic rhinitis does appear to be associated with the development of sinus disease, there is no evidence that histamine should be implicated as an important pathophysiological factor. It therefore does not seem plausible that antihistamines would be useful in the treatment of sinusitis. In fact, the anticholinergic properties of traditional antihistamines could reduce nasal secretions and might even impair appropriate sinus drainage. Given these considerations, future studies of the possible benefits of antihistamines in sinusitis should focus on nonsedating antihistamines (which lack anticholinergic activity) or on novel antihistamines with other properties such as indirect anti-inflammatory effects, for example cetirizine, azelastine, and ketotifen.

The use of alpha-adrenergic decongestants as an adjunct to antimicrobials in treating sinus disease remains controversial (45,46). Possible beneficial effects include the reduction of nasal mucosal edema and concomitant decrease in nasal airway resistance. At the same time, decongestants decrease local blood flow and hence can decrease local tissue delivery of antibiotics and potentially create a worsening anaerobic environment (47,48). Until adequate prospective studies can be completed, it would seem that decongestants are most useful early in the treatment of sinusitis to help enhance delivery of other ancillary treatments such as corticosteroids, and to help relieve symptoms.

Since nasal cromolyn appears to have both indirect and direct antiinflammatory properties and has been shown to be efficacious in allergic rhinitis, it would appear to be a useful adjunct for the treatment of sinusitis. This specific issue has yet to be appropriately studied in children with underlying allergic rhinitis. Other studies have failed to show any efficacy for cromolyn in the treatment of other inflammatory nasal conditions including eosinophilic nonallergic rhinitis and postviral nasal hyperreactivity (49,50).

In contrast to cromolyn, corticosteroids have demonstrable efficacy in a wider range of underlying inflammatory conditions (51). At the same time, corticosteroids would appear to be an ideal adjunctive treatment since they do not adversely affect human ciliary function or mucociliary clearance (52,53). So far, the best study of the possible utility of topical corticosteroids as an adjunctive treatment in sinusitis was a study comparing flunisolide to placebo along with a 3 week course of amoxicillin/potassium clavulanate 500 mg three times daily (54). Although the global assessment of improvement favored flunisolide in this study, objective improvement in sinus radiographs and symptoms after 3 weeks was comparable in both groups. Overall, the data would suggest the topical corticosteroids might be a useful ancillary treatment, but further prospective studies clearly need to be performed. Analogous research assessing a possible role of systemic corticosteroids as a short-term adjunctive treatment in refractory sinusitis also needs to be completed. Such studies would be particularly valuable in the younger child in whom topical corticosteroids are frequently ineffective or difficult to deliver, or in adults with significant nasal polyposis.

Nasal saline irrigation is a process that might appear to improve mucociliary clearance. Although few well-designed studies exist, research would suggest that nasal saline irrigation can be a useful adjunct by helping to remove directly infected secretions and inflammatory exudate (55,56). From a practical standpoint, the efficacy of saline irrigation is limited by the ability of a younger child to cooperate with Water Pik or bulb syringe delivery.

IX. SURGICAL THERAPY

Before considering surgical intervention for treating refractory sinus disease, the clinician should verify that medical treatment has been maximal. Such therapy includes prolonged appropriate antibiotics, and adjunctive treatments that might be useful in improving sinus ostial patency or enhancing mucociliary clearance. If this approach fails, or if the child continues to have significant recurrent chronic disease despite prophylactic therapy, surgical intervention should be strongly considered. At this point a coronal sinus CT is strongly recommended to verify the extent and anatomical areas that are diseased. This is particularly true since ethmoid surgery might be contemplated. At the same time, it is important to verify that the child is not immunodeficient, since surgical results have been disappointing in children with selective antibody defects.

The first level of surgical intervention has traditionally involved antral lavage, consideration of the placement of antral windows, and possible adenoidectomy. Based on current knowledge concerning the importance of the ethmoid region, more extensive disease may require ethmoidectomies and measures to enhance aeration of the ostiomeatal complex. These measures can be performed endoscopically in the least invasive way possible.

After surgery, in addition to close follow-up with the otolaryngologist, it is imperative that aggressive medical treatment be employed to help prevent recurrence of sinus ostial occlusion. For a child with allergic rhinitis, treatment may include more aggressive environmental control, regular antihistamines and topical nasal corticosteroids, and even consideration of immunotherapy. In addition, antibiotic prophylaxis after surgery should be strongly considered, particularly in the child for whom optimal surgical treatment has not been possible due to the size of the nasal vault and limited endoscopic access.

X. SINUSITIS AND ASTHMA

The association of sinus disease and bronchial asthma has been noted for many years. In fact, studies 60 and 70 years ago emphasized the importance of sinusitis as an exacerbating factor of asthma (57–59). Over the years, this concept was challenged, however, with the belief that sinus disease simply reflected more broad spectrum changes of the respiratory tract rather than sinusitis having an indirect effect on worsening lower airway function.

Recent research suggests that sinusitis can be an important trigger for asthma. Rachelefsky et al. have shown that children with "difficult to control asthma" experience marked improvement when they receive appropriate medical treatment for sinusitis (60). In this study of 48 asthmatic children with sinusitis, 7 required sinus lavage while the remainder received prolonged medical therapy. Almost 80% of the children with resolved sinusitis were able to discontinue regular use of bronchodilators and two-thirds demonstrated normal pulmonary function. Similar results were reported from the University of Pittsburgh's study of asthmatic children with sinus disease (61).

Further evidence of an association between sinusitis and asthma is apparent in Slavin's study at St. Louis University (62,63). This study focused on adults with corticosteroid-dependent asthma and sinusitis largely refractory to maximal medical management. Subsequent surgical intervention led to significant improvement in chronic asthma in two-thirds of the patients.

A variety of mechanisms have been suggested as a way to explain the apparent relationship between sinusitis and asthma. Among these theories, the most plausible include exacerbation of asthma secondary to the presence of eosinophils, inflammatory mediators, or the sinobronchial reflex. A striking study by Harlin et al. has demonstrated extensive infiltration with eosinophils into the sinus tissue of patients with sinusitis who also had chronic asthma (64). In contrast, patients without asthma and chronic sinusitis alone did not show eosinophils. Further studies demonstrated a correlation between the presence of eosinophil-derived major basic protein and both sinus and bronchial mucosal damage. This suggests that the eosinophil can act as an effector cell in both upper and lower chronic airway disease.

Another possible way in which sinusitis could aggravate asthma would be the production of inflammatory mediators that could irritate receptors locally in the sinuses (and create reflex bronchospasm) or actually be aspirated into the lower airway (and directly create bronchospasm). Radionuclide studies would suggest that aspiration of mediators from the upper to lower airway is extremely unlikely (65). Other studies at the time of maxillary sinus surgery suggest that the local levels of inflammatory mediators including histamine, leukotrienes, and prostaglandin D_2 (PGD_2) are much higher than those seen in uncomplicated allergic rhinitis (66). All of these mediators were at a level typically associated with irritant receptor stimulation.

The possibility of a sinobronchial neurologic reflex is an intriguing explanation for how sinusitis might exacerbate asthma (67). Indirect evidence for such a pathway is suggested from a variety of studies in which irritation of the upper airway with sulfur dioxide or silica particles increased lower airway resistance (68). This effect could be blocked by the administration of atropine, suggesting a cholinergic pathway (69). We assume that this could occur as stimulated trigeminal nerve sinus afferents trigger a response in bronchial vagal parasympathetic efferents.

XI. RESEARCH

As we begin to appreciate the clinical spectrum of sinus disease in children, a variety of research questions remain unanswered. Good prospective studies need to be initiated to look at the incidence of sinus disease in allergic and nonallergic children. If there is indeed an association between atopy and sinusitis, to what degree does aggressive treatment of allergy reduce the risk of sinus disease?

The role of ancillary treatments for sinusitis needs to be clarified, particularly with antihistamines, topical decongestants, and corticosteroids. In children with recurrent disease, the value of antimicrobial prophylaxis needs to be assessed.

Finally, the apparent relationship between sinusitis and asthma needs to be studied further. This should include further prospective investigations on the value of aggressive medical and surgical management for sinusitis in asthmatic patients and animal studies to help elucidate further a possible mechanism for this apparent link.

REFERENCES

1. Graney DO. Anatomy. In: Cummings CW, Frederickson JM, Harker LA, Krause CJ, Schuller DE, eds. Otolaryngology-Head and Surgery, vol 1. St. Louis: CV Mosby, 1986;845–50.
2. Drettner B. Pathophysiology of paranasal sinuses with clinical implications. Clin Otolaryngol 1980;5:272–84.
3. Rachelefsky GS, Katz RM, Siegel SC. Diseases of paranasal sinuses in children. Curr Prob Pediatr 1982;12:1–57.
4. Aust R, Falck B, Svanholm H. Studies of the gas exchange and pressure in the max illary sinuses in normal and infected humans. Rhinology 1979;17:245–51.
5. Carson JL, Collier AM, Hu SS. Acquired ciliary defects in nasal epithelium of children with acute viral upper respiratory infections. N Engl J Med 1985; 312:463–68.
6. Friday G, Fireman P, Sukanich A, Steinberg M. Sinusitis. In: Napitz CK and Tinkelman DG, eds. Childhood Rhinitis and Sinusitis. New York: Marcel Dekker, 1990:199–215.
7. Wald ER, Guevra N, Byers C. Upper respiratory tract infections in young children: duration of and frequency of complications. Pediatrics 1991;87:129–33.
8. Gwaltney JP Jr, Sydnor A Jr, Sando MA. Etiology and antimicrobial treatment of acute sinusitis. Ann Otol Rhinol Laryngeal 1981;90:68–71.
9. Virant FS. Chronic sinus disease in children. Pediatr Asthma Allergic Immunol 1988;185–90.
10. Flowers BK, Naclerio RM. The nose. In: Naspitz CK, Tinkelman DG, eds. Childhood Rhinitis and Sinusitis. New York: Marcel Dekker, 1990:147–92.
11. Shapiro GG. Role of allergy in sinusitis. Pediatr Infect Dis 1985;4:55–58.
12. Hisamatsu K, Canbo T, Nakazawa T, Murakami Y, Gleich GJ, Makiyama K, Koyama H. Cytotoxicity of human eosinophil granule major basic protein to human nasal sinus mucosa in vitro. J Allergy Clin Immunol 1990;86:52–63.
13. Pelikan Z, Pelikan-Filipek M. Role of nasal allergy in chronic sinusitis maxillaris (CSM)—diagnostic value of nasal challenge with allergen (NPT). J Allergy Clin Immunol 1990;86:484–91.
14. Wald ER, Milmoe GJ, Bower A, et al. Acute maxillary sinusitis in children. N Engl J Med 1981;304:749–54.
15. Kogutt MS, Swischuk LE. Diagnosis of sinusitis in infants and children. Pediatrics 1973;52:121–4.
16. McLean DC. Sinusitis in children. Lessons from twenty-four patients. Clin Pediatr 1970;9:342–5.
17. Hoshaw TC, Nickman NJ. Sinusitis and otitis in children. Arch Otolaryngol 1974;100:194–5.
18. Evans FO, Syndor B, Moore WEC, et al. Sinusitis of the maxillary antrum. J Laryngol Otol 1963;77:1009–13.
19. Berger W, Weiss J. A comparison of A-mode ultrasound and x-ray for the screening of maxillary sinus disease (abstract). J Allergy Clin Immunol 1985;75:187.
20. Shapiro GG, Furukawa CT, Pierson WE, et al. Blinded comparison of maxillary sinus radiography and ultrasound for diagnosis of sinusitis. J Allergy Clin Immunol 1986;77:59–64.

21. Zinreich SJ, Kennedy DW, Rosebaum AE, et al. Paranasal sinuses: CT imaging requirements for endoscopic surgery. Radiology 1987;163:769–75.
22. Babbel R, Harnsberger HR, Nelson B, Sonkens J, Hunt S. Optimization of techniques in screening CT of the sinuses. AJR 1991;157:1093–98.
23. Gross GW, McGeady SJ, Kerut T, Ehrlich SM. Limited-slice CT in the evaluation of paranasal sinus disease in children. AJR 1991;156:367–69.
24. Fernbach SK, Naidich TP. CT diagnosis of orbital inflammation in children. Neuroradiology 1981;22:7–13.
25. Lusk RP, Polmar SH, Muntz HR. Endoscopic ethmoidectomy and maxillary antrostomy in immunodeficient patients. Arch Otolaryngol Head Neck Surg 1991; 117:60–63.
26. Rachelefsky GS, Katz RM, Siegel SC. Chronic sinusitis in the allergic child. Ped Clin North Am 1988;35:1091–101.
27. Polmar SH. Sinusitis and immune deficiency. In Lusk RP, ed. Pediatric Sinusitis. New York: Raven Press, 1992:53–58.
28. Shapiro GG, Virant FS, Furukawa CT, Pierson WE, Bierman CW. Immune defects in patients with refractory sinusitis. Pediatrics 1991;87:311–6.
29. Umetsu DT, Ambrosino DM, Quinti I, Silber GR, Geha RS. Recurrent sinopulmonary infections and impaired antibody response to bacterial capsular polysaccharide antigens in children with selective IgG subclass deficiency. N Engl J Med 1985;313:1247–51.
30. Eibl MM, Wedgwood RJ. Intravenous immunoglobulin: a review. Immunodefic Rev 1989;1(suppl):1–42.
31. Silk HJ, Ambrosino D, Geha RS. Effect of intravenous gammablobulin therapy in IgG2 deficient and IgG2 sufficient children with recurrent infections and poor response to immunization with *Haemophilus influenzae* type b capsular polysaccharide antigen. Ann Allergy 1990;64:21–5.
32. Wald ER, Reilly JS, Casselbrant M, et al. Treatment of acute maxillary sinusitis in childhood: a comparative study of amoxicillin and cefaclor. J Pediatr 1984; 104:297–302.
33. Rodriguez RS, De La Torre C, Sanchez C, et al. Bacteriology and treatment of acture maxillary sinusitis in children: a comparative study of erythromycin-sulfisoxazole and amoxicillin. Abstracts of the Interscience Conference of Antimicrobial Agents and Chemotherapy (328), Los Angeles, CA 1988.
34. Tinkelman DG, Silk HG. Clinical and bacteriolgic features of chronic sinusitis in children. Am J Dis Child 1989;143:938–41.
35. Goldenhersh MJ, Rachelefsky GS, Dudley J, Brill J, Katz RM, Rohr AS, et al. The microbiology of chronic sinus disease in children with respiratory allergy. J Allergy Clin Immunol 1990;85:1030–9.
36. Wald ER, Byers C, Guerra N, Casselbrant M, Beste D. Subacute sinusitis in children. J Pediatr 1989; 115:28–32.
37. Shapiro ED, Milmoe GJ, Wald ER, Rodnan JP, Bowen AD. Bacteriology of the maxillary sinuses in patients with cystic fibrosis. J Infect Dis 1982;146: 589–93.
38. Brook I. Bacteriolgic features of chronic sinusitis in children. JAMA 1981; 246:967–9.

39. Muntz HR, Lusk RP. Bacteriology of the ethmoid bullae in children with chronic sinusitis. Arch Otolaryngol Head Neck Surg 1991;117:179–81.
40. Wald ER, Chiponis D, Ledesma-Medina J: Comparative effectiveness of amoxicillin and amoxicillin-clavulanate potassium in acute paranasal sinus infections in children: a double-blind, placebo-controlled trial. Pediatrics 1986;77:795–800.
41. Rachelefsky GS, Katz RM, Siegel SC. Chronic sinusitis in children with respiratory allergy: the role of antimicrobials. J Allergy Clin Immunol 1982;69:382–7.
42. Marchant CD, Shurin PA, Turczyk VA, et al. A randomized controlled trial of cefaclor compared with trimethoprim sulfamethoxazole for treatment of acute otitis media. J Pediatr 1984;105:633–8.
43. Sydnor AJ, Gwaltney JM Jr, Cochetto DM, Sheld WM. Comparative evaluation of cefuroxime axetil and cefaclor for treatment of acute bacterial maxillary sinusitis. Arch Otolaryngol Head Neck Surg 1989;115:1430–3.
44. Howie VM, Owen MJ: Bacteriologic and clinical efficcy of cefixime compared with amoxicillin in acute otitis media. Pediatr Infect Dis 1987;6:989–91.
45. Melen I, Friberg B, Andreasson L, et al. Effects of phenylpropanolamine on ostial and nasal patency in patients treated for chronic maxillary sinusitis. Acta Otolaryngol (Stockh) 1986;101:494–500.
46. Connell JT, Linzmayer MI. Comparison of nasal airway patency changes after treatment with oxymetazoline and pseudoephedrine. Am J Rhinol 1987;1:87–94.
47. Bende M. The effect of topical decongestants on blood flow in normal and infected nasal mucosa. Acta Otolaryngol (Stockh) 1983;96:523–7.
48. Saketkhoo K, Yergin BM, Januszkiewicz A, et al. The effect of nasal decongestants on nasal mucus velocity. Am Rev Respir Dis 1978;118:251–4.
49. Nelson BL, Jacob RL. Response of the nonallergic rhinitis with eosinophilia (NARES) syndrome to 4% cromolyn sodium nasal solution. J Allergy Clin Immunol 182;70:125–8.
50. Sederberg-Olsen JF, Sederberg-Olsen AE. Intranasal sodium cromoglycate in postcatarrhal hyperreactive rhinosinusitis: a double-blind placebo controlled trial. Rhinology 1989;27:251–5.
51. Siegel SC. Topical corticosteroids in the management of rhinitis. In: Settipane GA, ed. Rhinitis, 2nd ed. Providence: Oceanside Publications, 1991:231–40.
52. Dechateau GSMJE, Zuidema J, Merkus HM. The in vitro and in vivo effect of a new non-halogenated corticosteroid-budesonide-aersol on human ciliary epithelial function. Allergy 1986;41:260–5.
53. Holmberg K, Pipkorn U. Influence of topical beclomethasone dipropionate suspension on human nasal mucociliary activity. Eur J Clin Pharmacol 1986;30:625–7.
54. Meltzer EO, Busse WW, Druce HM, et al. Assessment of flunisolide nasal spray vs. placebo as an adjunct to antibiotic treatment of sinusitis (abstract). J Allergy Clin Immunol 1992; 89:301.
55. Majima Y, Sakakura Y, Matsubara T, et al. Mucociliary clearance in chronic sinusitis: related human nasal clearance and in vitro bullfrog palate clearance. Biorheology 1983;20:251–62.
56. Pavia D, Thomson ML, Clarke SW. Enhanced clearance of secretions from the human lung after the administration of hypertonic saline aerosol. Am Rev Respir Dis 1978;117:199–203.

57. Gottlieb MS. Relation of intranasal sinus disease in the production of asthma. JAMA 1925;85:105–9.

58. Bullen SS. Incidence of asthma in 400 cases of chronic sinusitis. J Allergy 1932;4:402–8.

59. Weille FL. Studies in asthma XIX. The nose and throat in 500 cases of asthma. N Engl J Med 1936;215:235–8.

60. Rachelefsky GS, Katz RM, Siegel SC. Chronic sinus disease with associated reactive airway disease in children. Pediatrics 1984;73:526–9.

61. Friedman R, Ackerman M, Wald E. Asthma and bacterial sinusitis in children. J Allergy Clin Immunol 1984;74:185–9.

62. Slavin RG. Relationship of nasal disease to sinusitis to bronchial asthma. Annals Allergy 1982;49:76–80.

63. Slavin RG, Cannon RE, Friedman WH, et al. Sinusitis and bronchial asthma. J Allergy Clin Immunol 1980;66:250–7.

64. Harlin SL, Ansel DG, Lane SR, et al. A clinical and pathological study of chronic sinusitis: the role of the eosinophil. J Allergy Clin Immunol 1988;81:867–75.

65. Borden PG, Van Hearden BB, Joubert JR. Absence of pulmonary aspiration of sinus contents in patients with asthma and sinusitis. J Allergy Clin Immunol 1990;85:82–8.

66. Stone BD, Georgitis JW, Matthews B. Inflammatory mediators in sinus lavage fluid (abstract). J Allergy Clin Immunol 1990;85:222.

67. Ogura JH, Harvey JZ. Nasopulmonary mechanisms, experimental evidence on the influence of the upper airway upon the lower. Acta Otolaryngol 1971;71:123–32.

68. Speizer FZ, Frank NR. A comparison of changes in pulmonary flow resistance in healthy volunteers acutely exposed to SO_2 by mouth and nose. Br J Ind Med 1966;23:75–9.

69. Kaufman J, Wright FW. The effect of nasal and nasopharyngeal irritation on airway resistance in man. Am Rev Respir Dis 1969;100:626–30.

8

Surgery of the Paranasal Sinuses in Adults

WILLIAM E. BOLGER
Uniformed Services University of Health Sciences
Bethesda, Maryland

DAVID W. KENNEDY
University of Pennsylvania Medical Center
Philadelphia, Pennsylvania

I. INTRODUCTION

Sinusitis is one of the most common reasons that patients seek medical advice in the United States (1). For successful treatment, it is imperative that the cause of each patient's sinonasal disease be identified. Infectious, irritative, allergic, and/or structural factors are important to consider. The majority of sinusitis cases can be successfully treated with medical therapy such as antibiotics, allergic management, and elimination of irritating environmental challenges. Surgery is therefore reserved for recalcitrant or complicated cases.

When sinus surgery is necessary, a variety of surgical approaches is available, ranging from functional to radical. Based upon animal experiments, Hilding deduced that sinus surgery should either restore normal function, or "amputate" the diseased sinus (2). Restoring sinus function was difficult in the past because of limitations in visualizing the sinus region during surgery; therefore, procedures that "amputated" disease were advocated. Recent developments such as sinus endoscopes now permit excellent intraoperative

---

The opinions or assertions contained herein are the private views of the authors and are not to be construed as official or as reflecting the views of the United States Air Force or the Department of Defense.

107

visualization of the region while advances in imaging techniques, such as computed tomography (CT), allow for accurate localization of regional areas that contribute to the causative pathologic change and demonstrate in detail the complex sinus anatomy. Through the use of CT and endoscopy, a surgical approach has been developed called functional endoscopic sinus surgery (FES) that removes disease, preserves normal nasal structure, restores normal nasal function and reduces the need for extirpative surgery (3–7).

Experience with FES has underscored the importance of the anterior ethmoid and middle meatus as local areas involved in the pathophysiology of sinusitis and studies have demonstrated that this is the most common area of disease in patients with chronic sinusitis (8,9). It is now widely accepted that disease in the anterior ethmoid and/or middle meatal region can impair ventilation and mucociliary clearance of the maxillary, ethmoid, and frontal sinuses and lead to sinus infection in these regions. The anterior ethmoid/middle meatal region is considered the most important pathophysiological region and has been named the ostiomeatal complex (OMC) (10). The FES approach specifically addresses the OMC while restoring normal function and preserving normal structures.

An overview of sinus surgery in adults is presented here. The perspective of the currently popular endoscopic surgical approach is highlighted, although the discussion has broad applicability to all surgical approaches to the sinuses.

II. PREOPERATIVE EVALUATION

A. History

The evaluation of sinus disease begins with a thorough clinical history. A general assessment of the nature of the sinus condition, whether chronic sinus infection or recurrent attacks of acute sinus infection, is ascertained. Specific symptoms, such as nasal congestion, facial discomfort, postnasal drip, malaise, headache referrable to the paranasal sinuses, or cough, are then outlined. An assessment of the severity of the symptom complex and its effect on the patient's well-being is also made. Thereafter, an attempt is made to determine the cause of the sinus condition through a review of the patient's medical history. Allergy or recent viral upper respiratory infection are common antecedent factors that should be considered. Other predisposing medical factors such as vasomotor rhinitis, sarcoidosis, acquired immunodeficiency syndrome, Churg-Strauss disease, or recent chemotherapy are important to consider. A history of reactive airway disease is also noteworthy in the overall care of the patient with sinusitis, especially if airway reactivity increases or becomes poorly controlled with concurrent sinus infection.

In patients selected for surgery, it is important to rule out any family history of bleeding, liver disease, chronic renal failure, bleeding with prior surgery, or use of medications that can predispose the patient to excessive bleeding with surgery. A specific inquiry should be made as to the use of aspirin or aspirin-containing over-the-counter products or other medications that affect platelet activity. Since excessive intraoperative bleeding that obscures visualization appears to be the most common cause of intraoperative complications, it is essential to ensure preoperatively that the patient's hemostatic system is intact. It is also prudent to review the patient's ophthalmologic history, as well as perform a gross check of visual acuity. If significant visual acuity problems, visual field defects, or diplopia are present, it is important to ascertain this prior to surgery.

B. Endoscopic Examination

Physical examination of the nose and paranasal sinuses has not been a significant part of the sinusitis evaluation performed by most clinicians. It also played only a minor role in otolaryngologists' evaluations, since standard inspection with a head light and nasal speculum allowed only for examination of the anterior portion of the nasal cavity and provided a limited view of the deeper, critical areas for sinus pathologic involvement (Fig. 1).

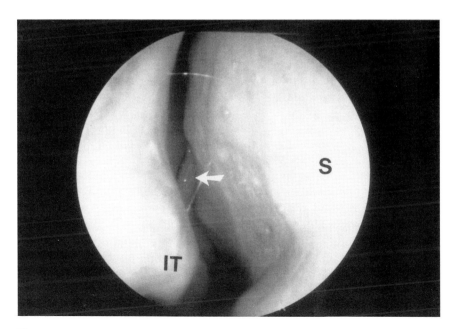

Figure 1 View customarily provided by traditional anterior rhinoscopy (headlight and nasal speculum). The exam reveals only a deviated nasal septum (5). No findings of sinusitis are apparent. IT, inferior turbinate (used with permission, from ref. 1).

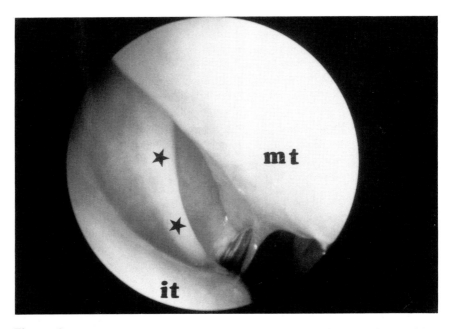

Figure 2 Typical view possible with a sinus endoscope. The telescope is passed between the right middle turbinate (mt) and inferior turbinate (it) where mucopurulent discharge (stars) is noted passing from the middle meatus into the nose. The discharge was arising from the inferior hiatus semilunaris (used with permission, from ref. 1).

Recent advances in fiberoptic technology have lead to the development of flexible and rigid nasal endoscopes that provide excellent intranasal illumination and allow for extensive examination of the nasal cavity (Fig. 2). Endoscopic examination is well tolerated by the awake patient, and is easily performed in the office setting. The entire nasal cavity, including the accessible components of the ostiomeatal complex region, can be closely inspected. Although the endoscopic findings in inflammatory sinusitis vary greatly (3,4), signs of mucosal edema, inflammation, pathologic drainage, or polyp formation signify underlying sinus pathologic involvement and the need for further evaluation and treatment. Endoscopically guided cultures of mucopurulent material directly from the ostia or recess of the affected sinus can be obtained. New evidence suggests that the endoscopic method is more accurate than a traditional random nasal culture (11). Anatomical variants such as a massive concha bullosa or an enlarged ethmoidal bulla that can interfere with mucociliary clearance and predispose patients to recurrent sinusitis can also be identified on endoscopic examination (12).

Endoscopic examination is helpful in evaluating the patient's responses to a variety of medical treatments such as topical nasal steroids, antibiotics, oral steroids, and antihistamines. Through serial endoscopic examinations, resolution of polyps, pathologic secretions, mucosal edema, and inflammatory changes can be evaluated. These objective data, combined with the patient's subjective response, is valuable in determining the need for further treatment. Nasal endoscopy may greatly reduce, and in many cases eliminate, the need for repeated radiographic examination during and after medical or surgical therapy.

Although diagnostic nasal endoscopy was originally used primarily for the evaluation of sinusitis, it has several other applications including the evaluation of cerebrospinal fluid (CSF) rhinorrhea, nasolacrimal duct obstruction, or injury; the examination of intranasal tumors; and surveillance following tumor resection. Following surgery for chronic sinusitis, endoscopy is useful for long-term follow-up. Endoscopic examination provides early objective data regarding recurrence of polyps, hyperplastic mucosa, and chronic infection, often long before symptoms occur. The widespread adoption of diagnostic nasal endoscopy is clearly the single greatest advance in the management of sinusitis in recent years (13).

The equipment needed for diagnostic nasal endoscopy includes 30 degree 4 mm endoscope, 30 degree 2.7 mm endoscope, Freer elevator, light source, fiberoptic cable, and an assortment of suction tips. Most diagnostic endoscopy can be performed with these few basic pieces of equipment, making it easily affordable for most otolaryngologists.

Diagnostic nasal endoscopy is typically performed in an orderly fashion, with the patient sitting or supine. The nasal cavities are sprayed with a topical decongestant and local aesthetic. Topical cocaine (4%) on a nasal applicator is applied to the inferolateral surface of the middle turbinate and to other sites where passage of the endoscope may exert pressure. The patient is placed in either the sitting or supine position with the head turned to the right while the examiner sits on the right side of the patient. The examiner should always take appropriate precautions when dealing with secretions and blood. Gloves, mask, and eye protection are recommended.

A complete examination can be successfully accomplished with three passes of the endoscope. In the adult, the 4 mm 30 degree telescope is usually selected first since it provides an excellent overall view of the nose and nasopharynx and is well tolerated by most patients. The endoscope lens is treated with a thin film of antifog solution at the start of the examination. The telescope is held lightly in the left hand by the shaft with the thumb and first two fingers and is introduced slowly, under direct vision. Undue pressure can be easily detected and patient discomfort minimized. The telescope is initially passed along the floor of the nose. From this site, the overall anatomy, presence of pathologic secretions or polyps, and the condition of nasal mucosa may be identified. In some cases it may also be possible to examine the inferior meatus as the telescope is passed posteriorly. The presence of a patent antrostomy also allows easy visualization of the antral mucosa. However, if the horizontal part of the inferior turbinal bone is small and the vertical portion is long or laterally directed, entrance into the inferior meatus may be difficult (14). Thereafter, the scope is advanced through the nasal cavity towards the nasopharynx to inspect for secretions passing posteriorly on the lateral wall into the nasopharynx. Drainage from the ostiomeatal area usually passes below the tubal orifices, and that from the posterior ethmoid and sphenoid passes above the torus (15). If disease is present, the thickened pathologic secretions may pass directly over the tubal orifice (1,15).

The second pass of the telescope is made between the middle and inferior turbinates. While one is directing the scope posteriorly, the inferior portion of the middle meatus, fontanelles, and accessory maxillary ostia can be examined. The scope is then passed medial to the middle turbinate and advanced posteriorly to examine the sphenoethmoidal recess. Rotating the scope superiorly and slightly laterally allows for visualization of the superior turbinate and meatus as well as the slitlike or oval ostia of the sphenoid sinus. Should access be difficult due to the narrow confines of these spaces, the 2.7mm telescope is ideally suited.

The third pass of the examination is made as the telescope is withdrawn. As the scope is brought back anteriorly, it can frequently be rotated laterally under the middle turbinate into the posterior aspect of the middle meatus. The bulla ethmoidalis, hiatus semilunaris, and infundibular entrance are inspected. Withdrawing the telescope further can provide an excellent view of the middle turbinate, uncinate process, and surrounding mucosa.

C. Radiographic Evaluation

Although plain sinus radiographs are useful in evaluating patients with acute sinusitis, they are of limited benefit in evaluating patients with chronic sinus disease since they fail to image the pathophysiologically important OMC region well and provide little information on the cause of the sinus condition. Advances in imaging techniques such as computed tomography now permit excellent demonstration of the fine structures in the anterior ethmoid/ostiomeatal complex region. In contrast to standard sinus radiographs, CT images mucosal membrane thickening and bony anatomical variations of the paranasal sinuses quite well.

To select patients for CT, the physician should consider if the patient's symptoms are related to the sinuses, are severe, and persist despite adequate medical therapy. In general, a clinical history and nasal endoscopy are used as a screening test for CT since they involve no radiation exposure and may provide the necessary information required for diagnosis and initiation of treatment. Patients who have evidence of persistent disease following medical therapy are selected for CT, in addition to those patients with a well-documented history of recurrent infections. In select clinical settings, such as when a patient has an outstanding history of severe facial pain or headaches and normal endoscopic findings, CT is recommended since it is possible to have significant, symptomatic ostial obstruction without changes on endoscopy or plain radiographs. CT is therefore used primarily to define the regional anatomy before surgery in patients who have already been diagnosed as having chronic or recurrent sinusitis based on nasal endoscopic findings and clinical history (16). CT is used secondarily to demonstrate the location of causative pathologic changes and thereby help direct the exact site of surgical intervention.

For optimal demonstration of the OMC, scanning is recommended in the coronal plane and a standardized scan technique is available (17). Scanning in the axial plane can be helpful if significant work is required in the sphenoid sinus or when performing revision surgery. Since it is desirable to visualize the underlying cause of disease rather than the secondary changes, CT is best performed after the patient has received appropriate medical therapy. A minimum of 2–3 weeks of antibiotic therapy, effective against the standard flora of chronic sinusitis, is recommended. In chronic disease, CT is ideally performed 6–8 weeks after optimal medical therapy is instituted. Surgery should not be recommended solely on the basis of CT findings since minor mucosal changes are frequently observed on CT in asymptomatic patients (9,18–20). It is important to corroborate CT findings with the patient's history and endoscopic findings, for accurate diagnosis.

In addition to using CT in the diagnosis of sinusitis and in pinpointing the location of pathology, CT is extremely useful in imaging the subtle anatomical variations between patients. By studying the CT before surgery, the surgeon can identify anatomical variations and avoid complications. Several important areas that should be reviewed in a ''check-list'' fashion for every patient.

The relationship of the uncinate process to the lamina papyracea is an important area to evaluate closely prior to surgery. If the uncinate process is displaced near or against the lamina papyracea, caution should be used in incising the lateral nasal wall to prevent incision through the uncinate and into the orbit. This is especially important in cases of an atelectatic infundibulum or hypoplastic maxillary sinus (21,22).

The ethmoid roof should also be examined: this area may vary in its orientation and shape from almost horizontal to almost vertical. The cribriform plate may lie up to 16 mm below the central aspect of the ethmoid roof (23), in which case the medial aspect of the ethmoid roof will be formed by the lateral lamellae of the cribriform plate, a bone noted in anatomical studies to be quite thin

(0.05 mm on average) (24). Excessive dissection in this region should be avoided to reduce the chance of spinal fluid leak. Each ethmoid roof is compared for asymmetry as well as for dehiscences that can occur congenitally, from chronic sinus disease, or due to previous surgery.

Careful preoperative CT analysis is crucial to avoid complications in the sphenoid and posterior ethmoid regions. The degree of pneumatization of the posterior ethmoids should be ascertained, particularly with regard to the vertical height from the medial aspect of the roof of the maxillary sinus to the skull base to provide the surgeon with an idea of the available working distance in this area. If, in the posterior ethmoid, an Onodi cell is extensively pneumatized, it will extend the posterior ethmoid cellular structures superior and lateral to the anterior wall of the sphenoid. The optic nerve and even a portion of the carotid artery can lie in the posterior ethmoids in such cases, covered only by thin bone (25,26).

Special attention should be directed to patients with previous sinonasal surgery. Normal landmarks, such as the middle turbinate or its remnant, should be sought. The skull base and lamina papyracea must be diligently examined for the presence of defects from prior surgery (Fig. 3).

D. Preoperative Medical Therapy

Clinical experience indicates that it is beneficial to prescribe medical therapy that reduces inflammation prior to surgical intervention. If chronic infection is present, a preoperative course of oral antibiotics will help reduce tissue inflammation and vascularity. If long-term antibiotic therapy has been used prior to surgery, oral vitamin K may help restore clotting factors reduced by the effect of the antibiotics on intestinal flora. In patients with sinonasal polyposis, a short course of oral corticosteroid therapy can reduce polyp size and vascularity. In patients with reactive nasal mucosa, tissue vascularity can be reduced by stabilizing the mucosa with steroids before surgical intervention. By initiating medical therapy and thereby decreasing inflammation and tissue vascularity, bothersome hematogenous oozing from mucosal surfaces can be diminished and visualization can therefore be improved, resulting in thorough and safe surgery.

III. INDICATIONS

In acute sinusitis, surgery is recommended if medical therapy fails to halt the progression of the disease, or if disease has spread outside the confines of the paranasal sinuses, causing a complication. In general, for cases of acute sinusitis that do not respond to medical management and for complications of sinusitis, traditional surgical approaches are recommended since the role of FES in these disorders is as yet undetermined and evolving. However, surgeons with exten-

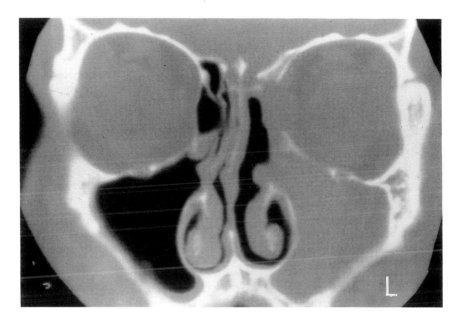

Figure 3 Preoperative analysis of the CT scan is especially important in patients undergoing revision surgery. In a patient referred for persistent disease following endoscopic surgery on the left, CT reveals absence of the lamina papyracea on the left and persistent sinus disease. The patient had suffered and orbital hematoma and diplopia following the initial procedure (used with permission, from Complications in Head and Neck Surgery, Chicago: Mosby-Year Book, 1992).

sive experience in FES are now employing the endoscopic approach with success for a variety of acute problems such as ethmoiditis with associated subperiorbital abscess and mucoceles of the frontal and ethmoid region (27,28).

For patients with chronic sinusitis that is significantly symptomatic and persists despite appropriate and adequate medical therapy, surgery is indicated. For patients with recurrent sinusitis, surgery is recommended when it is reasonably certain that the bony or mucosal abnormalities of the ostiomeatal complex noted on CT and endoscopy are predisposing the patient to frequent episodes of sinusitis. Surgery is not indicated on the basis of CT findings alone, since many asymptomatic patients have mucosal thickening or bony anatomical variations on CT (18). It is important to reiterate that CT findings *must* be corroborated by the patient's symptoms and endoscopic findings.

Surgery is recommended for patients with sinonasal polyposis when medical management fails to control polyp growth and significant obstruction of nasal airflow, or obstruction of the ostiomeatal complex with accompanying significant recurrent or chronic sinusitis results. However, many of these patients appear to have an underlying tendency to mucosal hyperreactivity that will persist following surgery. Endoscopic follow-up and often long-term medical therapy are required if late recurrence is to be avoided. If asthma is present in patients with sinonasal polyposis and/or chronic sinusitis, surgery may be considered if asthma control becomes very difficult due to sinus infections. In our experience the degree of improvement obtained in the asthma is somewhat variable following sinus surgery. Performing surgery on the sinuses when the sinus complaints are minimal is probably not often warranted, even when CT demonstrates sinus mucosal hypertrophy. On the other hand, when asthma is associated with sinus infections that are prolonged or difficult to treat, surgery can significantly improve both sinus and asthma complaints.

Recent experience with FES in patients with mucoceles of the frontal and ethmoid sinuses has shown this to be a very effective surgical approach (27). Indeed the functional endoscopic approach would appear to be the operative approach of choice for this problem and to avoid future complications from mucocele expansion.

IV. SURGICAL TECHNIQUE

The techniques for the various traditional sinus surgical methods differ greatly, as do those of the endoscopic approach. In this text, the technique of the functional endoscopic approach is outlined (5).

Surgery is performed with the patient in the supine position with the head slightly elevated and turned toward the surgeon. The nasal cavity is sprayed with a 0.05% solution of oxymetazoline and after an appropriate time has passed for decongestion, topical cocaine flakes on nasal applicators are applied to the nasal mucosa in the anterior ethmoid region, sphenopalatine region, posterior end of the middle turbinate, and middle meatus. After approximately 5 min, the lateral nasal wall is injected with 1% lidocaine with 1:100,000 epinephrine solution, specifically, just anterior to the root of the middle turbinate and at the inferior aspect of the anterior middle meatus just above the inferior turbinate. If dissection into the posterior ethmoids or sphenoid is required, additional vasoconstriction can be achieved by injecting the sphenopalatine artery region; a sphenopalatine injection can be performed via the greater palatine foramen or intranasally, through the ground lamella.

Surgery begins with an infundibulotomy by incising the mucosa immediately posterior to the anterior attachment of the uncinate process (Fig. 4). The uncinate process is then subluxed medially, grasped with a forceps, and removed. The extent of surgery is then guided by the location of disease noted on the preoperative evaluation. The ethmoid bullae is then usually opened and its contents inspected. If disease is present, the anterior ethmoid cells are opened by infrac-

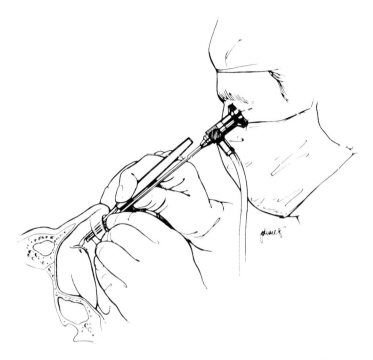

Figure 4 A surgeon using the nasal endoscope to guide the intranasal dissection (used with permission, from ref. 3).

turing their delicate walls with forceps and removing the bony septae. The medial orbital wall is identified, skeletonized, and preserved. The dissection proceeds from anterior to posterior, through the inferomedial aspect of the basal lamellae to enter the posterior ethmoid cells. If disease is noted in this region, the bony septae are removed to facilitate drainage. If sphenoidotomy is required, the sinus is entered inferiorly and medially to avoid injury to the laterally positioned optic nerve or carotid artery. While in the posterior ethmoid, the skull base can be more easily identified since the posterior ethmoid cells are usually fewer in number and larger than the anterior ethmoid cells. Retrograde dissection is then performed along the skull base. The anterior ethmoid artery is identified and small angled forceps used to enter the frontal recess. Care is taken to avoid traumatizing the mucosa of the internal os of the frontal sinus. The maxillary sinus ostium is then identified visually and if the opening is stenotic, it is widened with a curette and a back-biting forceps (Fig. 5). If hematogenous oozing is present at the end of surgery, a small hemostatic sponge is inserted into the operative cavity.

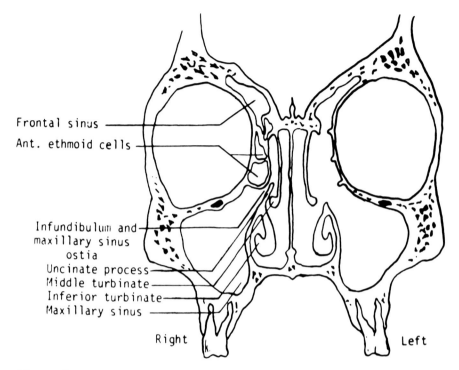

Figure 5 Coronal illustration of paranasal sinus anatomy before (right) and after (left) functional endoscopic sinus surgery. The improved ventilation and drainage of the sinuses are depicted on the left following FES (used with permission, Aviat Space Environ Med 1990;61:148–156).

V. POSTOPERATIVE CARE

A. Surgical Care: Sinonasal Debridement

One of the most common diagnostic and therapeutic uses of nasal endoscopy in the clinic setting is postoperative care after FES. During the weeks that follow FES, nasal endoscopic examinations and cavity debridement are essential to promote healing of the ethmoid cavity. Postoperative endoscopic care begins on the first or second day following surgery. Under appropriate topical anesthesia, clot, mucus, and fibrin are removed from the nasal and ethmoid cavities, while the openings to the maxillary, sphenoid, and frontal sinuses are cleared of obstructive tissue under direct endoscopic visualization. The maxillary and frontal sinuses are then suctioned free of blood and mucus with a curved suction instrument. In subsequent follow-up, small pieces of residual osteitic ethmoidal cell walls are removed to smooth out the cavity and promote remucosalization.

Should synechiae form following FES, despite good postoperative care, most can be lysed easily in the office setting using endoscopy. The frequency of follow-up during the healing period is dependent on the severity of disease and the postoperative endoscopic findings.

Patients who develop late recurrent disease typically appear to have early endoscopic evidence of persistent or recurrent disease; therefore, painstaking postoperative endoscopic care is vital to successful management. Endoscopic examination of these patients may reveal spicules of osteitic bone in association with regenerating hypertrophied polypoid mucosa and persistent low grade mucosal edema and inflammation. Removal of osteitic bone can reduce foci of inflammation and further promote healing. Occasionally a "missed" ethmoidal cell is identified during postoperative examination and can be resected under local anesthesia in the clinic setting (8).

Postoperative endoscopic care is important to ensure that the middle meatal antrostomy remains patent and functions as intended. Stenosis of the maxillary ostia can develop following endoscopic middle meatus antrostomy, although this is rare (29,30). Should this occur, the antrostomy should be reopened and enlarged. A more common problem found in the presence of persistent maxillary sinus disease after surgery is a middle meatal antrostomy that does not communicate with the natural ostium. Should this problem be identified on postoperative endoscopy, it can usually be corrected under local anesthesia in the office.

Stenosis of the frontal sinus ostia following FES and recurrence of sinus disease within the frontal recess are common problems requiring endoscopic evaluation and treatment for successful management. Fibrin, synechiae, fibrotic tissue, and regenerating polypoid mucosa should be removed under local anesthesia to re-establish ventilation and promote remucocilization and mucociliary clearance. If frontal stenosis persists despite good local therapy and medical management, open surgery of the sinus and fat obliteration are still occasionally required.

B. Medical Therapy

Postoperative medical therapy is important to promote healing of the surgical cavity. Patients typically receive broad-spectrum antibiotic coverage in the early postoperative period. In the presence of endoscopic evidence of persistent inflammation, antibiotic therapy is maintained and may be electively intensified, depending on the results of endoscopically obtained aerobic and anaerobic mucosal cultures. If regenerating mucosa becomes polypoid in appearance, oral steroid therapy can be initiated early when mucosal changes are still reversible. Endoscopic examination is a more sensitive indicator of persistent or recurrent disease than patient symptoms, enabling early medical treatment.

VI. COMPLICATIONS

Complications can occur with FES, as with any type of sinus surgery. Possible complications include hemorrhage, orbital injury, and CSF leak. The following section outlines these complications and proposes strategies for their prevention and management.

A. Bleeding

It is important to minimize bleeding during endoscopic sinus surgery to avoid the possible need for blood transfusion with its inherent risks and to decrease the risks of iatrogenic injury due to poor visualization of the surgical field. Bleeding can be minimized in a variety of ways. However, first is the use of meticulous surgical technique. Introduction of the endoscope and dissecting instruments must be accomplished slowly, in a controlled fashion, and under direct visualization to avoid mucosal trauma and resultant bleeding. Careful application of topical and infiltrative vasoconstrictive agents is vital to reduce intraoperative bleeding and adequate time must be allowed to achieve maximal vasoconstriction before beginning surgery. When general anesthesia is used, the use of anesthetics that cause marked peripheral dilation should be avoided and mild hypotension should be considered. As previously mentioned, it is also important to establish preoperatively that patients' hemostatic systems are intact, that they are not taking medications that would predispose them to bleeding, and that they receive appropriate preoperative medications to reduce tissue inflammation and vascularity.

The risk of significant bleeding can be reduced by identifying the anterior and posterior ethmoid arteries and avoiding surgical trauma to these vessels and their branches. The anterior ethmoid artery can travel along a bony mesentery, in some cases 1–3mm beneath the roof and can be mistaken for a bony septae of an ethmoid cell (24). The risk of inadvertently traumatizing the artery is reduced under local anesthesia since the accompanying nerve is very sensitive to manipulation.

Hemorrhage can also be avoided by limiting dissection in the region of the sphenopalatine artery and its branches. Enlarging the sphenoidotomy too far inferiorly with the sphenoid punch or resecting the posterior aspect of the middle turbinate are two surgical maneuvers that are associated with bleeding from sphenopalatine branches.

Should excessive bleeding occur during FES, the application of cotton moistened with vasoconstrictive agent is effect in most cases, although occasionally the use of oxidized cellulose, gelatin sponge, or microfibrillar collagen may be necessary. Unipolar electrocautery is ideal for persistent bleeding in the sphenopalatine region; however, bipolar electrocautery should be used for areas close to the dura or the orbital apex because of the possibility of current spread when working with a unipolar device.

If, during surgery, bleeding persists so that it interferes with visualization, it is safer to stop the procedure and, if necessary, return later using an alternative approach. Poor visualization attributable to bleeding appears to be a primary cause of major complications.

B. Orbital Complications

Several types of orbital injuries may occur during FES. Injuries can range from simple violation of the lamina papyracea without sequelae to injury of vital intraorbital structures such as the medial rectus muscle with diplopia or optic nerve with total visual loss. The frequency of orbital injury is low; however, it should be noted that injuries may occur more frequently early in a surgeon's endoscopic experience (31,32).

Several principles regarding prevention and management of orbital injuries during FES are important. The eyes should be routinely checked during the procedure for signs of lid edema, ecchymosis, or proptosis and therefore should not be covered. Early identification of the lamina papyracea during surgery is essential to prevent orbital injury. After the infundibulotomy incision, the anterior ethmoid cells are entered and the lamina papyracea should be identified. Bony septae of ethmoid cells are entered and the lamina papyracea to demonstrate widely this important landmark. It is carefully followed and skeletonized as the dissection continues posteriorly. Within the lateral aspect of the most posterior ethmoid cells and the lateral aspect of the sphenoid, dissection should only be performed with caution and under direct visualization. This is extremely important in cases where an Onodi cell is present or the posterior ethmoids are generously pneumatized.

If an orbital dehiscence is suspected during surgery, palpation of the eye while examining through the endoscope will highlight the area of dehiscence. If the lamina papyracea is violated during FES, further dissection should be terminated in the immediate region. If orbital fat has been exposed, it should not be removed. The lamina papyracea should be positively identified and skeletonized in the region adjacent to the dehiscence. The fat can be gently replaced and held in place with a small piece of gelfilm to avoid prolapse into the sinus cavity during the procedure. Thereafter, dissection may continue if the lamina can be clearly visualized and respected throughout the remainder of the dissection. Wide exposure, positive identification of the surgical landmarks, and careful dissection help prevent additional injury. The patient should be monitored for signs of an orbital hematoma such as lid edema, ecchymosis, and proptosis. In all cases in which the lamina papyracea has been violated, tight packing of the ethmoid cavity is prohibited since this can increase intraorbital pressure; whenever possible, no packing should be used in such cases.

To avoid orbital complication it is also crucial to identify and preserve the anterior ethmoid artery. Should this artery be inadvertently divided during surgery, the lateral aspect of the vessel can retract within the orbit and bleed. In dramatic fashion an orbital hematoma can result, necessitating emergency measures to prevent visual loss. If orbital hematoma occurs, sinus surgery should be terminated and treatment for orbital hematoma initiated without delay.

C. CSF Rhinorrhea

During endoscopic sinus surgery, penetration of the skull base can occur, result in CSF leak, and create the potential for meningitis. The complication occurs infrequently; however, the incidence is related to the experience level of the surgeon. Stammberger reports only 2 cases of CSF leak in more than 4,000 patients, yet Stankiewicz found that the incidence is higher among surgeons early in their endoscopic experience (12,31).

To prevent skull base injury and CSF leak, early identification of the ethmoid roof is recommended in cases in which significant superior dissection is necessary. When dissecting along the ethmoid roof, caution should be used in clearing tissue from the medial aspect of the roof, especially in the region of the anterior ethmoid artery. Anatomical studies have demonstrated that this is the most frequent site for CSF leak (24) (Fig. 6). Performing intranasal ethmoidectomy with the patient awake and under local anesthesia can significantly reduce the possibility of intracranial penetration, since there is an increased sensitivity to pain in the region of the anterior and posterior ethmoid nerves. Complaints of pain by the patient may alert the surgeon to encroachment in these areas and provide a further safety check.

The management of skull base injury with CSF leak is dependent partly on location but, in general, the source of the leak should be explored and immediate closure by mucosal flap or free tissue graft attempted.

Several general principles must be considered in dealing with intraoperative CSF leak management. Intraoperative neurosurgical consultation provides an additional perspective and is helpful in postoperative management. In addition to closure of the leak, placement of a lumber drain at the time of surgery may facilitate early leak closure. If general anesthesia was employed during the procedure, deep extubation is recommended to prevent excessive straining and coughing. Bedrest, elevation of the head of bed, stool softeners, and restriction from activity that might increase CSF pressure are also advisable. Any patient experiencing an intraoperative leak, even one that is stopped im-

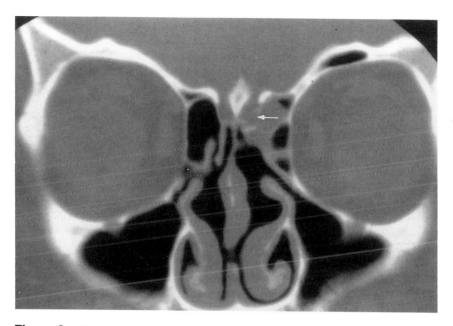

Figure 6 CT scan of a patient referred for closure of a CSF leak. The lateral lamella of the cribriform plate has been violated (arrow). At endoscopic leak closure it was apparent that the injury occurred from resection of the middle turnate. The scissor had been directed too far superiorly (used with permission, from Complications in Head and Neck Surgery, Chicago: Mosby-Year Book, 1992).

mediately, should undergo an early postoperative CT scan if there is any possibility of intracranial bleeding; frequently a later CT scan is indicated to check for infection. If ethmoid surgery is terminated in the presence of a leak, the nose should be only light packed or not packed at all. The use of tight packing as an alternative to a graft, in an attempt to stem the flow of fluid, increases the risk of meningitis and may not increase the probability of leak closure. In these cases, initial prophylactic antibiotic coverage is indicated. Occasionally, CSF leaks that do not respond to initial closure with a free mucosal graft from below and spinal drainage may require neurosurgical exploration from above.

D. Recurrence

Results with FES are encouraging: 83–93% of patients have reported substantial symptomatic improvement in studies with 1–2 year postoperative follow-up (7,33–35). Recurrence of sinusitis after FES and subsequent revision surgery occurs in approximately 7–10% of patients (7,33). At similar follow-up times, FES compares favorably with classic sinus surgery (33,36).

Recurrent or persistent sinus disease, scarring, and stenosis are important sequelae that the otolaryngologist must consider following sinus surgery. However, early objective diagnosis of these phenomena is almost impossible unless endoscopic evaluation or detailed radiologic imaging is performed. The limitations of anterior rhinoscopy and routine radiologic evaluation of the sinuses are never more apparent than in evaluation of the patient who has been previously operated on. In the absence of an acute sinus infection, routine evaluation may be unremarkable even in the presence of persistent disease and may seriously affect perceived results. Proctor pointed out long ago the importance of residual ostiomeatal disease in the failure of therapy directed at other sinuses (37). However, persistent disease in this area is frequently asymptomatic for a considerable period of time and the postoperative improvement in symptoms may be such that the reduced symptoms that persist are relatively unnoticed. Thus persistent disease frequently remains unrecognized for many years unless endoscopic evaluation is utilized. By the time the patient develops recurrent symptoms, disease may be widespread and extensive revision surgery necessary. In addition, following frontal sinus obliteration and some instances of radical removal of maxillary sinus mucosa, further evaluation of residual disease is made difficult by postoperative opacification, even with the use of advanced radiologic imaging.

Recurrence of sinusitis following sinus surgery is possible after both classic and endoscopic sinus surgery. However, endoscopic examination and cavity debridement following surgery are believed to be essential in promoting favorable healing of the surgical cavity without synechiae or stenosis that can lead to recurrence. Patients who develop late recurrent disease typically appear to have early endoscopic evidence of persistent or recurrent disease; therefore, painstaking postoperative endoscopic care is vital to successful management.

VII. CLASSIC SINUS SURGERY

The traditional open surgical approaches still have their role in the care of the patient with sinusitis and offer distinct advantages in certain clinical situations. In general, these surgical approaches remain the mainstay of treatment for acute sinusitis with intracranial or intraorbital complications or osteomyelitis. The transeptal approach to the sphenoid sinus offers the safest approach to the sphenoid sinus and is particularly useful in lesions in the midline of the sphenoid sinus. The Caldwell-Luc procedure has been largely surplanted by the middle meatal antrostomy; however, the former maintains a limited role in the treatment of irreversible membrane disease of the maxillary sinus and in the biopsy of tumors of this region. Frontal sinus obliteration has an important role in the treatment of persistent frontal recess stenosis. Frontal recess stenosis is a common problem following endoscopic sinus surgery, and osteoplastic fat obliteration is time-tested, effective method of treatment for this problem.

VIII. FUTURE DIRECTIONS IN TREATMENT

A. Advances in Medical Therapy

Sinusitis is primarily a medical disease and the overwhelming majority of cases respond to medical therapy. Recent advances in antibiotic therapy have further improved the medical armamentarium. The quinoline agents now offer an effective oral treatment for sinusitis caused by *Pseudomonas*. A host of cephalosporin agents are now available for oral administration that are effective against the usual organisms in sinusitis, and excellent coverage of anaerobic organisms is easily achievable. With continued advances in antibacterial therapy it is hoped that medical therapy will become even more effective.

New roles for existing medications may become apparent with continued study. Perhaps there is a role for prophylactic broad-spectrum antibiotic therapy during and shortly after upper respiratory tract infections to reduce the frequency of sinus infections in patients with recurrent sinusitis. Topical nasal steroid sprays and oral decongestants might prove beneficial in reducing sinus symptoms and infections in patients with hyperreactive nasal mucosa. Mucolytic agents might have a role in facilitating mucus flow through the sinus ostia, thereby reducing the likelihood of sinus infection after an upper respiratory tract infection.

B. Advances in Surgical Therapy

Although sinus endoscopy is most commonly used in the diagnosis and treatment of sinusitis, other uses are rapidly being reported. Sinus endoscopy is now considered an excellent tool in the diagnosis and treatment of CSF leak, intranasal encephalocele, nasolacrimal duct obstruction, and epitaxis. Recently, an endoscopic approach to the sella for transphenoidal hypophysectomy was reported, further extending the applications of endoscopic surgery (38). As innovations in the basic instrumentation occur, additional applications for the endoscopic approach should follow.

C. Staging and Classification

Although several significant advances have been made in sinonasal diseases in the past decade, numerous areas remain to be explored. One area of particular importance is the staging and classification of sinus disease. Sinus disease is presently classified only as acute, chronic, or recurrent. This method of classification does not address different pathophysiological mechanisms involved in sinusitis, nor does it address the extent of disease or prognosis for recovery.

Clinical experience and experimental data indicate that to classify sinusitis as acute, chronic, and recurrent is a gross oversimplification. In patients with polyposis, several subclassifications are already becoming apparent on a histologic level (39). In patients with chronic inflammatory sinonasal polyposis who do not have any known systemic disease, polyps have been noted to have a thick basement membrane and an abundance of eosinophils, whereas patients with cystic fibrosis polyps have been noted to lack eosinophils and have a thin basement membrane. However, patients with Kartagener's and Young's syndromes have polyps that lack eosinophils yet contain an abundance of lymphocytes. Therefore, several distinct pathologic processes exist, each with its own clinical course and response to treatment.

Several factors have been cited to influence treatment, such as immunoglobulin deficiency, asthma, environmental and food allergy (40–42). In general, based on radiographic and clinical data, it appears that prognosis is most strongly related to extent of disease, radiographic data and clinical disease (43).

REFERENCES

1. Kennedy DW. First-line management of sinusitis: a national problem? Overview. Otolaryngol Head Neck Surg 1990;103:847.
2. Hilding AC. Physiologic basis of nasal operations. Calif Med 1950;72:103–7.
3. Kennedy DW, Zinreich SJ, Rosenbaum AE, et al. Functional endoscopic sinus surgery: theory and diagnostic evaluation. Arch Otolaryngol 1985;111:576–82.
4. Stammberger H. Endoscopic endonasal surgery—concepts in treatment of recurring rhinosinusitis. Part I. Anatomic and pathophysiologic considerations. Otolaryngol Head Neck Surg 1986;94:143–7.
5. Kennedy DW. Functional endoscopic sinus surgery: technique. Arch Otolaryngol 1985;111:643–9.
6. Stammberger H. Endoscopic endonasal surgery—concepts in treatment of recurring rhinosinusitis. Part II. Surgical technique. Otolaryngol Head Neck Surg 1986;94:174–56.
7. Hoffmann DF, May M, Mester RTR. Functional endoscopic sinus surgery—experience with the initial 100 patients. Am J Rhinol 1990;4:129–32.
8. Kennedy DW, Zinreich SJ. The functional endoscopic approach to inflammatory sinus disease: current perspectives and technique modifications. Am J Rhinol 1988;2:89–96.
9. Bolger WE, Butzin C, Parsons DS. CT analysis of bony and mucosal abnormalities for endoscopic sinus surgery. Laryngoscope 1991;101:56–71.
10. Naumann H. Patholische anatomic der chronischen rhinitis und sinusitis. In: Proceedings, VIII International Congress of Oto-rhino-laryngology. Amsterdam: Excerpta Medica, 1965:80.

11. Orobello PW, Park RI, Belcher LJ, et al. Microbiology of chronic sinusitis. Arch Otolaryngol Head Neck Surg 1990;117:980–3.

12. Stammberger H, Wolf G. Headaches and sinus disease: the endoscopic approach. Ann Otol Rhinol Laryngol 1988;97(suppl. 134):3–23.

13. Kennedy DW. First-line management of sinusitis: a national problem? Surgical update. Otolaryngol Head Neck Surg 1990;103:884–6.

14. Stammberger H. Functional Endoscopic Sinus Surgery: The Messerklinger Technique. Philadelphia: B.C. Decker, 1991.

15. Stammberger H. An endoscopic study of tubal function and diseased ethmoid sinus. Arch Otolaryngol 1986;243:254–9.

16. Zinreich SJ. First-line management of sinusitis: a national problem? Paranasal sinus imaging Otolaryngol Head Neck Surg 1990;103:863–9.

17. Zinreich SJ, Kennedy DW, Rosenbaum AE, et al. Paranasal sinuses: CT imaging requirements for endoscopic surgery. Radiology 1987;163:769–75.

18. Calhoun K, Waggenspack GA, Simpson CB, et al. CT evaluation of paranasal sinuses in symptomatic and asymptomatic populations. Otolaryngol Head Neck Surg 1991;104:480–43.

19. Havas TE, Motbey JA, Gullane PJ. Prevalence of incidental abnormalities on computed tomographic scans of the paranasal sinuses. Arch Otolaryngol 1988; 114:856–9.

20. Diament MJ, Senac MO, Gilsanz V, et al. Prevalence of incidental paranasal sinuses opacification in pediatric patients: a CT study. J Comput Assist Tomogr 1987; 11:426–31.

21. Bolger WE, Woodruff WW, Morehead J, Parsons DS. Maxillary sinus hypoplasia: classification and description of associated uncinate hypoplasia. Otolaryngol Head Neck Surg 1990;103:759–65.

22. Furin MJ, Zinreich SJ, Kennedy DW. The atelectatic maxillary sinus. Am J Rhinol 1991;5:79–83.

23. Keros P: Uber die praktische beteudung der Niveau-Unterschiede der lamina cribrosa des ethmoids. In: Naumann HH. Head & Neck Surgery, vol 1 (Face and Facial Skull). Philadelphia: W.B. Saunders, 1980:392.

24. Kainz J, Stammberger H. The roof of the anterior ethmoid: a place of least resistance in the skull base. Am J Rhinol 1989;3:191–9.

25. Kennedy DW, Zinreich SJ, Hassab MH. The internal carotid artery as it relates to endonasal sphenoethmoidectomy. Am J Rhinol 1990;4:7–12.

26. Banssberg SF, Harner SG, Forbes G. Relationship of the optic nerve to the paranasal sinuses as shown by computed tomography. Otolaryngol Head Neck Surg 1987;96:331–5.

27. Kennedy DW, Josephson JS, Zinreich SJ, Mattox DE, Goldsmith MM. Endoscopic sinus surgery for mucoceles: a viable alternative. Laryngoscope 1989;99:885–95.

28. Draf W. Endonasal micro-endoscopic frontal sinus surgery: the Fulda concept. Oper Tech Otolaryngol Head Neck Surg 1991;2:234–40.

29. Davis WE, Templer JW, Lamear WR, et al. Middle meatal antrostomy: patency rates and risk factors. Otolaryngol Head Neck Surg 1991;104–467–72.

30. Kennedy DW, Zinreich SJ, Kuhn F, et al. Endoscopic middle meatus antrostomy: theory, technique and patency. Laryngoscope 1987;97:1–9.

31. Stankiewicz JA. Complications of endoscopic intranasal ethmoidectomy. Laryngoscope 1987;97:1270–3.
32. Vleming M, Middelweerd RJ, de Vries N. Complications of endoscopic sinus surgery. Arch Otolaryngol Head Neck Surg 1992;118:617–23.
33. Levine HL. Functional endoscopic sinus surgery: evaluation, surgery, and follow-up of 250 patients. Laryngoscope 1909;100:79–83.
34. Rice D. Endoscopic sinus surgery results at 2 year follow-up. Otolaryngol Head Neck Surg 1989;101:476–9.
35. Schaeffer SD, Close LG. Endoscopic management of frontal sinus disease. Laryngoscope 1990;100:155–60.
36. Amedee RG, Mann WJ, Gilsbach JM. Microscopic endonasal surgery: clinical update for treatment of chronic sinusitis with polyps. Am J Rhinol 1990;4:203–5.
37. Proctor DF. The nose, paranasal sinuses and pharynx. In: Walters W, ed. Lewis-Walters Practice of Surgery, Boston: Little Brown, 1982:7–42.
38. Jankowski R, Auque J, Simon C, Marchal JC, Hepner H, Wayoff M. Endoscopic pituitary surgery. Laryngoscope 1992; 102:198–202.
39. Settipane GA. Nasal polyps: epidemiology, pathology, immunology, and treatment. Am J Rhinol 1987;1:119–26.
40. Lusk R, Polmar SH, Muntz HR. Endoscopic ethmoidectomy and maxillary antrostomy in immunodeficient patients. Arch Otolaryngol Head Neck Surg 1991;117:60–3.
41. Lawson W. The intranasal ethmoidectomy: an experience with 1,077 procedures: Laryngoscope 1991;101:367–71.
42. Sogg A. Long-term results of ethmoid surgery. Ann Otol Rhinol Laryngol. 1989:98:699–701.
43. Kennedy DW. Prognostic factors, outcomes and staging in ethmoids sinus surgery. Laryngoscope 1992;102(Supp. 57):1–18.

9

Surgical Management of Pediatric Sinusitis

RODNEY P. LUSK
St. Louis Children's Hospital
Washington University
St. Louis, Missouri

The literature evaluating the surgical management of pediatric sinusitis is confusing. This is due, at least in part, to the multifactorial causes of sinusitis and the difficulty in making the diagnosis. Neither the signs and symptoms nor the physical examination are diagnostic for chronic condition, and many disease processes resemble sinusitis. Our assessments of the severity of sinusitis were previously based on plain films, which we now know to be inaccurate in assessing the extent and location of pediatric sinusitis (1). We continue to lack an accurate staging mechanism for the severity of pediatric sinusitis and therefore lack a standard for comparing our results.

This chapter discusses the existing methods of surgical management of pediatric chronic sinusitis and indicates, where possible, the most viable options.

I. PHYSICAL EXAMINATION

Maxillary sinusitis is difficult to detect by physical examination, signs, or symptoms alone (2–4). In children, regardless of the examination method used, only anterior rhinoscopy can be accomplished. In our experience, the otoscope remains the best instrument for examining the child's nose. The middle meatus is frequently not well visualized, but if it is clear, one can be encouraged, although not assured, that the ostiomeatal complex is free of disease (Fig. 1). If purulence is seen in this region, (Fig. 2) one should be suspicious that an infection is present.

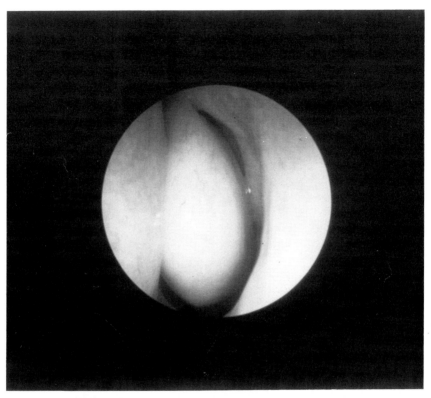

Figure 1   View of the middle meatus in a normal child.

II. FOREIGN BODY REMOVAL

Foreign bodies are not an infrequent cause of unilateral purulent nasal discharge (Fig. 3). Except when it is caused by a foreign body, purulent rhinorrhea is almost always bilateral. Removal of the foreign body results in resolution of symptoms, usually with no sequelae.

III. ADENOTONSILLECTOMY AND/OR ADENOIDECTOMY

Adenoid hypertrophy may cause nasal obstruction and present with many of the same symptoms as chronic sinusitis. The reported incidence and severity of diseased tonsils and adenoids associated with chronic sinusitis vary with the investigator and the methods of diagnosis. Almost all of these studies are retrospective, with poor documentation of both the severity of sinusitis and the indications for the tonsillectomy or adenoidectomy, and usually with inadequate follow-up.

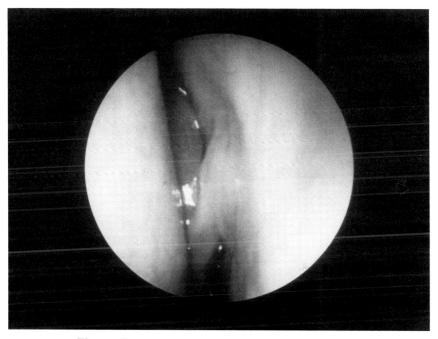

Figure 2 Purulence from the middle meatus of a child.

Much of the confusion regarding surgical management lies in the fact that purulent rhinorrhea is common in children (5) and neonates (6), but does not necessarily reflect sinusitis (2,7,8). It may, for example, be caused by adenoidal obstruction. When there is sinusitis, the frequency may be related to the size of the adenoids (3,9,10). Merck (9) noted diseased antra in 13% of children with small adenoid pads, 24% of those with medium-sized adenoid pads, and 34% of those with large adenoid pads. Birrell (3) found maxillary sinus disease in 27% of the 580 patients who underwent tonsillectomy and adenoidectomy. Carmack (11) attempted to exclude patients with sinusitis or allergy and still found that 14.2% of the children undergoing "routine tonsillectomy and adenoidectomy" had maxillary sinusitis found by antral lavage. Stevenson (12) said that he had never seen a case of maxillary sinusitis that did not have an adenoid pad present, but obviously this does not mean that the adenoid pad caused the disease. Some association between sinusitis and the size or the degree of disease of the adenoid pad does seem likely, however. But Walker (13) found that the degree of infection of the tonsils was more of a factor in sinusitis than the size of the adenoid pad. The causal relationship is not clear.

The role of tonsillectomy and/or adenoidectomy (T&A) in treating sinusitis is not clear. The older literature supports it as a treatment modality, but the

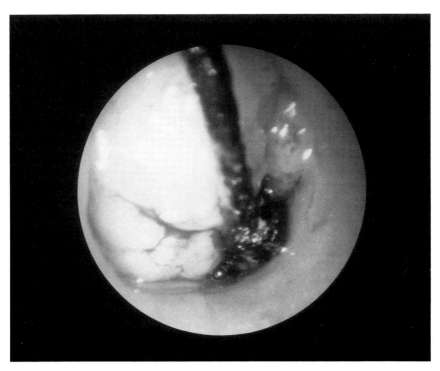

Figure 3   Foreign body in the anterior nose. Removal resulted in resolution of purulent nasal discharge.

indications are not well defined. More recent studies show that T&A has not consistently cured chronic pediatric sinusitis (8,11–15). Paul (8) found that T&A did not always clear purulent rhinorrhea and that antibiotics alone were almost as effective. His study did not specify duration of follow-up, but it does indicate the inability of T & A alone to cure all cases of sinusitis. Fujita (16) found that adenoidectomy "improved" nasal sinusitis in 56% of children, but 24% improval improvement occurred in the nonadenoidectomy-treated group.

Our current state of knowledge does not allow us to predict which children with sinusitis will experience an improvement or resolution of their disease with adenoidectomy alone. If the child has an enlarged adenoid pad (Fig. 4), performing an adenoidectomy may be a prudent first step. How large the adenoids must be before the obstruction causes symptoms or contributes to infection remains a matter of judgment (Fig. 5). If the adenoid pad is not obstructive, our experience indicates that adenoidectomy does not alter the course of the sinusitis. The studies regarding the efficacy of adenoidectomy should be re-

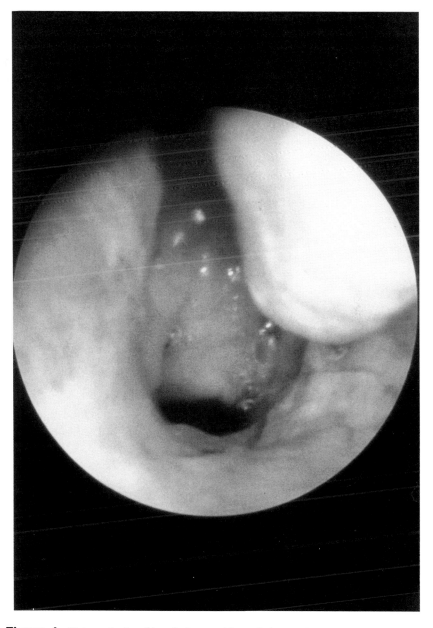

Figure 4   Enlarged adenoid pad that could result in nasal airway obstruction and
mimic or cause chronic sinusitis.

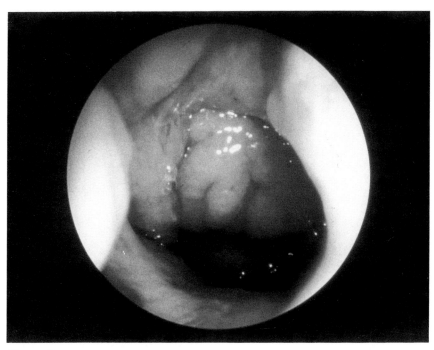

Figure 5 Medium-sized adenoid pad. It is questionable whether removal would result in symptomatic improvement.

peated using coronal computed tomographic (CT) scans as one of the criteria for diagnosing sinusitis.

IV. ANTRAL LAVAGE

Antral lavage is frequently recommended for the treatment of chronic sinusitis, the rationale being to suction debris out of the maxillary sinus or to force debris out through the natural ostium. A telescope can be placed through the puncture into the sinus to examine its contents. The maxillary sinus can be irrigated through the natural ostium, the inferior meatus, or the canine fossa (anterior) puncture. Since irrigation and sinusotomy can be directed only to the maxillary sinus, this modality of surgical management can be effectively used only in patients with maxillary sinus disease. We now know that most children also have ethmoid disease (1).

Perhaps the oldest technique of antral lavage is through the natural ostium of the maxillary sinus. This is usually combined with another procedure such as T & A. A curved cannula is rotated laterally and anteriorly behind the uncinate process. Frequently the cannula engages the natural ostium, and the maxillary sinus can be aspirated or lavaged with warm saline solution until clear. The cannula cannot be introduced in all patients (17,18).

Lund (19) credits Gooch with the first description of an intranasal inferior meatal puncture in the 1770s. Mikulicz (20) preferred the inferior meatal puncture because the middle meatal approach is not always anatomically possible, the sphenopalatine artery could cause troublesome bleeding, and cannulating the natural ostium could result in orbital complications. He was also concerned about damage to the ostium of the maxillary sinus (21). This method has the disadvantage of not being useful in young children because the floor of the maxillary sinus has not developed below the insertion of the inferior turbinate, and the maxillary sinus therefore cannot be entered.

The canine fossa puncture is performed by going through the bone of the anterior antral wall. It is the most direct route to the sinus. This procedure is easier and safer than the other two techniques but difficult to perform under local anesthesia. In children the anterior wall to the maxillary sinus may be thick and difficult to penetrate. Complications that can occur with maxillary puncture are that the permanent teeth can be traumatized, a false passage can be created into the nose through the middle meatus or the ostium, and the trocar can be passed through the roof of the maxillary sinus into the orbit or through the posterior maxillary sinus wall into the pterygopalatine fossa. If these spaces are irrigated, significant complications can occur.

Lavage has also been combined with the use of cannulas of different types for irrigating the maxillary sinus. Some authors (11,12,22,23) have recommended leaving the sinus cannulated for multiple irrigations. Over time these methods of treatment have proved unsuccessful (in part because only the maxillary sinus is addressed) and are now rarely used. For this reason Stammberger (24) does not recommend canine fossa puncture in children younger than 9 years old. Lavage combined with sinoscopy has been used as a standard to measure the accuracy of plain radiographs. Kim (25) found that sinoscopy revealed the correct status of the maxillary sinusitis more frequently than did plain sinus films.

Antral lavage has had mixed reviews in the literature. Rarely is antral lavage successful with one intervention, and several authors (12,26–28) recommend multiple lavage before proceeding to a Caldwell-Luc procedure. Crooks (27) recommended weekly lavage until the patient's sinuses were clear and reported as many as 10 lavage procedures before abandoning this mode of therapy. Stammberger (24) does not believe that multiple lavages are necessary if an adequate local decongestant is applied to the ostiomeatal complex.

Antral lavage continues to be practiced today, and in selected patients it probably has merit. No good prospective studies allow us to predict which patients will respond to antral lavage. In today's medical environment it is unlikely that parents, pediatricians, or otolaryngologists will tolerate frequent local lavage, and the need for multiple general anesthetics would meet with equal resistance. Antral lavage may be appropriate at the time of another procedure, such as T&A. Its overall efficacy requires further delineation.

V. INFERIOR MEATAL ANTROSTOMY

Inferior meatal antrostomy has become a popular surgical technique in the management of maxillary sinusitis (19). Despite of its many advocates, however, there has been little scientific investigation of its efficacy. This procedure gained popularity until introduction of the Caldwell-Luc procedure, which was actively preferred for several years but recently has become less popular (19).

A crucial factor in the success of the inferior meatal antrostomy is the patency of the "window" over time. Lund (19) found that 50% of windows were patent, 45% were closed, and 5% could not be assessed. Of the 15 patients younger than 16 years, 13 had closed antrostomies. The patent antrostomies were in patients 14 and 15 years old. In a prospective study Lund concluded that the antrostomy had to be greater than 1 cm to remain patent. It is difficult, if not impossible, to make an antrostomy of this size in children, and this is probably the reason for poor window patency. Muntz and Lusk (29) performed a retrospective evaluation of 39 children (mean age, 6.3 years) who had chronic sinusitis and had undergone bilateral inferior meatal antrostomies. They found that symptoms were not controlled in 60% of the children at 1 month and in 73% 6 months postoperatively. Repeated inferior meatal antrostomies failed to control symptoms in seven patients.

It was thought that the inferior position of the meatus and ventilation would cure the sinusitis (30). We now understand that mucociliary clearance patterns continue to transport the secretions to the natural ostium of the sinus (31–33). If there continues to be obstruction at the natural ostium, secretions will accumulate and the sinus will remain infected.

As with antral lavage, some children benefit from inferior meatal windows, but there are no prospective data to assist us in patient selection. We, therefore, have abandoned the procedure as a primary mode of therapy (29), with one exception. Children with ciliary dyskinesia have abnormal ciliary function, and the inferior meatal antrostomies allow gravity to help evacuate secretions from the maxillary sinus. The problem of window patency, however, remains.

VI. MIDDLE MEATAL ANTROSTOMY

Another mechanism for ventilating and draining the antrum is through the middle meatus and the natural ostium of the maxillary sinus. This procedure has become central to our current treatment of chronic maxillary sinusitis. As we have already noted, an early approach to irrigation of the sinus was through the natural ostium of the maxillary sinus. Wilkerson (34) was the first in the United

States to recommend limited middle meatal windows even though this approach was thought to be technically more difficult and to have a higher incidence of complications than the inferior meatal antrostomy (20). Proetz (21) opposed middle meatal antrostomy, as did Hilding (35), based on his series of experiments on the maxillary sinus in rabbits. Using three animals in each of three groups, Hilding found that when the natural ostium was enlarged all three rabbits became infected, whereas only two of three animals became infected when the opening was made in the inferior portion of the sinus. From this work, Hilding concluded that an antrostomy should be as far from the natural ostium as possible. The concept of middle meatal antrostomy subsequently fell into disrepute until Wilkerson (34) rekindled interest in surgery on the middle meatus.

Clinical research evaluating the effectiveness of middle meatal antrostomy is sparse, but does suggest a high patency rate with this approach. Kennedy et al. (31) retrospectively evaluated 117 middle meatal antrostomies in 75 adult patients. Of 95 procedures followed-up for more than 4 months, 98% of the antrostomies were patent. Lavelle and Harrison reported a 94% patency rate in 150 patients (36).

Middle meatal antrostomy involves removal of ostiomeatal disease or anatomical abnormalities that may predispose the patient to chronic maxillary sinus disease. It retains the orientation of the mucociliary transport, and re-establishes physiological drainage. This approach has significant theoretical advantages and is a cornerstone in our current management of pediatric chronic sinusitis.

VII. ETHMOIDECTOMY

None of the surgical procedures described previously addresses the ethmoid sinuses. The anterior ethmoid sinuses are diseased almost as often as the maxillary sinuses. Removing diseased tissue from the ethmoid sinuses can be accomplished in a number of ways. External ethmoidectomy, which has been used for a number of years to treat complicated sinus disease, is thought to give maximum visualization and safety. Intranasal ethmoidectomy (without the aid of a telescope) in children is not recommended because of the small size of the ethmoid cavity and the increased potential for complications. The transantral approach to the ethmoid has not gained popularity because of fear of traumatizing the teeth and the small size of the maxillary sinus. Because of these limitations, the endoscopic approach is particularly attractive in children. It allows resection of disease in the ethmoid sinuses without scarring the face and involves very little morbidity if the surgeon stays within the bounds of the ethmoid cavity. The failure of tonsillectomy, adenoidectomy, antral lavage, and inferior meatal windows to control symptoms of chronic sinusitis has led to the choice of endoscopic ethmoidectomy (partial or total) combined with middle meatal antrostomy as the preferred surgical treatment. This procedure is safe in experienced hands, but is not yet widely performed in children.

VIII. RADIOGRAPHIC EXAMINATION

In the pediatric population, the sinuses are developing and are difficult to visualize accurately. It is unfortunate that plain films both over- and underread the amount of disease located in the ethmoid sinuses and cannot be used as a screening device to select children for full CT scans. CT scans in the pediatric population are more difficult to perform because younger children frequently require intravenous (IV) sedation. The spiral CT scanner is much faster and significantly decreases the time required to perform the study. As a matter of practicality, if the child's symptoms are severe enough and of sufficient duration that the surgeon and the parents would choose surgical intervention, it is reasonable to proceed with a CT scan. Sinusitis is a disease that waxes and wanes, and the CT scan cannot be used as the sole criterion for surgical intervention. One cannot infer anything about the chronicity of opacification seen on CT scans. One of the ways to help determine the chronicity of the infection is to treat the patient with adequate medical therapy before performing the CT scan. If disease continues to be present, one may infer that it is chronic.

IX. ANTIBIOTIC THERAPY

We currently use full-dose antibiotic therapy (amoxicillin/potassium clavulanate [Augmentin], erythromycin/sulfisoxazole [Pediazole], or cefuroxime axetil [Ceftin]) and topical nasal steroid sprays for 4 weeks before the CT scan is taken. No good prospective studies define the efficacy of long-term antibiotic therapy or the use of topical nasal steroid sprays. Even if disease is noted on the CT scan after the patient has been on appropriate therapy for 4–6 weeks, one cannot assume that the disease is irreversible and warrants surgical intervention.

It is our belief that surgical intervention should be undertaken only after maximum medical management has failed. Maximal medical management has not been defined with prospective studies but at this time would include 4–6 weeks of an appropriate antibiotic and topical nasal steroid sprays. Clinicians will have to use their best judgment to decide the best course of action. Although the use of prophylactic antibiotics in sinusitis has not been studied, this modality will probably have a place in the medical management of recurrent sinusitis.

X. SURGICAL INTERVENTION

If the CT scan shows no evidence of sinus disease while the patient is receiving full-dose antibiotics, surgical intervention is probably not warranted. In this capacity prophylactic antibiotic treatment is most likely to be efficacious. If the CT scan shows "pansinusitis," surgical intervention is probably warranted: however, it is not absolutely necessary because we do not know the natural history of pediatric sinusitis and therefore cannot predict with certainty the outcome of longer medical management. The hardest judgments to make are those regarding surgical intervention in children with minimal disease after prolonged medical management. When in doubt, it is best to continue medical management and evaluate the child's symptoms. With time, the best course will become clear.

As a basic principle, sinus surgery in children should be as conservative as possible yet correct the underlying problem. In some children this may require only an anterior ethmoidectomy and maxillary antrostomy, while in others it may require more aggressive surgery.

In the pediatric age group, disease is located primarily in the anterior ethmoid and maxillary sinuses (1). Stammberger (32,37,38) notes that the anterior ethmoid, especially the infundibulum, holds the key to recurrent sinusitis. Since we know that in the majority of children the disease is located in the anterior ethmoid and maxillary sinuses, I have adopted the Messerklinger technique, which has been so carefully clarified by Stammberger (32,38–40) and Kennedy (31,41–43). This approach removes only the diseased tissue and maximizes preservation of mucosa.

Regardless of the technique, intranasal endoscopic surgery has two goals: maximal preservation of all normal mucosa, and to secure communication between the nasal cavity and the paranasal sinuses via the natural channels. This does not require removal of all of the cells or mucosa but does require opening the areas of obstruction. As Wigand states (44), intranasal endoscopic operations on the paranasal sinuses for chronic sinusitis are mainly limited to opening the narrow bony points to restore ventilation and internal drainage. The operation should be tailored to the individual and the extent of the chronic sinusitis.

I have tried to standardize the endoscopic ethmoidectomy procedure as much as possible in an effort to minimize the risk of complications and yet perform an adequate operation.

XI. ANATOMY

Surgery of the pediatric sinuses cannot be safely performed without a thorough knowledge of the anatomy of the nose. An extensive discussion of the lateral nasal anatomy is not presented here because there are excellent articles and books on this subject (24,44–46). Figure 6 is an axial diagram of the middle turbinate and the middle anterior ethmoids. This diagram will be used to help explain the surgical procedure. It is important to note that all the anatomical structures of the sinuses are present in pediatric patients. The pediatric ethmoid labyrinth is smaller than in the adult, and the surgery must therefore be precise, with careful identification of anatomical landmarks.

XII. ENDOSCOPIC PROCEDURE

An abbreviated description of how the endoscopic ethmoidectomy is performed is presented here. A thorough discussion of the procedure is described in the surgical chapter of a book devoted exclusively to pediatric sinusitis (47).

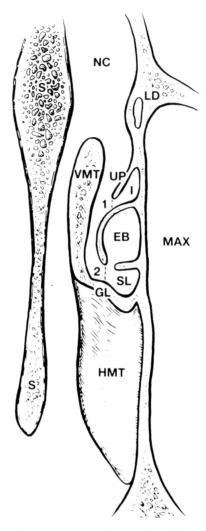

Figure 6 Axial view of the anterior ethmoid complex. NC, nasal cavity; LD, lacrimal duct; VMT, vertical middle turbinate; UP, uncinate process; I, infundibulum; EB, ethmoid bulla; SL, sinus lateralis; GL, ground (basal or grand) lamella; HMT, horizontal lamella; S, septum; MAX, maxillary sinus; 1, inferior hiatus semilunaris; 2, superior hiatus semilunaris.

A general anesthetic is always required in children. Because the myocardium is sensitized with halothane, it is our recommendation that halothane be stopped before vasoconstriction is started. We have evaluated three different vasoconstricting agents during functional endoscopic sinus surgery in 57 children (48).

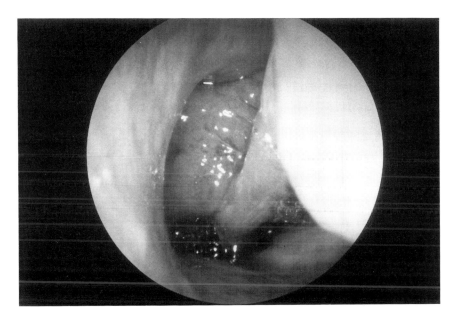

Figure 7 Purulence from the posterior ethmoid cavity.

Oxymetazoline 0.05%, phenylephrine 0.25%, or cocaine 4% was applied to the nasal mucosa in a prospective, randomized, double-blind fashion. Oxymetazoline 0.05% proved to be the most effective vasoconstrictor and was associated with the fewest complications. In two patients receiving 0.25% phenylephrine the surgical procedure had to be aborted because of bleeding severe enough to compromise visualization.

The nasal cavity is inspected after the nose is vasoconstricted, and sites of purulent nasal discharge are noted (Fig. 7). Evidence of purulent discharge will give a clue to the location of disease. Usually an obstructive adenoid pad would have already been noted, and the decision about adenoidectomy would have been made preoperatively. Examination of the sphenoid recess in children is difficult even with a 2.7 mm telescope because of the very narrow channel (Fig. 8).

The uncinate process is identified and removed in a controlled manner with a sickle knife and forceps (Fig. 9). The hypoplastic sinus can be clearly identified on coronal CT scans (Fig. 10); in these patients the uncinate process may be very difficult to identify.

Once the uncinate process is removed, any residual uncinate bone is removed at its lateral attachment. It is crucial to make sure that all the uncinate process is removed to improve access, to give adequate exposure to the natural ostium of

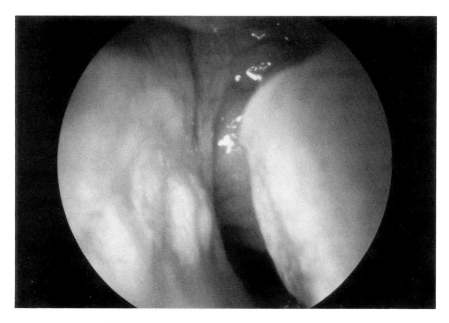

Figure 8   Narrow space in the sphenoid recess.

the maxillary sinus, to enlarge the middle meatus, and to prevent scarring and a narrowed middle meatus postoperatively.

It is now my impression that the ostium is easiest to identify and to enlarge at the beginning of the procedure when the bleeding is less. The size of the ostium and the degree of obstruction can be most accurately assessed with a 30 degree telescope. The small ostium is enlarged through the posterior fontanel and less aggressively anteriorly to prevent trauma to the lacrimal duct. An effort is made to preserve mucosa along the lower border of the ostium and this flap of mucosa is rolled into the nose. If this flap can be created, the ostium will remain patent and heal quickly (Fig. 11).

It is important to make sure that the opening into the maxillary sinus is connected to the natural ostium. If it is not, there will be an accumulation of secretions that will result in persistent symptoms (Fig. 12).

The ethmoid bulla is then entered in a controlled manner (Fig. 13). If there is a disease in the bulla it is cultured for anaerobic, aerobic, and fungal organisms. All movements within this cavity must be performed under direct visualization with deliberate, calculated movements. Most frequently an anterior ethmoidectomy is performed.

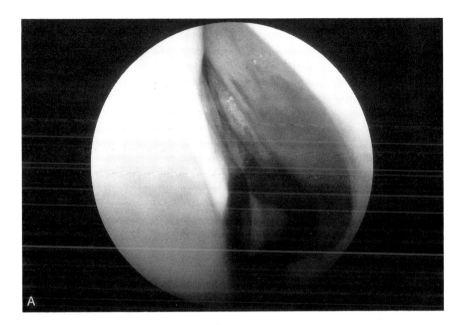

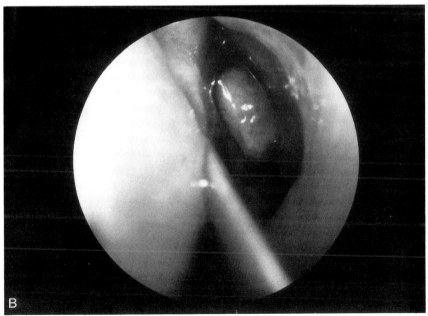

Figure 9 (A) Incision of the uncinate process. (B) Ethmoid bulla after removal of the uncinate process.

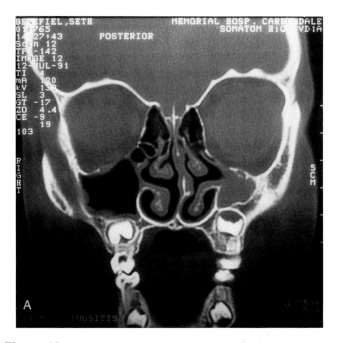

Figure 10   (A) Hypoplastic sinus CT scan. (B) Endoscopic view.

In an anterior ethmoidectomy, the entire ethmoid bulla should be removed. The lamina papyracea should be clearly identified and the mucosa preserved if possible (Fig. 14). This boundary defines the limits of the dissection and can be followed into the posterior ethmoid cells.

If there is disease in the posterior ethmoid cells, they are opened. The posterior cells are larger than the anterior cells, and the roof of the ethmoid is easier to identify posteriorly (Fig. 15). The mucosa from the posterior cells should be removed carefully in an attempt to leave as much as possible.

The sphenoid sinus is not as frequently diseased in children as in adults and therefore is not frequently opened. In children the opening must be made through the ethmoid cells because there is not enough room to open the sinus in the space medial to the middle turbinate.

On the coronal CT scan the sphenoid sinus is located directly behind the posterior ethmoid with the roof usually lower than the ethmoid (Fig. 16). When performing the operation, the surgeon finds the sphenoid lower and more medial than one would anticipate from the CT scan. If there is sphenoid disease it is

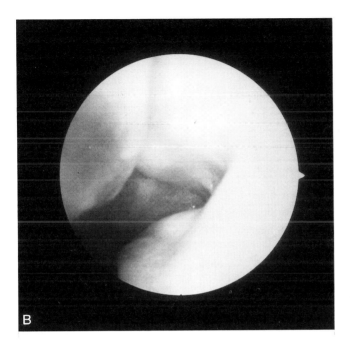

frequently helpful to have a few axial CT cuts to help define the anatomy of the lateral walls of the sinus.

Once the level of the roof of the ethmoid has been identified in the posterior cells, this plane can be followed into the anterior ethmoid cells. If the mucosa along the roof is normal, every effort should be made to leave it intact.

The appropriate management of the developing frontal recess and frontal sinus is not clear. It would seem prudent to be very conservative in the frontal recess until more is known about its development (Fig. 17).

XIII. POSTOPERATIVE CARE

The usual postoperative care for patients undergoing sinus endoscopy must be modified because of poor patient cooperation in the pediatric age group. Even anterior rhinoscopy cannot be performed in some children postoperatively. We currently stent the ethmoid cavity with Gelfilm (Upjohn, Kalamazoo, MI) (Fig. 18).

Experience has taught us that the Gelfilm should be removed under a general anesthetic approximately 2 weeks postoperatively. Some granulation tissue is also removed from the frontal recess and the ostium of the maxillary sinus,

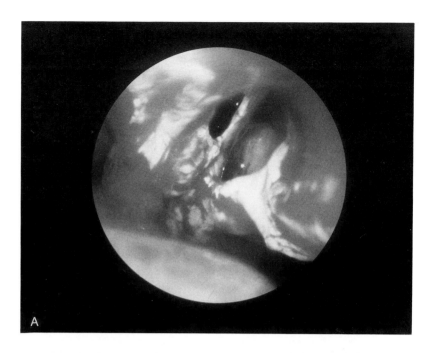

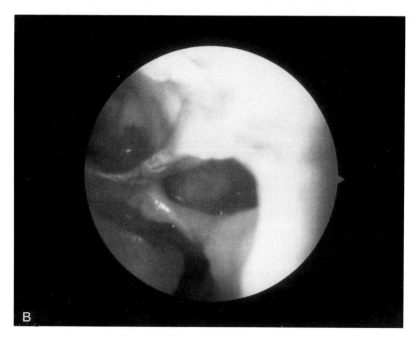

Figure 11 (A) Inferior flap created at the maxillary antrostomy. (B) Well-healed maxillary ostium 2 weeks postoperatively.

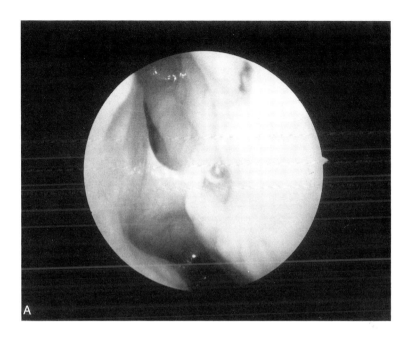

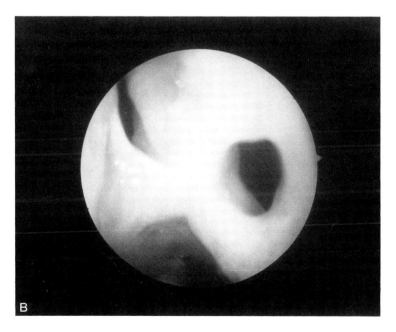

Figure 12 (A) Secretions accumulating at the site of the natural ostium that had not been adequately opened. (B) Visualization of the ostium with secretions removed.

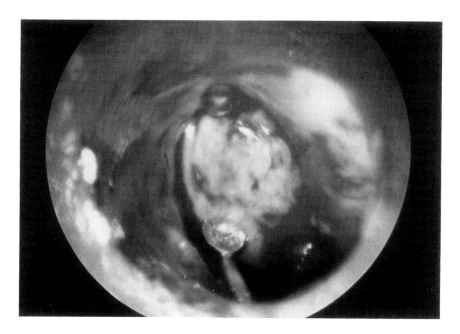

Figure 13 J curette entering the ethmoid bulla.

although no effort is made to remove all of it because this is thought to be part of the normal healing process. Another half roll of Gelfilm is then placed back into the middle meatus and allowed to absorb over the next 2 or 3 weeks. During the postoperative phase the patient remains on full-dosage antibiotics. Scarring has been limited using this method (Fig. 19). When we have deviated from this routine, scarring has been a problem (Fig. 20).

A. Follow-Up and Results

The success of the surgical intervention is best assessed by observing the patient's symptoms and examining a follow-up CT scan. Unfortunately, routine follow-up CT scans are not possible in children, so the final measure of efficacy must be the resolution of symptoms.

Our surgical results to date have been very encouraging (49). Our pilot data show that endoscopic ethmoidectomy can be performed safely and that 74% of all parents believe that their children are "normal" 1 year after the surgical procedure. In none of the children were symptoms worsened, and surgical complications were insignificant.

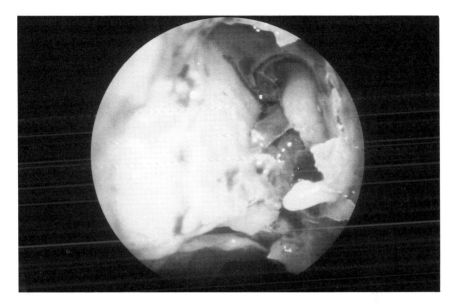

Figure 14 Lamina papyracea clearly defined in a cadaver specimen.

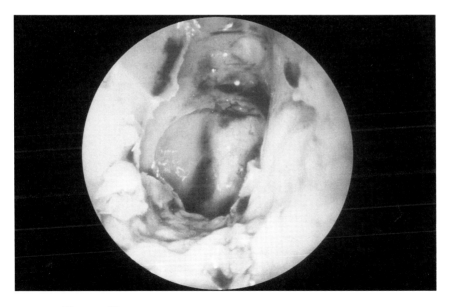

Figure 15 Large posterior ethmoid cells in a cadaver specimen.

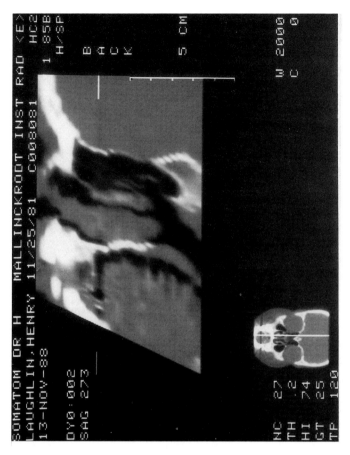

Figure 16 Computed tomographic scan of sphenoid sinus located posterior to the ethmoid cells.

B. Surgical Complications

Although the risk of complications may be higher in children because of the smaller anatomical spaces in which the surgeon must work, surgical complications in pediatric disease so far have been few. Stankiewicz (50) showed the importance of acquiring experience in endoscopic techniques and demonstrated that such experience decreases the complication rate (51). An accurate knowledge of the anatomy and prudent judgment further decrease risks to an acceptable level. Hemorrhage may be considered a complication but is rarely a problem in the pediatric population.

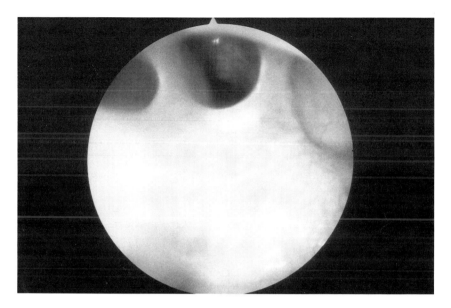

Figure 17 View of the frontal recess.

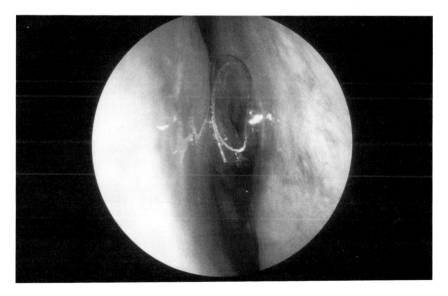

Figure 18 Gelfilm in the ethmoid cavity in the immediate postoperative period.

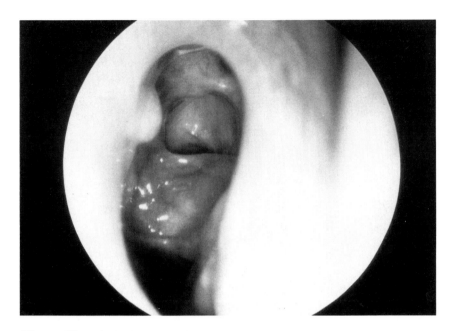

Figure 19 Middle meatus and healed ethmoid cavity without evidence of scarring.

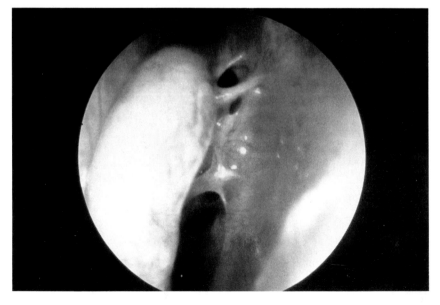

Figure 20 Scarring in the superior middle meatus.

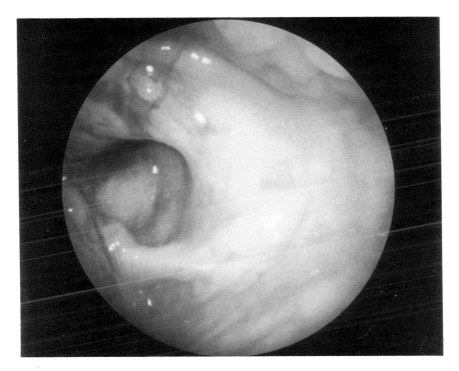

Figure 21 Sphenoid sinus of a 7-year-old child; the optic nerve is clearly seen along the lateral wall.

The complications can be classified into two broad categories: orbital and intracranial. Orbital complications can occur in the form of blindness secondary to direct injury to the optic nerve or secondary to retrobulbar hemorrhage, diplopia secondary to trauma to the orbital muscles or secondary fibrosis, and epiphora secondary to trauma to the lacrimal duct. Congenital dehiscences are sometimes noted in the wall of the orbit, in the lamina papyracea, or over the posterior ethmoid cells. If these are recognized preoperatively, the chance of trauma is reduced.

Blindness, secondary to direct optic nerve injury, is rare but has occurred (52,53). Trauma is most likely to occur in the sphenoid sinus or Onodi cell (the posteriormost ethmoid cell) in adults. These cells are less developed in children, but even in the young child the optic nerve can be exposed (Fig. 21). Visual loss during a retrobulbar hemorrhage is probably secondary to compromise of the central retinal artery flow (54–56) and posterior ciliary artery that supply the artery to the optic nerve (56,57). Recovery of vision is unlikely if retinal ischemia persists for more than 100 min (58).

During surgery, the eyes should be protected with a lubricating agent but not taped so that movement can be easily seen and any developing proptosis quickly visualized. If visualization is not satisfactory or if the surgeon is unsure of the position within the ethmoid cavity, it is prudent to terminate the procedure. Freedman and Kern (59) noted an increase in the number of complications on the right side. Stankiewicz (53), therefore recommended operating on this side first. It has been our experience, however, that the periorbital area is exposed with equal frequency on the left.

A last predisposing factor for orbital complications is the use of packing. Packing is rarely, if ever, needed. Persistent bleeding is easy to control with Avatine and a short duration of packing, which is removed before the patient is woken. If packing is used with a dehiscence in the orbit, pressure can cause hemodynamic compromise of the retina (53).

In the event of an orbital bleed, decompression of the orbit into the ethmoid cavity through an external incision is probably the quickest and most effective way of decompressing the orbit. The periorbit should be incised if there is evidence of surgical trauma (52,53).

The major intracranial complication that can occur is a cerebrospinal fluid (CSF) leak. This is relatively rare (51,53). The cause is usually penetration of the fovea ethmoidalis. A most important principle is to stay lateral to the middle turbinate. The dissection must be meticulous by using small bits, taking care not to penetrate the roof of the ethmoid cavity.

REFERENCES

1. McAlister WH, Lusk RP, Muntz HR. Comparison of plain radiographs and coronal CT scans in infants and children with recurrent sinusitis. *Am J Roentgenol* 1989;153:1259–64.
2. Shone GR. Maxillary sinus aspiration in children. What are the indications. *J Laryngol Otol* 1987;101:461–4.
3. Birrell JF. Chronic maxillary sinusitis in children. *Arch Dis Child* 1952;27:1–9.
4. Maresh MM, Washburn AH. Paranasal sinuses from birth to late adolescence. *Am J Dis Child* 1940;60:841–61.
5. Preston HG. Maxillary sinusitis in children, its relation to coryza, tonsillectomy and adenoidectomy. *Va Med Monogr* 1955;82:229–32.
6. Wilson TG. Surgical anatomy of ENT in the newborn. *J Laryngol Otol* 1955;69:229.
7. Clark WD, Bailey BJ. Sinusitis in children. *Tex Med* 1983;79:44–7.
8. Paul D. Sinus infection and adenotonsillitis in pediatric patients. *Laryngoscope* 1981;91:997–1000.
9. Merck W. Relationship between adenoidal enlargement and maxillary sinusitis. *HNO* 1974;6:198–9.

10. Nickman NJ. Sinusitis, otitis and adenotonsillitis in children: a retrospective study. *Laryngoscope* 1978;88:117–21.
11. Carmack JW. Sinusitis in children. *Ann Otol Rhinol Laryngol* 1931;40:515–21.
12. Stevenson RS. The treatment of subacute maxillary sinusitis especially in children. *Proc R Soc Med* 1947;40:854–8.
13. Walker FM. Tonsillectomy and adenoidectomy: unsatisfactory results due to chronic maxillary sinusitis. *Br Med J* 1947;908–10.
14. Hoshaw TC, Nickman NJ. Sinusitis and otitis in children. *Arch Otolaryngol* 1974;100:194–5.
15. Cleminson FJ. Nasal sinusitis in children. *J Laryngol Otol* 1921;36˙505–13.
16. Fujita A, Takahashi H, Honjo I. Etiological role of adenoids upon otitis media with effusion. *Acta Otolaryngol Suppl* (Stockh) 1988;454:210–3.
17. Van Alyea OE. Nasal Sinus and Anatomical and Clinical Considerations. Baltimore, MD: Williams & Wilkins, 1942.
18. Myerson MC. The natural orifice of the maxillary sinus. *Arch Otolaryngol* 1932;80–91.
19. Lund VJ. Inferior meatal antrostomy. Fundamental considerations of design and function. *J Laryngol Otol Suppl* 1988;15:1–18.
20. Mikulicz J. Zur operativen Behandlung das KEmpyens der Highmorshohle. *Lagenbecks Arch Klin Chir* 1887;34:626–34.
21. Proetz AW. *Essays on the Applied Physiology of the Nose.* St. Louis: Annals Publishing Co; 1941:356.
22. Alden AM. A new procedure in the treatment of chronic maxillary sinus suppuration in children. *Arch Otolaryngol* 1926;4:521–5.
23. Asherson N. Intubation of the maxillary antrum for acute empyema. *Lancet* 1937;1399–400.
24. Stammberger H. *Functional Endoscopic Sinus Surgery.* Philadelphia: B. C. Decker, 1991.
25. Kim HN, Kim YM, Choi HS. Diagnostic and therapeutic significance of sinoscopy in maxillary sinusitis. *Yonsei Med J* 1985;26:59–67.
26. StClair T, Negus VE. *Diseases of the Nose and Throat.* London: 1937:232.
27. Crooks J, Signy AG. Accessory nasal sinusitis in childhood. *Arch Dis Child* 1936;11:281–306.
28. Maes JJ, Clement PA. The usefulness of irrigation of the maxillary sinus in children with maxillary sinusitis on the basis of the Water's x-ray. *Rhinology* 1987;25:259–64.
29. Muntz HR, Lusk RP. Nasal antral windows in children: A retrospective study. *Laryngoscope* 1990;100:643–6.
30. Hajek M. *Pathology and Treatment of the Inflammatory Diseases of the Nasal Accessory Sinuses.* St. Louis: CV Mosby, 1926.
31. Kennedy DW, Zinreich SJ, Shaalan H, Kuhn F, Naclerio R, Loch E. Endoscopic middle meatal antrostomy: theory, technique and patency. *Laryngoscope* 1987;97:1–9.
32. Stammberger H. Endoscopic endonasal surgery—concepts in treatment of recurring rhinosinusitis. Part I. Anatomic and pathophysiologic considerations. *Otolaryngol Head Neck Surg* 1986;94:143–7.

33. Hilding AC. Role of ciliary action in production of pulmonary atelectasis, vacuum in paranasal sinuses and in otitis media. *Ann Otol Rhinol Laryngol* 1943; 52:816–33.

34. Wilkerson WW. Antral window in the middle meatus. *Arch Ophthalmol* 1949; 49:463–89.

35. Hilding AC. Experimental sinus surgery: effects of operative windows on normal sinuses. *Ann Otol Rhinol Laryngol* 1941;50:379–92.

36. Lavelle RJ, Harrison MS. Infection of the maxillary sinus: the case for the middle meatal antrostomy. *Laryngoscope* 1971;81:90–106.

37. Stammberger H. Unsere endoskopische Operationstechnik der lateralen Nasenwand—ein endoskopisch-chirurgisches Konzept zur Behandlung entzundlicher Nasennebenhohlenerkrankungen. *Laryngol Rhinol Otol (Stuttg)* 1985;64:559–66.

38. Stammberger H. Nasal and paranasal sinus endoscopy. A diagnostic and surgical approach to recurrent sinusitis. *Endoscopy* 1986;18:213–18.

39. Stammberger H. Endoscopic endonasal surgery—concepts in treatment of recurring rhinosinusitis. Part II. Surgical technique. *Otolaryngol Head Neck Surg* 1986;94:147–56.

40. Stammberger H. Endoscopic surgery for mycotic and chronic recurring sinusitis. *Ann Otol Rhinol Laryngol* 1985;119:1–11.

41. Kennedy DW. Serious misconceptions regarding functional endoscopic sinus surgery [letter]. *Laryngoscope* 1986;96:1170–1.

42. Kennedy DW, Kennedy EM. Endoscopic sinus surgery. *AORN J* 1985;42:932–4.

43. Kennedy DW, Zinreich SJ, Rosenbaum AE, Johns ME. Functional endoscopic sinus surgery. Theory and diagnostic evaluation. *Arch Otolaryngol* 1985; 111:576–82.

44. Wigand ME. *Endoscopic Surgery of the Paranasal Sinuses and Anterior Skull Base*. New York: Thieme Medical Publishers, 1990.

45. Lang J. *Clinical Anatomy of the Nose, Nasal Cavity and Paranasal Sinuses*. New York: Thieme Medical Publishers, 1989:50.

46. Messerklinger W. *Endoscopy of the Nose*. Baltimore-Munich: Urban & Schwarzenberg, 1978.

47. Lusk RP. Surgical management of chronic sinusitis. In: Lusk RP, ed. *Pediatric Sinusitis*. New York: Raven Press, 1992:77–126.

48. Riegle EV, Gunter JB, Lusk RP, Muntz HR, Weiss KL. Comparison of vasoconstrictors for functional endoscopic sinus surgery in children. *Laryngoscope* 1992;102:820-3.

49. Lusk RP, Muntz HR. Endoscopic sinus surgery in children with chronic sinusitis— a pilot study. *Laryngoscope* 1990;100:654–8.

50. Stankiewicz JA. Complications of endoscopic intranasal ethmoidectomy. *Laryngoscope* 1987;97:1270–3.

51. Stankiewicz JA. Complications in endoscopic intranasal ethmoidectomy: an update. *Laryngoscope* 1989;99:686–90.

52. Buus DR, Tse DT, Farris BK. Ophthalmic complications of sinus surgery. *Ophthalmology* 1990;97:612–19.

53. Stankiewicz JA. Blindness and intranasal endoscopic ethmoidectomy: prevention and management. *Otolaryngol–Head Neck Surg* 1989;101:320–9.

54. Heinze JB, Hueston JT. Blindness after blepharoplasty: mechanism and early reversal. *Plas Reconstr Surg* 1978;61:347–54.

55. Hartley JH, Lester JC, Schatten WE. Acute retrobulbar hemorrhage during elective blepharoplasty. Its pathophysiology and management. *Plas Reconstr Surg* 1973; 52:8–15.

56. Anderson RL, Edwards JJ: Bilateral visual loss after blepharoplasty. *Ann Plast Surg* 1980;5:288–92.

57. Walter RR. Is blindness a realistic complication in blepharoplasty procedures? *Ophthalmology* 1978;85:730–5.

58. Hayreh SS, Weingeist TA. Experimental occlusion of the central artery of the retina. IV: Retinal tolerance time to acute ischaemia. *Br J Ophthalmol* 1980; 64.818–25.

59. Freedman HM, Kern EB. Complications of intranasal ethmoidectomy: a review of 1,000 consecutive operations. *Laryngoscope* 1979;89:421–34.

10

Sinusitis and Asthma

MICHAEL R. BORTS and RAYMOND G. SLAVIN
Saint Louis University School of Medicine
St. Louis, Missouri

I. ASSOCIATION OF SINUSITIS AND ASTHMA

The association of paranasal sinus disease and asthma has been recognized for many years. Whether sinusitis alone can induce asthma has been debated since the early 20th century, and remains a point of controversy despite many years of observation.

The earliest studies of a relationship between the upper airway (the nose, nasopharynx, and sinuses) and the bronchi began with Kratchmer in 1870, who demonstrated that chemical irritation of the nasal mucosa of cats and rabbits with ether, cigarette smoke, and sulfur dioxide resulted in bronchoconstriction (1). In succeeding years investigators showed that mechanical and electrical stimulation of the nasal mucus membrane resulted in reflex bronchoconstriction (2).

There was great interest in the early 20th century in the association between the upper and lower airway. By 1932 reports on the incidence of sinusitis in asthma numbered over 4,000 (3–7). Various studies have cited the incidence of sinusitis in asthmatics between 12% (3) and 90% (4). Sluder (8) attributed this association to a nasal reflex in humans, based on observations in animals such as Kratchmer's experiments (1). Gottlieb (9) expanded on the reflex hypothesis and postulated four possible mechanisms for the association: mucopurulent postnasal drainage leading to continuous infection of the trachea and bronchi;

absorption of toxic products from retained purulent material in the sinuses triggering an immunologic response manifest as asthma; nasal obstruction leading to mouth breathing of cold, dry air with resultant bronchospasm; and nerve reflex bronchospasm through irritation of the nasal ganglion. These postulates still form the foundation of our understanding of this relationship today (10).

Following these early clinical observations, there was little mention of sinusitis and asthma in the literature until the 1970s. Phipatanakul and Slavin reported five nonatopic asthmatic patients whose lower airway disease improved dramatically after diagnosis and treatment of paranasal sinus disease (11). These encouraging results stimulated others to look for sinusitis in association with asthma.

II. DIAGNOSIS AND EPIDEMIOLOGY OF SINUSITIS

The ability to substantiate a causative association between sinusitis and asthma is predicted on the ability to diagnose sinusitis conclusively. Sinusitis may be defined as inflammation of the mucous membranes that line the paranasal sinuses (12). This may be infectious in nature, or related to hyperplastic changes in the mucosa associated with eosinophil infiltration. Since sinus membrane biopsy is not readily available, it is difficult to decide what findings correlate with pathologic conditions of the sinuses. Symptoms such as headache, fever, and facial pain are often absent in sinusitis (13). The most commonly used imaging test is plain sinus radiography. Maxillary sinus mucosal thickening greater than 6 mm has been demonstrated to correlate with high incidence of recovery of pathogens on needle aspiration of the maxillary sinus (14). The reliability of mucosal thickening in the ethmoid region on plain films is less certain (15). Plain sinus films can both overestimate the incidence of maxillary sinus disease and underestimate ethmoid disease. Although more expensive than plain films, computed tomography is the diagnostic test of choice to define anatomical pathologic change in the sinuses (16). Nevertheless, most studies have employed plain sinus films to investigate the association between upper and lower airway disease. A-mode ultrasonography has been used, but is reliable only in detecting fluid in the maxillary sinus cavity (17). Fiberoptic rhinoscopy can be useful if pus is evident at the sinus ostia (18), but its reliability is dependent on the skill of the endoscopist as well as his or her ability to recognize pathologic changes.

Some individuals demonstrate abnormal sinus radiographs in absence of any evident disease process. Fascenalli found abnormal sinus films in 25% of healthy, asymptomatic airmen (19). However, only 16% of these (4% of the total) had significant abnormalities defined as opacification or mucosal thickening of greater than 5 mm.

A number of studies have confirmed a higher incidence of abnormal sinus films in asthmatic subjects. Berman and Matheson in a study involving nasal antral puncture, lavage, and culture of sinus fluid contents, confirmed a high incidence of abnormal sinus radiographic findings in a group of asthmatic subjects asymptomatic for sinus disease (20). Twenty-one of 52 patients had abnormal maxillary sinus radiographs. Recovery of bacteria was low compared to the incidence of radiographic abnormality. Of four with complete opacification, only three yielded mucus on antral puncture. Of the remaining 17 with mucoperiosteal thickening, only 3 yielded mucus. Overall, over 20% of sinus aspirations yielded bacterial growth, a smaller percentage than the 40–65% that had previously been reported (21). One explanation for a high incidence of negative cultures on aspiration is the presence of a pathogen such as a mycoplasma or virus (22).

The association between sinusitis and asthma has been noted not only in adults but also in children. Rachelefsky and co-workers found that 53% of children with asthma had abnormal sinus radiographs (23). Adinoff described a similar incidence of sinus radiograph abnormalities in asthmatic children admitted to National Jewish Hospital (24). Fifty-two percent of 42 had abnormal sinus radiographs. A retrospective review by Adinoff and co-workers of asthmatic children 1–8 years of age admitted to National Jewish over a 5 year period demonstrated 72 of 98 (73%) with abnormal sinus films (25).

Kovatch and co-workers studied the incidence of abnormal sinus radiographs in a group of unselected children (26). Criteria for an abnormal maxillary sinus radiograph were defined as an air-fluid level, partial or complete opacification, or mucous membrane thickening of at least 4 mm. Eight of 14 children (57%) with signs and symptoms of upper respiratory inflammation had abnormal sinus radiographs. Only 2 of 31 children (7%) had abnormal radiographs in the absence of signs or symptoms of upper respiratory inflammation. In both adults and children, the incidence of sinus radiograph abnormalities in a clinically normal individual is very low. The incidence is significantly greater in individuals with a history of asthma.

Although many studies have supported the association, not all demonstrate a correlation between the severity of asthma and the severity of sinus radiograph abnormalities. Zimmerman and others found the overall prevalence of sinus radiograph abnormalities to be greater in children with asthma than in controls with dental problems; however, the percentage of patients with abnormalities found on sinus radiographs was the same whether the asthma was mild (requiring minimal medication) or severe (requiring multiple medications) (27).

III. MICROBIOLOGICAL BASIS OF SINUSITIS AND ASTHMA

Studies of the microbiological basis of sinusitis have been made in adults and children, and are discussed in greater detail elsewhere (14,28). Isolation of pathogenic bacteria and viruses has been accomplished by aspiration of the maxillary antra and by direct antral swabbing (29,30). Material swabbed from the nares and the posterior pharynx is contaminated with resident nasal flora and is of doubtful significance (29).

In acute sinusitis in adults, the most common bacterial isolates are nontypable *Hemophilus influenzae* and *Streptococcus pneumoniae*. Other bacteria include *Streptococcus pyogenes* and alpha-hemolytic streptococci. Viruses isolated include rhinovirus, influenza virus type A, and parainfluenza virus. In acute sinusitis in children, Wald found *S. pneumoniae*, nontypable *H. influenzae*, and *Moraxella catarrhalis* to be the major organisms recovered from maxillary sinus aspirates (30). Anaerobes are more common in chronic sinusitis, and include alpha-hemolytic streptococci, *Bacteroides*, *Veillonella*, and *Corynebacterium*. Staphylococci are also observed. Fungal infections represent a less common but treatable cause of chronic sinus inflammation (31–33). The earliest reports were of actinomycetes, *Nocardia*, *Candida*, *Mucor*, and *Aspergillus* in immunocompromised hosts. Recently reports have been increasingly common in patients without other underlying immunologic deficiency.

IV. POSTULATED MECHANISMS OF AIRWAY HYPERREACTIVITY IN SINUSITIS

The relationship between the upper and lower airway is complex. This is evidenced by the lack of consistent findings in various studies. Some investigators believe that sinusitis can be a trigger of asthma: that once the sinusitis is removed, so is the need for bronchodilators. Others believe that sinusitis and asthma are both manifestations of the same underlying disease, either allergic inflammation in both areas or infection in two locations within the same respiratory tract. Potential mechanisms for the association between sinusitis and asthma are reviewed below.

A. Aspiration of Infected Material

Production of mucopurulent material is a typical finding in sinusitis. This may either be expressed as nasal discharge or postnasal drainage. Silent aspiration of this material has been considered to "seed" the lower airways with infection, and consequent inflammation of the lower airway. Children with immunodeficiency and asthma treated with intravenous immunoglobulin demonstrate clinical improvement in asthma (34). This would seem to support the role of infection in asthma; however, such observations do not prove an infectious component directly related to the sinusitis. Nor does it account for the other immunomodulating actions of intravenous immunoglobulin.

Whether nasopharyngeal secretions are aspirated at all has been a subject of conflicting results in studies. Winfield and colleagues could not demonstrate aspiration after instilling barium sulfate or propyliodone into the nasopharynx of normal sleeping individuals (35). Huxley and others found aspiration in 45% of normal subjects by injection of a radionuclide into the nasopharynx (36). Bardin and colleagues attempted to mimic what is postulated in asthmatics with sinusitis (37). They instilled radionuclide in the maxillary sinus of four patients with maxillary sinusitis and nine patients with sinusitis and asthma during therapeutic needle puncture of the sinus. In all patients the radionuclide could be demonstrated in the sinus, nasopharnyx, and gastrointestinal tract over the ensuing 24 hr, but not in the lower airway. This elegant negative study suggests that aspiration is not a factor in the coexistence of sinusitis and asthma.

B. Cellular and Soluble Factors

Similarities in the histopathologic findings among nasal, sinus, and bronchial tissue in subjects with asthma was noted in 1929 by Hansel (38). He found that both tissues were extensively infiltrated by eosinophils. Tissue eosinophilia is consistently associated with exacerbations of both upper and lower respiratory tract diseases (39,40). There is evidence that major basic protein (MBP) plays a major role in mediating injury to respiratory epithelium. MBP, a protein stored in the eosinophil, is cytotoxic to the respiratory epithelium. It is found in toxic concentrations in sputum specimens from patients with asthma (41). Harlin and others found a histopathologic picture in the sinuses very similar to that in the lungs, with the presence of Creola bodies (clusters of exfoliated respiratory epithelial cells), Charcot-Leyden crystals (cellular eosinophil lysophospholipase), and mucus plugs in the paranasal airways (42,43). Although the effect of MBP would appear to be a local phenomenon, the factors that regulate the eosinophil in the sinuses are likely to affect the eosinophil in the lower airways. A number of factors (eosinophil-activating factors derived from mast cells, monocytes, and T lymphocytes) regulate whether this pathologic process occurs in an individual (44). Other eosinophil proteins such as eosinophil peroxidase, eosinophil-derived neurotoxin, and eosinophil cationic protein are also released locally and can cause tissue damage in the upper and lower airway (45–47).

C. Inhalation of Cold, Dry Air

Mucosal edema and secretions associated with sinusitis can result in significant nasal obstruction, and consequent mouth-breathing. This can interfere with the nose's normal function of warming and humidifying air. In normal individuals the respiratory tract is efficient in heating and humidifying inhaled cold air. Some patients with asthma complain of increased symptoms when exposed to cold air. There appears to be marked individual intolerance to cold air in some asthmatics. Wells demonstrated that exposure to cold air produced increased airways resistance in 15 patients with a history of cold air intolerance, in contrast to controls and patients with chronic obstructive pulmonary dysfunction without a history of cold air intolerance (48). In recent years, McFadden demonstrated that the combination of cold air and hyperpnea, whether produced by exercise or isocapnic hyperventilation, is a potent stimulus for bronchoconstriction in asthmatic persons (49). The essential stimulus for this bronchoconstriction is heat loss from the airway mucosa. This is not seen in all asthmatic patients, and appears to be related to individual tolerance to cold air.

D. Nasobronchial Reflex

The existence of a nasobronchial reflex has been proposed for many years. Sluder first postulated asthma as a reflex in 1919 (8). He demonstrated worsening asthma with direct irritation of the mucosa in the region of the sphenoid sinus. This theory suggests that stimulation of neural receptors in the nose and sinuses can activate the afferent fibers that form part of the trigeminal nerve. Collaterals from the trigeminal nerve fibers enter the reticular formation, where connection is made with the dorsal vagal nucleus. Parasympathetic fibers then proceed to the bronchial musculature causing bronchospasm. Surgical interruption of the vagus nerve in animals has been demonstrated to preclude a change in airway resistance following a stimulus to the upper airway (50).

Kaufman and Wright demonstrated the existence of such a reflex in humans without asthma (51). Silica particles placed on the nasal mucosa for 150 sec caused a significant increase in measured airway resistance in all challenged subjects. Prior injection of up to 0.8 mg of atropine prevented any increase of resistance after a similar challenge. Yan and Salome initiated nasal obstruction in asthmatics with nasally applied histamine at a concentration too small to have a systemic effect (52). Besides a uniform increase in nasal airway resistance, half of the subjects had a greater than 20% fall in forced expiratory volume in 1 sec (FEV_1). This finding was independent of the degree of bronchial hyperreactivity demonstrated by histamine challenge. Nolte and Berger performed a similar experiment in asthmatics in which the stimulus was a single cold stimulus in the nose (53). This stimulus triggered an increase in lower airway resistance that could be blocked by prior intrabronchial application of an anticholinergic drug. The increase in airway resistance was not due to the direct effects of the cold stimulus on the lower airway. In their experiment, laryngectomized patients had an identical response when nasally challenged with cold.

In contrast to these findings are several studies that fail to demonstrate the existence of a nasobronchial reflex. Hoehne and Reed produced symptoms of allergic rhinitis, but no fall in FEV_1, by application of ragweed pollen or histamine to the nasal mucosa (54). Rosenberg and colleagues obtained similar negative results with intranasal allergen challenge (55). Schumacher and colleagues, in a placebo-controlled, double-blind study, were unable to demonstrate a nasobronchial reflex in nasal challenge with both histamine and allergen in normal subjects and subjects with stable asthma and allergic rhinitis (56). The fact that the nasal reflex cannot be demonstrated in all subjects suggests that we do not have a full understanding of this phenomenon in humans.

E. Diminished Beta-Adrenergic Responsiveness

Szentivanyi hypothesized that asthmatic individuals have an autonomic nervous system imbalance in airways due to an inherent beta-adrenergic blockade (57). There is evidence to support diminished beta-adrenergic function from both in vitro and in vivo studies. Busse utilized lysosomal release from neutrophils to serve as a model of cellular beta-adrenergic responsiveness (58). Studies of responsiveness to isoproterenol from asthmatics during upper respiratory infections demonstrated decreased response. He suggested that respiratory viruses alter the inhibitory response to a beta-agonist, which normally prevents mediator secretion (59). This virus-induced beta-blockade therefore results in greater granulocyte lysosomal product release and further local inflammation. It is proposed that sinusitis is associated with augmented beta-adrenergic hyporeactivity in a similar manner; however, such studies have not been performed in asthmatics with documented bacterial sinusitis. This postulated mechanism remains speculative in bacterial sinusitis.

V. TREATMENT

A. Medical Treatment

In its general principles, treatment of sinusitis in a patient with asthma need not differ significantly from uncomplicated sinusitis. Goals of treatment include treatment of bacterial infection present in the sinus cavities; reduction of swelling at the sinus ostia; drainage of sinus secretions; and promotion of continued sinus drainage after resolution of symptoms (60). This often requires treatment with a 21 day course of a broad-spectrum antibiotic, a topical nasal steroid (61), a decongestant–mucolytic agent (62), and saline nasal wash. The choice of antibiotic is mostly dependent on whether the subjective and objective findings suggest acute sinusitis, for which amoxicillin is generally adequate, or chronic sinusitis, for which coverage for anaerobic bacteria and staphylococci may be needed.

An important issue in treatment is whether the outcome of treatment for sinus disease includes improvement in asthma. Early results by Slavin were encouraging (63). He reported on 33 adults with sinus disease and asthma. Atopy was present in 36%, nasal polyps in 90%, aspirin intolerance in 52%, and clinical signs of sinusitis in only 45%. The asthma in 28 of the 33 patients improved with therapeutic measures directed at the sinusitis, which included antibiotics in

2 patients, antrostomy in 2, bilateral Caldwell-Luc procedures in 3, and bilateral intranasal sphenoethmoidectomy in 26. Rachelefsky demonstrated similar results in children (64). In a study of 79 children with sinusitis and asthma, 48 were able to discontinue taking bronchodilators after their sinusitis resolved with antimicrobial therapy. Friedman and co-workers demonstrated improved asthma symptom diary scores and pulmonary function in children not responding to conventional bronchodilator therapy after diagnosis and medical treatment of radiographically evident sinus disease (65).

B. Surgical Treatment

Surgical management of sinusitis that is severe, persistent, and refractory to medical treatment has been advocated by Friedman and others (66). They performed intranasal sphenoethmoidectomy on 50 patients who were not allergic. Anatomical factors such as mucosal hypertrophy, blocked sinus ostia, and fluid accumulation contributed to disease refractory to medical therapy. Surgical techniques included nasoantral window in the inferior meatus, polypectomies, ethmoidectomies, and sphenoid resections. Of the 50 patients receiving the procedure, reduction or elimination of sinusitis, relief of upper airway obstruction, and improvement in asthma occurred in 45. Twenty-six of 28 steroid-requiring patients were able to reduce or discontinue use of systemic corticosteroids.

VI. ASPIRIN SENSITIVITY, RHINOSINUSITIS, AND ASTHMA

A. Definition

Shortly after the introduction of aspirin in the late 19th century, Gilbert recognized that aspirin could precipitate an acute attack of asthma (67). Reports of greater numbers of affected patients by Cooke (68) and Van Leeuwen (69) soon followed. In 1937 Prickman and Buchstein reported 62 patients who were aspirin-sensitive, 43 of whom had asthma (70). In 1967 Samter and Beers suggested the clinical triad of asthma, nasal polyposis, and aspirin sensitivity (71). In more general terms, the triad consists of upper respiratory inflammation, manifest as vasomotor rhinitis, sinusitis, nasal or sinus polyps, lower respiratory inflammation manifest as asthma, and intolerance to aspirin or related compounds. This triad is often referred to as the Samter syndrome (72).

B. Incidence

The reported incidence varies relative to the population studied. The incidence is as low as 3% in asthmatics evaluated in a general practice (73) and 20% in patients with severe asthma evaluated in a referral center (74). Although the syndrome can present at any time of life, it most commonly presents in the third or fourth decade of life. It affects both men and women. Although most reports have been in adults, it has been well described in children (75–80).

C. Clinical Manifestations

The initial symptom is usually an intermittent, watery rhinorrhea that "runs like a faucet." The patient often seeks medical attention at this point either for the profuse rhinorrhea or accompanying nasal obstruction. Sinusitis or nasal polyps are often found. The frequency of polyposis in this triad is reported to be from 50 to 95% Although most reports describe sinusitis as a manifestation of this syndrome, there is no good estimate of the incidence of sinusitis associated with aspirin sensitivity. The typical patient is often described as a middle-aged white subject with vasomotor rhinitis, perennial bronchial asthma, eosinophilia, negative skin tests to inhalant allergens, and intolerance to aspirin.

The nature of asthma in the triad is variable. Although some patients deny asthma symptoms until ingestion of aspirin, most have a history of bronchial hyperreactivity prior to an aspirin trigger. Severity ranges from mild to steroid-resistant asthma. There is no direct correlation between the degree of underlying bronchial hyperreactivity and the degree of aspirin sensitivity (81).

The intolerance to aspirin generally manifests within 15 min–3 hr after ingestion. Symptoms include profuse rhinorrhea, nausea, vomiting, abdominal cramping, diarrhea, and bronchospasm. Epinephrine is the most effective treatment acutely. Most patients recover with 2 hr, but bronchial hyperreactivity may persist for several days. The natural history of the disease is variable. The rhinitis, nasal polyposis, and sinusitis, if present, do not resolve spontaneously without medical or surgical intervention. Aspirin sensitivity can, however, change over time (82).

Intolerance to aspirin often extends to related compounds, most notably nonsteroidal anti-inflammatory drugs. Indomethacin is highly cross-reactive in aspirin-sensitive patients (83). Others such as sulindac appear to have a lower potential for an adverse reaction. Nonacetylated salicylates such as sodium salicylate, salicylic acid esters, and choline salicylate are generally tolerated without adverse reactions. Acetaminophen is generally considered safe in these patients as well, although there have been reports of adverse reactions when it is given at high dosages (84,85).

D. Mechanism

Aspirin and cross-reactive nonsteroidal drugs lack structural similarity, which detracts from the likelihood of an immunologic mechanism. However, all of these compounds share the functional ability to alter arachidonic acid metabolism by inhibiting cyclo-oxygenase. Shunting arachidonic acid metabolism toward the lipoxygenase pathway results in preferential production of potent bronchoconstricting leukotrienes (86). Although aspirin can irreversibly acety-late cyclo-oxygenase in platelets, nucleated cells of the respiratory tract nor-mally have the ability to synthesize new enzyme (87). In subjects with aspirin-sensitive asthma, platelet arachidonic acid metabolism is normal (88). However, cyclo-oxygenase from nasal polyp cells and arachidonic acid metabolism in stimulated alveolar macrophages has been found to be defective (89). It is pos-tulated that this defect is responsible for an overabundance of leukotrienes in aspirin-sensitive asthmatics.

E. Medical and Surgical Management

Treatment for patients with Samter's syndrome involves avoidance of aspirin, medical therapy for upper and lower respiratory inflammation, such as topical or systemic corticosteroids, consideration of surgical therapy of the upper airway, and aspirin desensitization.

   Surgical management includes polypectomy and surgery of the sinuses. Polyps are generally bilateral and generally arise from the diseased mucosa of the sinuses. They often obstruct the ostiomeatal complex and therefore block the normal ventilation and drainage of the sinuses. Simple polypectomy gener-ally does not control the tendency for polyp formation to recur. In addition, worsening of the asthma has been noted in older studies of patients undergoing polypectomy (90). Slavin and co-workers demonstrated that sphenoethmoidec-tomy was not only effective in relieving sinusitis but also prevented recur-rence of polyps and improved asthma in patients (91). McFadden reviewed 25 aspirin-sensitive patients with severe ethmoid disease who were treated over 11 years (92). Of 16 patients who initially underwent limited surgical procedures (bilateral intranasal ethmoidectomies), 6 required subsequent sur-gery for recurrent sinusitis. Nine patients initially had radiographic evidence of severe antral as well as ethmoid disease. This group with initially more severe disease underwent more aggressive initial surgical procedures, including bilat-eral Caldwell-Luc operations with intranasal and transantral sphenoethmoidec-tomies, and did not require further surgical treatment. All patients noted a reduction in asthma symptoms, reduced need for medications including steroids, and a reduction in subsequent sinus infections. Of 64 surgical procedures in this group, bronchospasm occurred only in one patient in whom preoperative steroids were omitted. This as well as Slavin's experience support that sinus surgery can safely be performed without jeopardizing control of asthma perioperatively.

F. Aspirin Desensitization

As much as sensitivity to aspirin is a vital attribute of this syndrome, so is the ability to establish tolerance with administration of repetitive doses of aspirin. The ability to ''desensitize'' was first described in 1922 (93). Once induced, tolerance can be maintained by daily administration of aspirin or a related com-pound (94–97). If the aspirin is stopped, the refractory period will last for be-tween 1 and 9 days. A number of studies have demonstrated some improvement in the rhinosinusitis and asthma with aspirin desensitization followed by aspirin (98–103).

Sweet and co-workers compared a group of 35 aspirin sensitive rhinosinus-itis–asthma patients who underwent aspirin-desensitization with continued as pirin treatment with 32 who were desensitized to aspirin and then discontinued its use, and 30 who did not undergo desensitization (104). Both groups who un-derwent desensitization demonstrated reduction in severity of asthma with lower corticosteroid requirements, reduced episodes of sinusitis, and reduced need for nasal polypectomies and sinus surgery compared with the control group. The group receiving was continuous aspirin able to reduce use of inhaled cortico-steroids significantly as well.

The current data support the finding that aspirin desensitization followed by daily aspirin be considered an option for patients with aspirin-sensitive rhino-sinusitis–asthma, particularly those who have poorly controlled asthma requir-ing high dosages of corticosteroids, patients who have required repeated surgery for nasal polyps or sinusitis, and patients who have a medical condition that re-quires the use of aspirin or a nonsteroidal anti-inflammatory drug. In these as in all patients, care must be taken to exclude a contraindication to aspirin, such as its anticoagulant or gastrointestinal effects, before embarking on a course of desensitization.

VII. SUMMARY

Despite a century of observation that upper airway disease has a deleterious ef-fect on asthma, most evidence for a link between sinusitis and asthma remains circumstantial. Nevertheless, when sinus disease is left untreated, asthma is dif-ficult to control. Multiple mechanisms have been proposed. The greatest evi-dence supports a nasobronchial reflex and involvement of cellular and soluble factors of inflammation. Such abnormalities cannot, however, be universally demonstrated in human subjects.

It is the responsibility of the clinician, particularly in difficult-to-control asthma, to be aware of the relationship between sinusitis and asthma and to look for occult sinusitis, nasal polyps, or aspirin sensitivity. Once these are recog-nized, highly effective medical and surgical treatment is available.

REFERENCES

1. Kratchmer I. cited by Allen W. Effect on respiration, blood pressure, and carotid pulse of various inhaled and insufflated vapors when stimulating one cranial nerve and various combinations of cranial nerves. Am J Physiol 1928; 87:319–25.

2. Dixon WE, Brodie TG. The bronchial muscles, their innervation and the action of drugs upon them. J Physiol 1903; 29:97–173.

3. Bullen SS. Incidence of asthma in 400 cases of chronic sinusitis. J Allergy 1932; 4:402–7.

4. Matthews J. Anaphylaxis and asthma. Med Rec 1913; 84:512–4.

5. Chobot R. The incidence of sinusitis in asthmatic children. Am J Dis Child 1930; 39:257–64.

6. Rackemann FM, Tobey HG. The nose and throat in asthma. Arch Otolaryngol 1929; 9:612–21.

7. Cooke RA. Infective asthma: indications of its allergic nature. Am J Med Sci 1932; 183:309–17.

8. Sluder G. Asthma as a nasal reflex. JAMA 1919; 73:589–91.

9. Gottlieb MS. Relation of intranasal disease in the production of bronchial asthma. JAMA 1925; 85:105–8.

10. Minor MW, Lockey RF. Sinusitis and asthma. South Med J 1987; 80:1141–7.

11. Phipatanakul CS, Slavin RG. Bronchial asthma produced by paranasal sinusitis. Arch Otolaryngol 1974; 100:109–12.

12. Van Alyea OE. Sinusitis: what it is and what it is not. Postgrad Med 1963; 34:473–8.

13. Slavin RG. Sinusitis in adults and its relation to allergic rhinitis, asthma and nasal polyps. J Allergy Clin Immunol 1988; 82:950–6.

14. Evans FO Jr, Sydner JB, Moore WEC, Moore GR, Manwaring JL, Brill AH, Jackson RT, Hanna S, Shaar JS, Holdeman LV. Sinusitis of the maxillary antrum. N Engl J Med 1975; 293:735–9.

15. McAlister WH, Lusk R, Muntz HR. Comparison of plain radiographs and coronal CT scans in infants and children with recurrent sinusitis. Am J Radiol 1989; 153:1259–64.

16. Zinreich SJ. Paranasal sinus imaging. Otolaryngol Head Neck Surg 1990; 103:863–9.

17. Rohr AS, Spector SL, Siegel SC, Katz RM, Rachelefsky GS. Correlation between A-mode untrasound and radiography in the diagnosis of maxillary sinusitis. J Allergy Clin Immunol 1986; 78:58–61.

18. Selner JC, Koepke JW, Rhinolaryngoscopy in the allergy office. Ann Allergy 1985; 54:479–82.

19. Fascenalli FW. Maxillary sinus abnormalities: radiographic evidence in an asymptomatic population. Arch Otolaryngol Head Neck Surg 1969; 95:190–3.

20. Berman SZ, Matheson DA, Stevenson DD, Usselman JA, Shore S, Tan E. Maxillary sinusitis and bronchial asthma: correlation of roentgenograms, cultures and thermograms. J Allergy Clin Immunol 1974; 53:311–7.

21. Grove RC, Farrior JB. Chronic hyperplastic sinusitis in allergic patients. J Allergy 1940; 11:271–6.

22. Spector SS, English GM, McIntosh K, Farr RS. Adenovirus in the sinuses of an asthmatic patient with apparent selective antibody deficiencies. Am J Med 1973; 55:227–31.

23. Rachelefsky GS, Goldberg M, Katz RM, et al. Sinus disease in children with respiratory allergy. J Allergy Clin Immunol 1978; 61:310.

24. Adinoff AD, Wood RW, Buschman D. Chronic sinusitis in childhood asthma: correlations of symptoms, x-rays, culture and response to treatment. Pediatr Res 1983; 17:264–8.

25. Adinoff AD, Cummings NP. Sinusitis and its relationship to asthma. Pediatr Ann 1989; 18:785–90.

26. Wald ER, Milmore GJ, Bowen A. Acute maxillary sinusitis in children. N Engl J Med 1981; 304:749–54.

27. Zimmerman B, Stringer D, Feanny S, Reisman J, Hak H, Rashed N, et al. J Allergy Clin Immunol 1987; 80:268–73.

28. Orobello PW Jr., Park RI, Belcher LJ, Eggleston P, Lederman HM, Banks JR, Modlin JF, Naclerio RM. Microbiology of chronic sinusitis in children. Arch Otolaryngol 1991; 117:980–3.

29. Frederick J, Braude AI. Anaerobic infection of the paranasal sinuses. N Engl J Med 1974; 290:135–7.

30. Wald ER, Milmoe W, Bowen AD, et al. Acute maxillary sinusitis in children N Engl J Med 1981; 304:749–54.

31. Goldstein MF, Atkins PC, Cogen FC, Kornstein MJ, Levine RS, Zweiman B. Allergic aspergillus sinusitis. J Allergy Clin Immunol 1985; 76:515–24.

32. Zieske LA, Kopke RD, Hamill R. Dematiaceous fungal sinusitis. Otolaryngol Head Neck Surg 1991; 105:567–77.

33. Manning SC, Schaefer, SD, Close LG, Vuitch F. Culture-positive allergic fungal sinusitis. Arch Otolaryngol 1991; 117:174–8.

34. Page R, Friday G, Stillwagon P, Skoner D, Caliguiri L, Fireman P. Asthma and selective immunoglobulin subclass deficiency: improvement of asthma after immunoglobulin replacement therapy. J Pediatr 1988; 112:127–31.

35. Winfield JB, Sande MA, Gwaltney JM. Aspiration during sleep. JAMA 1973; 233:1288.

36. Huxley EJ, Viroslav J, Gray WR, Pierce AK. Pharyngeal aspiration in normal adults and patients with depressed consciousness. Am J Med 1978; 64:564–8.

37. Bardin PG, Van Heerden BB, Joubert JR. Absence of pulmonary aspiration of sinus contents in patients with asthma and sinusitis. J Allergy Clin Immunol 1990; 86:82–8.

38. Hansel FK. Clinical and histopathologic studies of the nose and sinuses in allergy. J Allergy 1929; 1:43–70.

39. Burrows B, Hasan FM, Barbe RA, Halonen M, Lebowitz MD. Epidemiologic observations on eosinophilia and its relation to respiratory disorders. Am Rev Respir Dis 1980; 122:709–19.

40. Lowell FC. Clinical aspects of eosinophilia in atopic disease. JAMA 1967; 202:875–8.

41. Frigas E, Loegering DA, Solley GO, Farrow GM, Gleich GJ. Elevated levels of the eosinophil granule granule major basic protein in the sputum of patients with bronchial asthma. Mayo Clin Proc 1981; 56:345–53.

42. Harlin SL, Ansel DG, Lane SR, Myers J, Kephart GM, Gleich GJ. A clinical and pathologic study of chronic sinusitis: the role of the eosinophil. J Allergy Clin Immunol 1988: 81:867–75.

43. Hogg JC. The pathology of asthma. Clin Chest Med 1984; 5:567–71.

44. Thorne KJI, Richardson BA, Veith MC, Tai PC, Spry CJF, Butterworth AE. Partial purification and biological properties of an eosinophil-activity factor. Eur J Immunol 1985; 15:1083–91.

45. Jong EC, Klebanoff SJ. Eosinophil-mediated mammalian tumor cell cytotoxicity: role of the peroxidase system. J Immunol 1980; 124:1949–53.

46. Henderson WR, Chi EY, Jong EC, Klebanoff SJ. Mast cell-mediated tumor-cell cytotoxicity. J Exp Med 1981; 153:520–33.

47. Gleich GJ, Adolphson CR. The eosinophilic leukocyte: structure and function. Adv Immunol 1986; 39:177–253.

48. Wells R. Effects of cold air on respiratory airflow resistance in patients with respiratory tract disease. N Engl J Med 1960; 263:503–9.

49. Deal EC Jr, McFadden ER Jr, Ingram RH Jr, et al. Airway responsiveness to cold air and hyperpnea in normal subjects and in those with hay fever and asthma. Am Rev Respir Dis 1980; 121:621–8.

50. Nadel JA, Widdicombe JG. Reflex effects of upper airway function on total lung resistance and blood pressure. J Appl Physiol 1962; 17:861–5.

51. Kaufman J, Wright G. The effect of nasal and nasopharyngeal irritation on airway resistance in man. Am Rev Respir Dis 1969; 100:626–30.

52. Yan K, Salome C. The response of the airways to nasal stimulation in asthmatics with rhinitis. Eur J Respir Dis 1983; 64(suppl 128):105–8.

53. Nolte D, Berger D. On vagal bronchoconstriction in asthmatic patients by nasal irritation. Eur J Respir Dis 1983; 64(suppl 128):110–4.

54. Hoehne JH, Reed CE. Where is the allergic reaction in ragweed asthma? J Allergy Clin Immunol 1971; 48:36–9.

55. Rosenberg GL, Rosenthal RR, Norman PS. Inhalational challenge with ragweed pollen and ragweed-sensitive asthmatics. J Allergy Clin Immunol 1983; 71:302–10.

56. Schumacher MJ, Cota KA, Taussig LM. Pulmonary response to nasal-challenge testing of atopic subjects with stable asthma. J Allergy Clin Immunol 1986; 78:30–5.

57. Szentivanyi I. The beta-adrenergic theory of atopic abnormality in asthma. J Allergy 1968; 42:203–32.

58. Busse WW. Decreased granulocyte response to isoproterenol in asthma during upper respiratory symptoms. Am Rev Respir Dis 1977; 115:783–91.

59. Busse WW, Anderson CL, Dick EC, Warshauer D. Reduced granulocyte response to isoproterenol, histamine and prostaglandin E after in-vitro incubation with rhinovirus 16. Am Rev Respir Dis 1980; 122:641–6.

60. Druce HM, Slavin RG. Sinusitis: a critical need for further study. J Allergy Clin Immunol 1991; 88:675–7.

61. Druce HM. Adjuncts to medical management of sinusitis. Otolaryngol Head Neck Surg 1990; 103:880–3.

62. Melen I, Friberg B, Andreasson L, Ivarsson A, Jannert M, Johansseen C-J. Effects of phenylpropanolamine on ostial and nasal patency in patients treated for chronic maxillary sinusitis. Acta Otolaryngol 1986; 101:494–500.

63. Slavin RG. Relationship of nasal disease and sinusitis to bronchial asthma. Ann Allergy 1982; 49:76–80.

64. Rachelefsky GS, Katz RM, Siegel SC. Chronic sinusitis in children with respiratory allergy; the role of antimicrobials. J Allergy Clin Immunol 1982; 69:382–7.

65. Friedman R, Ackerman M, Wald E, Casselbrant M, Friday G, Fireman P. Asthma and bacterial sinusitis in children. J Allergy Clin Immunol 1984; 74:185–9.

66. Friedman WH, Katsantonis GP, Slavin RG, et al. Sphenoethmoidectomy: its role in the asthmatic patient. Otolaryngol Head Neck Surg 1982; 90:171–7.

67. Gilbert GB. Unusual idiosyncrasy to aspirin. JAMA 1911; 56:1262.

68. Cooke RA. Allergy in drug idiosyncrasy. JAMA 1919; 73:759–60.

69. Van Leeuwen WS. A possible explanation for certain cases of hypersensitivities to drug in men. J Pharmacol Exp Ther 1924; 24:25–32.

70. Prickman LE, Buchstein HF. Hypersensitivity to acetylsalicylic acid (aspirin). JAMA 1937, 108.445–51.

71. Samter M, Beers RF Jr. Concerning the nature of intolerance to aspirin. J Allergy 1967; 40:281–93.

72. Zeitz HJ, Jarmoszuk I. Nasal polyps, bronchial asthma, and aspirin sensitivity: the Samter syndrome. Compr Ther 1985; 11(6):21–6.

73. Walton CHA, Randle DL. Aspirin allergy. Can Med Assoc J 1957; 76:1016–8.

74. Farr RS. The need to re-evaluate acetylsalicylic acid (aspirin). J Allergy 1970; 45:321–8.

75. Fischer TJ, Guilfoile TD, Kesarwala HH, et al. Adverse pulmonary responses to aspirin and acetaminophen in chronic childhood asthma. Pediatrics 1983; 71:313–8.

76. Rachelefsky GS, Coulson A, Siegel SC, Stiehm ER. Aspirin intolerance in chronic childhood asthma: determined by oral challenge. Pediatrics 1975; 56:443–8.

77. Tan Y, Collins-Williams C. Aspirin-induced asthma in children. Ann Allergy 1982; 48:1–5.

78. Vedanthan PK, Menon MM, Bell TD, et al. Aspirin and tartrazine oral challenge: incidence of adverse response in chronic childhood asthma. J Allergy Clin Immunol 1977; 60:8–13.

79. Weinberger M. Analgesic sensitivity in children with asthma. Pediatrics 1978; 62:910–5.

80. Yunginger JW, O'Connell EJ, Logan GB. Aspirin-induced asthma in children. J Pediatr 1973; 82:218–21.

81. Kowalski ML, Grzelewska-Rzymowska I, Szmidt M, Rozniecki J. Bronchial hyperreactivity to histamine in aspirin sensitive asthmatics: relationship to aspirin threshold and effect of aspirin desensitization. Thorax 1985; 40:598–602.

82. Spector SL, Wangaard CH, Farr RS. Aspirin and concomitant idiosyncrasies in adult asthmatic patients. J Allergy Clin Immunol 1979; 64:500–6.

83. Vanselow NA, Smith Jr. Bronchial asthma induced by indomethacin. Ann Intern Med 1967; 66:568–72.

84. Settipane RA, Stevenson DD. Cross sensitivity with acetaminophen in ASA-sensitive asthmatics. J Allergy Clin Immunol 1988; 81:180.

85. Smith AP. Response of aspirin-allergic patients to challenge by some analgesics in common use. Br Med J 1971; 2:494–6.

86. Pleskow WW, Stevenson DD, Mathison DA, et al. Aspirin-sensitive rhinosinusitis/asthma: spectrum of adverse reactions to aspirin. J Allergy Clin Immunol 1983; 71:574–9.

87. Vane J. The evolution of nonsteroidal anti-inflammatory drugs and their mechanism of action. Drugs 1987; 33(suppl 1):18–27.

88. Bonne C, Moneret-Vautrin DA, Wayoff M. Arachidonic acid metabolism and inhibition of cyclooxygenase in platelets from asthmatic subjects with aspirin intolerance. Ann Allergy 1985; 54:158–60.
89. Szczeklik A. Analgesics, allergy and asthma. Drugs 1986; 32(suppl 4):148–63.
90. Samter M. Intolerance to aspirin. Hosp Pract 1973; 8(12):85–90.
91. Slavin RG, Linford PA, Friedman WH. Sphenoethmoidectomy (SE) in the treatment of nasal polyps, sinusitis and bronchial asthma. J Allergy Clin Immunol 1983; 71:156.
92. McFadden EA, Kany RJ, Fink JN, Toohill RJ. Surgery for sinusitis and aspirin triad. Laryngoscope 1990: 100:1043–6.
93. Widal WF, Abrami P, Lermoyez J. Anaphylaxie et idiosyncrasie. Presse Med 1922; 30:189.
94. Zeiss CR, Lockey RF. Refractory period to aspirin in a patient with aspirin-induced asthma. J Allergy Clin Immunol 1976; 57:440–8.
95. Bianco S, Robuschi M, Petrini G. Aspirin-induced tolerance in aspirin-asthma detected by a new challenge test. IRCS J Med Sci 1977; 5:129.
96. Stevenson DD, Simon RA, Mathison DA. Aspirin-sensitive asthma: tolerance to aspirin after positive oral aspirin challenge. J Allergy Clin Immunol 1980; 66:82–8.
97. Stevenson DD. Aspirin desensitization. N Engl Reg Allergy Proc 1986; 7:101.
98. Chiu JT. Improvement in aspirin-sensitive asthmatic subjects after rapid aspirin desensitization and aspirin maintenance (ADAM) treatment. J Allergy Clin Immunol 1983; 71:560–7.
99. Lumry WR, Curd JG, Zieger RS, Pleskow WW, Stevenson DD. Aspirin-sensitive rhinosinusitis: the clinical syndrome and the effects of aspirin administration. J Allergy Clin Immunol 1983; 71:580–7.
100. Nelson RP, Stablein JJ, Lockey RF. Asthma improved by acetylsalicylic acid and other nonsteroidal anti-inflammatory agents. N Engl Reg Allergy Proc 1986; 7:117.
101. Szczeklik A, Gryglewski RJ, Nizankowska E. Asthma relieved by aspirin and other cyclooxygenase inhibitors. Thorax 1978; 33:664–5.
102. Lockey RF. Aspirin-improved ASA triad. Hosp Pract 1978; 13(8):129–38.
103. Lockey RF, Rucknagel DL, Vanselow NA. Familial occurrence of asthma, nasal polyps, and aspirin intolerance. Ann Intern Med 1973; 78:57–63.
104. Sweet JM, Stevenson DD, Simon RA, Matheson DA. Long-term effects of aspirin desensitization-treatment for aspirin-sensitive rhinosinusitis-asthma. J Allergy Clin Immunol 1990; 85:59–65.

11

Sinusitis and Related Tissues

MICHAEL J. SCHUMACHER
Steele Memorial Children's Research Center
University of Arizona Health Sciences Center
Tucson, Arizona

Tissues and structures that lie in anatomical proximity to the paranasal sinuses commonly have effects on sinus function that lead to sinus infection, either from ostial obstruction or from direct spread of infection from adjacent tissue. It is also possible that some pathophysiological processes may affect the same respiratory epithelium that lines the cavities of the nose and the paranasal sinuses, without sinusitis necessarily being a result of obstruction of sinus drainage by nasal pathologic change. Anatomical proximity of the sinuses to the orbit and the cranial cavity explains the occurrence of serious infection in the orbit and central nervous system that may occur when sinusitis is not effectively treated. This chapter explores these relationships.

I. ANATOMY

The maxillary sinuses are situated between the palate and upper teeth inferiorly and the floor of the orbit superiorly, which explains how dental disease may lead to sinusitis and how maxillary sinusitis can spread to cause orbital cellulitis. Orbital cellulitis may also result from infection in the ethmoidal sinuses, because of their close proximity to the medial wall of the orbit. The superior walls of the frontal sinuses are within a few millimeters of the frontal lobes, and portions of their floor relate to the orbits. The sphenoidal sinuses are in close proximity to the pituitary, the cavernous venous sinus, the optic nerves, the internal carotid arteries, and, anteriorly, to the orbits. Infection in the frontal, sphenoidal, or ethmoidal sinuses may lead to intracranial infection by direct extension.

Drainage of fluid from the maxillary sinuses is found to be slow in subjects with small maxillary ostia (1). Therefore, interference with normal sinus draining through the ostia could lead to retention of secretions and sinusitis. This is particularly apt to occur when there is anatomical obstruction in the region of the middle meatus into which the maxillary sinus, frontal sinus, and anterior ethmoidal cells drain. This region, known as the ostiomeatal complex, may be obstructed by nasal polyps, cystic malformation of the middle turbinate (concha bullosa), and septal deviation. Older children are known to show a stronger association between sinusitis and septal deviations or bullous conchae than younger children (2). The anatomy of this area relevant to intervention by endoscopic surgery has been well described (3). Relationships between sinus disease and concha bullosa or septal deviation are readily demonstrable by coronal computed tomography (4). This topic, including effects of surgical correction of ostiomeatal obstruction, is discussed in Chapter 8.

II. PREDISPOSITION TO SINUSITIS BY PATHOLOGIC INVOLVEMENT IN ADJACENT TISSUES

It has long been suspected that chronic sinusitis may be a complication of chronic rhinitis, because of the likelihood that inflammatory edema of the nasal mucosa in the vicinity of the sinus ostia could impair sinus drainage, and because of a common finding of an association between the two conditions in clinical practice. The relationships between allergic rhinitis and sinusitis have been difficult to explore because of the high frequency of allergic rhinitis in the unselected general population. This problem is compounded by the difficulty in differentiating between chronic rhinitis and chronic sinusitis, because of their similar symptoms. No randomly selected population samples have been studied for the incidence of sinusitis and rhinitis. However, there is suggestive evidence of a relationship in studies of patients presenting for treatment at allergy or otolaryngology clinics. Two different questions can be asked. How common is allergic rhinitis in patients with sinusitis? How common is chronic sinusitis in patients with allergic rhinitis?

The first question was addressed in a retrospective study of adult patients presenting to a suburban otolaryngology clinic with nasal or sinus symptoms (5). Among 74 patients found to have chronic sinusitis, 54% also had allergic rhinitis as assessed by positive skin tests or a strongly positive history of allergy. It was also noted that allergen exposure frequently exacerbated ''sinus symptoms'' in patients with sinusitis. In a previous study by the same author, 56% of patients with sinusitis who required functional endoscopic sinus surgery had positive skin tests to aeroallergens, an incidence of atopy higher than that found in the general population (6). Friedman (7) noted that 94% of patients undergoing sphenoethmoidectomy for chronic hyperplastic sinusitis were atopic. Grove and Farrior investigated 200 patients who required operative treatment for chronic hyperplastic sinusitis, finding that 82% had asthma, 14% had hay fever, and 50% of the whole group had one or more positive allergen skin tests (8).

The second question (the incidence of chronic sinusitis in patients with allergic rhinitis), has been studied best in children seen in allergy clinics. In a prospective study of 70 children referred for evaluation of chronic respiratory symptoms, Rachelefsky (9) found that 27% had abnormal sinus radiographs. In another allergy clinic study, Shapiro (10,11) found the incidence of sinusitis in allergic children to be even higher. In this survey of 91 atopic children with cough, chronic rhinorrhea, and fatigue unresponsive to antihistamines and decongestants, 70% had sinusitis (as defined by mucosal thickening greater than 6 mm) or sinus opacification. However, selection of patients with rhinitis unresponsive to antihistamines may well have increased the incidence of sinusitis. De Cleyn et al. (12) studied 270 patients of all ages with asthma and/or rhinitis, finding abnormal sinus radiographs in 54%. Loss of translucency of the sinuses was more common in children. Sinus pathologic change was found to be strongly associated with asthma, but not with allergy as defined by history, skin testing, and results of radioallergosorbent assay testing (RAST). These conflicting findings concerning the relationship between allergic rhinitis and sinusitis indicate the need for further study, in randomly sampled populations.

In children with allergic rhinitis studied by Shapiro (10), middle ear abnormalities including effusion, negative middle ear pressure, or ventilating tubes were often found in children who also had sinusitis, confirming an association previously noted by Hoshaw and Nickman (13). Although it is unlikely that there is a direct causal relationship between sinusitis and otitis, it is likely that rhinitis could predispose to both of these conditions.

It is quite possible that chronic sinusitis may not be one disease. In some patients, there may be a chronic bacterial and/or fungal infection that results from impairment of sinus drainage or introduction of foreign material into the sinuses. In other patients, inflammation and hypersecretion occurring in the sinuses may be reflections of the same pathologic process occurring in the nasal cavities. Moreover, the demonstration that unilateral nasal allergen challenge can induce glandular secretion in the contralateral nasal cavity by reflex mechanisms (14) suggests the possibility that deposition of allergen in the nasal cavity could cause reflex glandular secretion in the sinuses. Once sinusitis is established, cholinergically induced nasal secretion contains subnormal amounts of protective proteins including secretory IgA and lysozyme (15). If reflex mucus secretion does occur in the sinuses, this could also result from a reflex response to late phase nasal inflammatory response to allergens. This hypothesis has not yet been tested. Direct penetration of the sinus ostia by large amounts of allergens appears to be unlikely. However, in allergic fungal sinusitis, it is probable that spores or fungi including *Aspergillus*, *Alternaria*, and other fungi do induce inflammation in the sinuses directly, through immunologic mechanisms similar to those occurring in bronchopulmonary aspergillosis.

Although inflammatory mechanisms leading to obstruction of ostia in nonallergic rhinitis have been proposed as a cause for chronic sinusitis (16), sinusitis was found to be relatively uncommon in adults with perennial nonallergic rhinitis (17). To demonstrate unequivocally a causative relationship between allergic or nonallergic rhinitis and sinusitis, prospective studies of prevention of sinusitis with anti-inflammatory treatment of rhinitis (topical corticosteroids) and the response of sinusitis to nasal corticosteroid treatment in allergic and nonallergic rhinitis are needed.

The association of acute sinusitis with viral rhinitis and the association of chronic sinusitis with cystic fibrosis, ciliary dyskinesia, immunodeficiency, and aspirin sensitivity with nasal polyposis are well known and discussed in Chapters 14 and 15. Atrophic rhinitis may also lead to sinusitis, and when this occurs, there are bony changes including a reduction in the size of the maxillary sinuses with simultaneous expansion of the nasal cavities (18).

It has been known for many years that maxillary sinusitis may result from infection surrounding maxillary teeth (19). This association, termed the endoantral syndrome because of the spread of endodontic infection to the maxillary sinus (either spontaneously or as a complication of dental surgery), has been reviewed (20). In one large survey of patients with chronic maxillary sinusitis, 40% of the patients were found to have a dental cause, mostly marginal periodontitis and periapical granuloma. In that study, it was rare to find a dental cause of chronic maxillary sinusitis in patients under the age of 30 years (21). Although direct penetration of a periapical abscess into the maxillary sinus may occur, direct invasion of oral flora through the mucous membranes surrounding the teeth may also occur (22). Orofacial infections of dental origin are usually from anaerobic gram-negative bacteria including *Fusobacterium nucleatum* (23). Chronic maxillary sinusitis due to *Aspergillus* infection may also result from dental infection or its treatment. For example, radiopaque foreign bodies have been found in the maxillary sinuses of patients with maxillary sinus aspergillosis. These were thought to be due to overfilling of maxillary teeth with dental paste containing zinc, and zinc is known to promote the growth of *Aspergillus fumigatus* (24). Foreign material may also enter the sinuses as the result of root canal surgery, carrying bacteria with it (20).

Anatomical considerations suggest that it is unlikely that adenoidal hypertrophy would cause sufficient obstruction to sinus drainage to predispose to chronic sinusitis. The few published studies of this question provide conflicting evidence. For example, Fukuda et al. (25) showed that when adenoidal hypertrophy was sufficient to cause snoring and nasal obstruction, it was not significantly more prevalent in children with sinusitis than in children without sinusitis. However, Takahashi et al. (26) found that sinusitis in children improved twice as frequently in children who underwent adenoidectomy. Additional studies are needed to confirm this observation.

III. EXTENSION OF SINUS INFECTION TO ADJACENT TISSUES AND STRUCTURES

Unrecognized or inadequately treated sinusitis may cause serious complications through extension into the orbit or the cranial cavity. Although orbital and intracranial infection following sinusitis has become an uncommon problem since a variety of effective antibiotics have become available, these complications continue to cause blindness, central nervous system (CNS) lesions, and death. Adequate treatment of acute and chronic sinusitis can usually prevent these serious complications: it is essential to recognize orbital and neurologic symptoms early and search for "silent" chronic sinusitis that may lead to these complications. Sphenoidal sinusitis is frequently asymptomatic and not diagnosed until intracranial complications occur (27–29). Orbital or facial cellulitis is often an early sign of intracranial extension.

Although there are no systematic, prospective studies of the orbital and intracranial complications of sinusitis, intracranial complications were observed in 3.7% of patients whose acute or chronic sinusitis was severe enough to require admission to the hospital (30). These complications included subdural empyema, cerebral abscesses, cavernous and sagittal sinus thrombosis, and osteomyelitis. It is possible that intracranial complications are more common in children with group C streptococcal sinusitis (31). If one excludes cyanotic congenital heart disease and ventricular shunts, the most common single underlying cause of cerebral abscess is acute frontal sinusitis (32). Neither the frontal sinusitis nor the intracranial complication is usually diagnosed correctly at first presentation, indicating the importance of suspecting both conditions in patients presenting with acute frontal headache and deteriorating consciousness (32). Frontal sinusitis may lead to a frontal lobe abscess without any focal and neurologic signs and may present with changes in behavior only (33). Occasionally frontal sinusitis extends to cause osteomyelitis and a subperiosteal abscess of the frontal bone, usually with frontal bone erosion and frontal cellulitis (Pott's puffy tumor). This frequently leads to orbital cellulitis and/or intracranial suppuration (34, 35).

In children, either brain abscess or extradural abscesses may be caused by either otitis media or sinusitis. Sinusitis is a much more common cause of extradural abscess, whereas brain abscesses in children are more often a complication of otitis (36–40). In the absence of immunodeficiency there is no reliable way to predict which patients with sinusitis will develop intracranial complications (41).

Anatomical proximity of the maxillary and ethmoidal sinuses to the floor and medial walls of the orbits suggests that orbital infection could readily occur as a complication of sinusitis. However, true orbital infection, as distinct from preseptal (periorbital) cellulitis, may be uncommon. There are no systematic studies of the incidence of orbital complications of sinusitis. Chandler et al. (42) proposed a clinical staging of orbital inflammation, listed in order of severity. These are inflammatory edema or preseptal cellulitis (stage 1), orbital cellulitis (stage 2), subperiosteal abscess (stage 3), orbital abscess (stage 4), and cavernous sinus thrombosis (stage 5). Orbital cellulitis and subperiosteal abscess usually result from extension of sinusitis, particularly involving the ethmoidal sinuses (42,43). On the other hand, periorbital cellulitis, a much more common condition than stage 2–5 orbital inflammation, is limited to the eyelids in the preseptal region and occurs much more commonly in children than in adults. This relatively benign condition is much less frequently caused by sinusitis (43–45). However, a systematic search for ethmoidal sinusitis should be made in children with periorbital cellulitis presenting with an elevated white cell count and a high fever (46).

Proptosis, chemosis, restricted eye movements, and decreased visual acuity differentiate true orbital cellulitis from preseptal cellulitis. Since orbital inflammation usually involves retrobulbar tissues, loss of vision is a serious and sometimes permanent complication (47). Although all patients with signs that are more extensive than those of simple preseptal infection require high-resolution CT scanning immediately, CT may not detect a cerebral abscess and surgical exploration may be required to prevent blindness. In particular, subperiosteal abscess of the orbit requires drainage to prevent blindness when it presents in children (48,49). Orbital inflammation occurring in association with sinusitis is not necessarily infective. Goldberg et al. (50) reported three cases of chronic sinusitis associated with orbital inflammation or optic neuropathy in patients with long-standing intranasal cocaine abuse. In two of the patients, the orbital cellulitis responded to steroid therapy.

REFERENCES

1. Aust R, Drettner B, Hemmingsson A. Elimination of contrast medium from the maxillary sinus. Acta Otolaryngol (Stockh) 1976; 81:468–74.
2. Van der Veken P, Clement PA, Buisseret T, Desprechins B, Kaufman L, Derde MP. [CAT-scan study of the prevalence of sinus disorders and anatomical variations in 196 children]. Acta Otorhinolaryngol Belg 1989; 43:51–8.
3. Becker SP. Anatomy for endoscopic sinus surgery. Otolaryngol Clin North Am 1989; 22:677–89.
4. Calhoun KH, Waggenspack GA, Simpson CB, Hokanson JA, Bailey BJ. CT evaluation of the paranasal sinuses in symptomatic and asymptomatic populations. Otolaryngol Head Neck Surg 1991; 104:480–83.

5. Benninger MS. Rhinitis, sinusitis, and their relationships to allergies. Am J Rhinol 1992; 6:37–43.
6. Benninger MS, Mickelson SA, Yaremchuk K. Functional endoscopic sinus surgery: morbidity and early results. Henry Ford Hosp Med J 1990; 38:5–8.
7. Friedman WH. Surgery for chronic hyperplastic rhinosinusitis. Laryngoscope 1975; 85:1999–2011.
8. Grove RC, Farrior JB. Chronic hyperplastic sinusitis in allergic patients. A bacteriologic study of two hundred operative cases. J Allergy 1940; 11:271–76.
9. Rachelefsky GS, Goldberg M, Katz RM, Boris G, Gyepes MT, Shapiro MJ, Mickey MR, Finegold SM, Siegel SC. Sinus disease in children with respiratory allergy. J Allergy Clin Immunol 1978; 61:310–4.
10. Rachelefsky GS, Shapiro GG. Diseases of paranasal sinuses in children. In: Bierman CW, Pearlman DS, eds. Allergic Diseases of Infancy, Childhood and Adolescence, 1st ed. Philadelphia: WB Saunders, 1980: 526–34.
11. Shapiro GG. Role of allergy in sinusitis. Pediatr Infect Dis 1985; 4:S55–8.
12. De Cleyn KM, Kersschot EA, De Clerck LS, Ortmanns PM, De Schepper AM, Van Bever HP, Stevens WJ. Paranasal sinus pathology in allergic and non-allergic respiratory tract diseases. Allergy 1986;41:313–8.
13. Hoshaw TC, Nickman NJ. Sinusitis and otitis in children. Arch Otolaryngol 1974; 100:194–5.
14. Raphael GD, Igarashi Y, White MV, Kaliner MA. The pathophysiology of rhinitis. V. Sources of protein in allergen-induced nasal secretions. J Allergy Clin Immunol 1991;88:33–42.
15. Jeney EVM, Raphael GD, Meredith SD, Kaliner MA. Abnormal nasal glandular secretion in recurrent sinusitis. J Allergy Clin Immunol 1990;86:10–8.
16. Druce HM. Chronic sinusitis and nonallergic rhinitis. In: Settipane GA, ed. Rhinitis, 2nd ed. Providence, RI: Oceanside Publications, 1991:185–90.
17. Enberg RN. Perennial nonallergic rhinitis: a retrospective review. Ann Allergy 1989;63:513–6.
18. Pace Balzan A, Shankar L, Hawke M. Computed tomographic findings in atrophic rhinitis. J Otolaryngol 1991;20:428–32.
19. Bauer WH. Maxillary sinusitis of dental origin. Am J Ortho Oral Surg (Oral Surg Sec) 1943;29:133–51.
20. Selden HS. The endo-antral syndrome: an endodontic complication. J Am Dent Assoc 1989;119:397–8, 401–2.
21. Melén I, Lindahl L, Andréasson L, Rundcrantz H. Chronic maxillary sinusitis. Definition, diagnosis and relation to dental infections and nasal polyposis. Acta Otolaryngol 1986;101:320–7.
22. Heimdahl A, Nord CE. Orofacial infections of odontogenic origin. Scand J Infect Dis 1983;Suppl 39:86–91.
23. Heimdahl A, von Konow L, Satoh T, Nord CE. Clinical appearance of orofacial infections of odontogenic origin in relation to microbiological findings. J Clin Microbiol 1985;22:299–302.
24. Legent F, Billet J, Beauvillain C, Bonnet J, Miegeville M. The role of dental canal fillings in the development of *Aspergillus* sinusitis. A report of 85 cases. Arch Otorhinolaryngol 1989;246:318–20.

25. Fukuda K, Matsune S, Ushikai M, Imamura Y, Ohyama M. A study on the relationship between adenoid vegetation and rhinosinusitis. Am J Otolaryngol 1989;10:214–6.

26. Takahashi H, Fujita A, Honjo I. Effect of adenoidectomy on otitis media with effusion, tubal function and sinusitis. Am J Otolaryngol 1989;10:208–13.

27. Finkelstein R, Honigman S, Doron Y, Braun Y. Sphenoid sinusitis presenting as chronic meningitis. Eur Neurol 1986;25:183–7.

28. Larranaga J, Fandino J, Gomez Bueno J, Rodriguez D, Gonzalez Carrero J, Botana C. Aspergillosis of the sphenoid sinus simulating a pituitary tumor. Neuroradiology 1989;31:362–3.

29. Leramo OB, Char G. Intrasellar abscess simulating a pituitary tumor. West Indian Med J 1989;38:171–5.

30. Clayman GL, Adams GL, Paugh DR, Koopmann CF Jr. Intracranial complications of paranasal sinusitis: a combined institutional review. Laryngoscope 1991;101:234–9.

31. Gallagher PG, Myer CM, Crone K, Benzing G. Group C streptococcal sinusitis. Am J Otolaryngol 1990;11:352–4.

32. Chalstrey S, Pfleiderer AG, Moffat DA. Persisting incidence and mortality of sinogenic cerebral abscess: a continuing reflection of late clinical diagnosis. J R Soc Med 1991;84:193–5.

33. Daya S, To SS. A 'silent' intracranial complication of frontal sinusitis. J Laryngol Otol 1990;104:645–7.

34. Gardiner LJ. Complicated frontal sinusitis: evaluation and management. Otolaryngol Head Neck Surg 1986;95:333–43.

35. Pender ES. Pott's puffy tumor: a complication of frontal sinusitis. Pediatr Emerg Care 1990;6:280–4.

36. Bannister G, Williams B, Smith S. Treatment of subdural empyema. J. Neurosurg 1981;55:82–8.

37. Yogev R. Suppurative intracranial complications of upper respiratory tract infections. Pediatr Infect Dis J 1987;6:324–7.

38. Harris LF, Haws FP, Triplett JN Jr, Maccubbin DA. Subdural empyema and epidural abscess: recent experience in a community hospital. South Med J 1987;80:1254–8.

39. Hoyt DJ, Fisher SR. Otolaryngologic management of patients with subdural empyema. Laryngoscope 1991;101:20–4.

40. McIntyre PB, Lavercombe PS, Kemp RJ, McCormack JG. Subdural and epidural empyema: diagnostic and therapeutic problems. Med J Aust 1991;154:653–7.

41. Nunez DA. Presentation of rhinosinugenic intracranial abscesses. Rhinology 1991;29:99–103.

42. Chandler JR, Langenbrunner DJ, Stevens DR. The pathogenesis of orbital complications in acute sinusitis. Laryngoscope 1970;80:1414–28.

43. Schramm VL, Curtin HD, Kennerdell JS. Evaluation of orbital cellulitis and results of treatment. Laryngoscope 1982;92:732–8.

44. Spires JR, Smith RJ. Bacterial infections of the orbital and periorbital soft-tissues in children. Laryngoscope 1986;96:763–7.

45. Jackson K, Baker SR. Periorbital cellulitis. Head Neck Surg 1987;9:227–34.
46. Weizman Z, Mussaffi H. Ethmoiditis-associated periorbital cellulitis. Int J Pediatr Otorhinolaryngol 1986;11:147–51.
47. Patt BS, Manning SC. Blindness resulting from orbital complications of sinusitis. Otolaryngol Head Neck Surg 1991;104:789–95.
48. Souliere CR Jr, Antoine GA, Martin MP, Blumberg AI, Isaacson G. Selective non-surgical management of subperiosteal abscess of the orbit: computerized tomography and clinical course as indication for surgical drainage. Int J Pediatr Otorhinolaryngol 1990;19:109–19.
49. Williams BJ, Harrison HC. Subperiosteal abscesses of the orbit due to sinusitis in childhood. Aust N Z J Ophthalmol 1991;19:29–36.
50. Goldberg RA, Weisman JS, McFarland JE, Krauss HR, Hepler RS, Shorr N. Orbital inflammation and optic neuropathies associated with chronic sinusitis of intranasal cocaine abuse. Possible role of contiguous inflammation. Arch Ophthalmol 1989;107:831–5.

12

Sinusitis and AIDS

JOHN J. ZURLO
Hershey Medical Center
Hershey, Pennsylvania

FLIOT W. GODOFSKY
Polyclinic Medical Center
Harrisburg, Pennsylvania

I. INTRODUCTION

The acquired immunodeficiency syndrome (AIDS) has now been identified for over 10 years since its initial recognition in 1981 (1,2). Over the course of the epidemic, a variety of previously uncommon opportunistic infections have been seen with ever-increasing frequency. We now recognize *Pneumocystis carinii*, *Toxoplasma gondii*, and *Mycobacterium avium*-complex as common agents that cause disease in patients with AIDS. We have learned to recognize their clinical presentations and, with experience, we have developed and continue to develop more effective therapeutic and prophylactic regimens against these organisms.

Some infectious complications such as those mentioned above are well described in the literature. Other infections, although they appear to occur frequently and cause considerable morbidity, are poorly described. Sinusitis is one such condition. Descriptions of sinusitis in patients infected with human immunodeficiency virus (HIV) date back to 1984, although most are in the form of case reports or small series (3–5). Only recently have two large case studies been published that shed some light on the clinical features of sinusitis in this population (6,7). This chapter is intended as a state-of-the-art review of sinusitis in HIV infection.

II. HIV INFECTION: IMPACT ON THE IMMUNE SYSTEM

A detailed description of the pathogenesis of HIV is beyond the scope of this chapter. The reader is referred to several excellent papers for more comprehensive reviews (8–10). HIV is a retrovirus, one of several known to cause disease in humans. Two distinct subtypes, HIV-1 and HIV-2, are known to occur and both produce a similar immunodeficiency illness. Although HIV-1 is the agent responsible for the vast majority cases of AIDS in the United States, HIV-2 is the prevalent subtype in western Africa (11). Like other retroviruses, HIV possesses the unique ability to convert its own viral, single-stranded RNA to double-stranded DNA for incorporation into the host cell genome. This process is catalyzed by the viral enzyme reverse transcriptase.

The principal target cell for the virus is the CD4 lymphocyte (T-helper cell). This key immunoregulatory cell is crucial to the normal functioning of the immune system. Among its many roles include modulation of antibody production, synthesis of immunoregulatory cytokines, and interaction with antigen-presenting cells to initiate the immune response against a variety of foreign antigens. Other cells have been found to be targets for HIV. Myeloid progenitor cells, gut epithelial cells, glial cells, and cells of the macrophage/monocyte lineage are just a few of the expanding list of cells from which HIV has been recovered (10).

Via two envelope glycoproteins, gp120 and gp41, HIV attaches to the CD4 molecule on CD4 lymphocytes. The virus is then internalized into the cell, at which time reverse transcriptase, part of the viral polymerase protein complex, catalyzes the conversion of viral RNA to DNA. The viral DNA is then transported into the nucleus where it is integrated into the host cell genome. Once incorporated, the virus remains in a latent stage until one of a variety of proposed stimuli, working through host cell-activating factors collectively called NF-κB proteins, triggers viral replication (12). Newly synthesized viral proteins are transported to the cytoplasm and are assembled into virions. The virions bud from the host cell within an envelope acquired from host cell membrane. This budding process results in cell death (9).

As CD4 cells are lysed and killed by replicative infection, the total number of CD4 cells measured in the peripheral blood decreases. As a result, the various immune functions in which CD4 cells play a role become progressively impaired. Yet even latently infected cells do not function normally, further compounding the overall immune defect (10). The end result is a severe, progressive immunodeficiency state in which virtually all arms of the immune system are affected, with cellular immune mechanisms being the hardest hit. Table 1 lists the common opportunistic infections seen in HIV-infected patients, all of which exploit the virally induced, cell-mediated immune defect.

Table 1 Common Opportunistic Infectious Complications in Patients with AIDS

Class	Organism	Syndrome
Protozoa		
	Pneumocystis carinii	Pneumonia
	Toxoplasma gondii	Focal encephalitis
	Cryptosporidium sp.	Diarrhea
Viruses		
	Varicella zoster	Cutaneous shingles
	Herpes simplex types I and II	Mucocutaneous disease
	Cytomegalovirus	Retinitis, colitis, esophagitis
Mycobacteria		
	M. avium-complex	Disseminated infection
	M. tuberculosis	Pulmonary, extrapulmonary
	M. kansasii	Pneumonia
Fungi		
	Candida albicans	Thrush, esophagitis
	Cryptococcus neoformans	Meningitis, fungemia
	Histoplasma capsulatum	Disseminated infection
Bacteria		
	Streptococcus pneumoniae	Pneumonia, bacteremia
	Haemophilus influenzae	Pneumonia, bacteremia

Other arms of the immune system also suffer as a result of HIV. Infection of macrophage/monocyte lineage cells impairs antigen presentation. Also immune surveillance wanes as evidenced by the high incidence of lymphomas seen late in the disease process. Finally, T-helper cell-dependent antibody production is adversely affected, resulting in humoral immune dysfunction (13–15).

III. SINUSITIS IN HIV-INFECTED PATIENTS

A. Epidemiology

The precise epidemiology of sinusitis in this population is sketchy. Incidence data, derived mainly from retrospective studies using various clinical and/or radiographic criteria, have reported rates of 7–16% (6,7,16–19). In two prospective studies, incidence rates of 30% and 68% were reported (19,20). An additional prospective study by Pon and associates reported a prevalence rate of 21% among 180 patients who underwent screening paranasal sinus plain films over 2 year period (21). As in non-HIV-infected patients, sinusitis is likely to have a seasonal predilection. In the same study, Pon and associates reported a 45% prevalence of disease during the winter months (21).

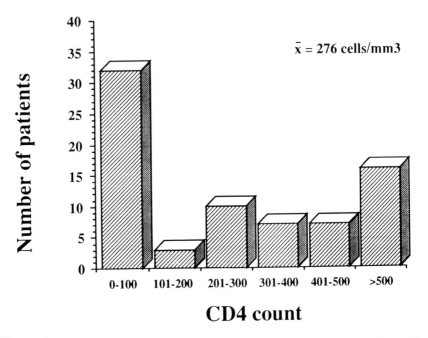

Figure 1 CD4 count distribution among 75 HIV-infected patients with radiographically documented sinusitis (reproduced, with permission, from ref. 7).

B. Pathogenesis

There is compelling evidence to suggest a relationship between sinusitis and the degree of underlying immunodeficiency in this group of patients. There are two aspects to this relationship. First, there is an association between the incidence of sinusitis and CD4 count: the lower the CD4 count the higher the incidence of sinusitis (6,7). Figure 1 illustrates this association, showing the distribution of CD4 counts among 75 HIV-infected patients with sinusitis. Of note, while the mean CD4 count for the group was 276 cells/mm^3, 43% had CD4 counts below 100/mm^3 (7). The mean CD4 count in 3 other series has ranged between 38 and 162 cells/mm^3 (6,17,22). Second, among patients with sinusitis, those with recurrent, extensive, or chronic disease tend to have the lowest CD4 counts (6,7,17). Godofsky and associates, for example, reported that 7 of 8 patients with CD4 counts above 200/mm^3 experienced resolution of disease while 41 of 56 patients with counts below 200/mm^3 had chronic disease (6).

Despite this well-recognized association of sinus disease with declining cell mediated immunity, the precise immunologic defect that predisposes patients to sinopulmonary infections is unclear. Several possible mechanisms may be im-

Table 2 Summary of Three Studies Evaluating IgG Subclasses in HIV-Infected
Patients

Study	No of patients	IgG$_1$	IgG$_2$	IgG$_3$	IgG$_4$
Aucouturier (26)	61	High	Low	High	Low
Parkin (28)[a]	72	High	Low	High	Normal
Kekow (27)	14	High	Low	Normal	Normal

[a]Patients with recurrent pyogenic infections had significantly lower levels of IgG$_2$ than those
without infection.

portant. As a preface to this discussion, there is clearly a subset of HIV-infected
patients who experience recurrent bacterial infections primarily with encapsulated organisms (23–25). Community-acquired pneumonias are particularly
well described (23). In two series, the most commonly isolated pathogens were
Streptococcus pneumoniae and *Haemophilus influenzae*, two pathogens also associated with sinusitis (23,24). A higher propensity to concurrent bacteremia
has also been described in these patients (23,24). This predisposition to bacterial infections may be related to humoral immune dysfunction.

1. Humoral Immune Dysfunction

Quantitative and qualitative defects in antibody production have been well described in HIV-infected patients (13–15). Early in the course of infection, there
is a polyclonal hypergammaglobulinemia consisting primarily of IgA and IgG
and, to a lesser extent IgM. Decreases in antibody concentration have also been
noted, particularly in patients with advanced disease. IgG subclass deficiencies
may be of particular importance. At least three investigators have quantified
IgG subclasses in HIV-infected patients (Table 2) (26–28). All three noted significantly increased levels of IgG$_1$ and generally low levels of IgG$_2$. Parkin and
associates found that patients with recurrent pyogenic infections had significantly lower levels of IgG$_2$ than those without infections (28). It is noteworthy
in this regard that antibodies directed against the polysaccharides of *Streptococcus pneumoniae* and *Haemophilus influenzae* have been shown to belong
mainly to the IgG$_2$ subclass (29–31). Thus quantitative IgG subclass deficiency
may be the underlying cause of sinusitis and other bacterial infections in a subset
of HIV-infected patients.

Qualitative antibody defects may also play a role. B cells in vitro demonstrate
a poor proliferative response to T-cell-dependent and T-cell-independent mitogens (13). An in vivo correlate to this observation is the poor antibody response
noted among HIV-infected patients receiving various polysaccharide and viral
vaccines (32–35). This abnormal response appears to worsen with declining
immunocompetence. It is likely that some patients do not develop specific

antibodies against bacterial and viral pathogens despite normal serum levels of immunoglobulin classes and subclasses.

The most conclusive way to delineate the role of humoral immune dysfunction in recurrent bacterial infections would be to demonstrate whether immunoglobulin infusion reduces the incidence or severity of infection. To date no large-scale trial in HIV-infected adults has been undertaken to answer this question. However in HIV-infected children, in whom recurrent bacterial infections are a major cause of morbidity and mortality, monthly intravenous immunoglobulin infusion clearly reduced the bacterial infection rate and increased the disease-free interval (36). Also, regular intravenous administration of immunoglobulin has been shown to reduce the incidence of bacterial infections in patients with chronic lymphocytic leukemia, a disease characterized by low circulating immunoglobulin levels (37). A well-designed trial of immunoglobulin infusion may be worthwhile in HIV-infected adults who demonstrate a propensity to recurrent bacterial infections.

2. Serum IgE and Atopy

An abnormality in IgE homeostasis may be another mechanism underlying the predisposition to sinusitis in this group. An overall association between IgE and HIV infection has been suggested by Wright and associates (38). They measured serum IgE levels among three groups of individuals: 67 HIV-infected men (primarily homosexual or bisexual), 27 uninfected heterosexual men, and 18 uninfected homosexual men. IgE levels were considerably higher in the infected subjects compared to either of the uninfected groups. Furthermore, the IgE level correlated inversely with the CD4 count, although it did not correlate with serum IgG or IgA levels. No correlation was noted between IgE level and the presence of atopic diseases (38).

Two other investigators have explored serum IgE levels and HIV infection in relation to allergic diseases and atopic manifestations. Sample and associates reported that among 47 consecutive HIV-infected patients evaluated as outpatients over a 4 month period, 87% reported new or worsening allergic symptoms. Upper airway inflammatory or allergic abnormalities were noted in 70% of the group and 30% had radiographic evidence of sinusitis. Fifty percent had elevated serum IgE levels (20). Parkin and associates evaluated six patients with AIDS whose atopic conditions worsened subsequent to infection with HIV. Although serum IgE levels were no different from a nonatopic control group of patients with AIDS, two patients experienced a dramatic improvement in symptoms after treatment with recombinant gamma-interferon, a cytokine that may not be synthesized adequately in HIV-infected patients with advanced infection (39). Small and associates in an as yet unpublished investigation noted two significant correlations. First, a group of HIV-infected patients with sinusitis had a significantly higher mean serum IgE level than a group of infected patients without sinusitis. Second, there was a strong correlation between IgE level and severity of sinus disease (Small, personal communication). It is therefore conceivable that IgE-mediated atopic disease is a principal underlying cause of sinus disease in a subgroup of HIV-infected patients.

3. Defective Mucus Production

Still another underlying factor in the development of sinusitis may be abnormal mucus production. It has been observed that nasal mucus is unusually thick and tenacious in some HIV-infected patients with recurrent sinus disease. Based on this observation, Tami and associates have begun a small placebo-controlled trial to assess the effectiveness of a high-dosage oral mucolytic agent, guaifenesin, to prevent recurrence of sinusitis in this group. Preliminary results suggest that the patients in the guaifenesin-treated group have had a decrease in the quantity and thickness of nasal secretions. Whether these effects will translate into a decreased frequency of sinusitis is yet to be determined (Tami, personal communication).

4. Other Considerations

Which of any of these factors may be important to the pathogenesis of sinusitis and upper airways disease is not at all clear at this time. Additional consideration should be given to abnormal granulocyte function, obstruction induced by nasopharyngeal lymphoid hyperplasia, chronic exposure to tobacco or inhaled cocaine, or even the contribution of periodontal disease, which occurs commonly in late-stage HIV infection (40).

C. Microbiological Considerations

1. Bacteria

Table 3 lists the principal bacterial pathogens that have been isolated from HIV-infected patients with sinusitis. As in community-acquired sinusitis in non-HIV-infected patients, *Streptococcus pneumoniae* and *Haemophilus influenzae* have been the principal isolates (6,17,41). Unlike in immunocompetent hosts, however, *Pseudomonas aeruginosa* has been reported by several investigators (4,6,17,22,42). *Staphylococcus aureus* has also been noted by some investigators and may be quite common (16). Coagulase-negative staphylococci and viridans streptococci have been reported frequently but are probably not pathogenic in most settings. Other gram-negative organisms likely to be important include *Moraxella catarrhalis* and enteric organisms such as *E. coli* and *Klebsiella pneumoniae*. Anaerobic organisms are also likely to be of importance in this population, especially in chronic sinusitis. A patient with sinusitis caused by *Legionella pneumophila* was described in a case report, although this pathogen is likely to be uncommon (43). *Mycobacterium avium*-complex (MAC) has

Table 3   Likely Pathogens in Sinusitis in HIV-Infected Patients

Bacteria (in approximate order of frequency)
  Streptococcus pneumonia
  Haemophilus influenzae
  Pseudomonas aeruginosa
  Staphylococcus aureus
  Anaerobes
  Branhamella catarrhalis
  E. coli
  Klebsiella pneumoniae
  Legionella pneumophila
Nonbacterial pathogens (in alphabetical order)
  Acanthamoeba castellani
  Alternaria alternaria
  Cryptococcus neoformans
  Cytomegalovirus
  Pseudallescheria boydii

also been recovered from a sinus aspirate along with other bacteria including *H. influenzae* in a patient with sinusitis (7). Whether MAC played a role in sinusitis in this case is unclear.

2. Nonbacterial Pathogens

Fungal pathogens isolated from HIV-infected patients with sinusitis have included *Pseudallescheria boydii*, *Alternaria alternaria*, and *Cryptococcus neoformans* (41,44,45). In the patient with *Alternaria alternaria*, the diagnosis was confirmed by biopsy. The patient was successfully treated with amphotericin B (44). The patient with cryptococcal sinusitis also had a confirmatory sinus mucosal biopsy during surgery and was successfully treated with a combination of amphotericin B and 5-flucytosine (45). *Acanthamoeba castellani*, a free-living ameba, has also been reported to cause sinusitis in an HIV-infected patient. The patient was treated with ketoconazole and rifampin but died subsequently from *Salmonella* septicemia (46). Cytomegalovirus (CMV) has been described in two patients with sinusitis, isolated as the sole pathogen (47). In one patient who was debrided and drained, treatment with gancyclovir resulted in symptomatic improvement despite the radiographic persistence of pansinusitis; the other patient, after becoming asymptomatic following surgical drainage, was treated with gancyclovir for 1 month and remained asymptomatic (47). Given the questionable significance of CMV isolated from late-stage HIV-infected patients, even with the appropriate histologic findings, it is unclear whether this virus is a true cause of sinusitis (48,49).

Table 4 Symptoms and Signs of Sinusitis in HIV-Infected Patients

Symptoms
  Fever
  Frontal headache
  Nasal congestion
  Postnasal drip
  Maxillary facial pain
  Periorbital pain/pressure
  Cough
Signs
  Hyperpyrexia
  Maxillary facial tenderness
  Purulent nasal or postnasal discharge
  Facial swelling
  Posterior oropharyngeal lymphoid hypertrophy

D. Clinical Features

1. Symptoms and Signs

In the two largest series that have looked at sinusitis in patients with HIV infection, the symptom complex has been similar to sinusitis observed in the normal population (Table 4). Fever, frontal headaches, and nasal congestion are most frequent, followed by postnasal drip and facial pain, typically over the maxillary area (6,7). Periorbital pain and pressure and pain referred to the upper molars may suggest maxillary sinusitis. Cough is not infrequent. One patient with severe pansinusitis experienced seizures that were refractory to antiepileptic therapy until he underwent surgical drainage (7). Signs of sinus disease include hyperpyrexia, maxillary facial tenderness, and facial swelling. Symptomatic sinusitis may be masked by other comorbid conditions. Fever and headache, for instance, are common presenting symptoms in both *Toxoplasma* encephalitis and cryptococcal meningitis. Therefore, a high level of suspicion is often required to diagnose sinusitis in patients with late-stage HIV infection.

Examination of the posterior oropharynx will often uncover purulent postnasal discharge and lymphoid hypertrophy. Transillumination has been reported by some investigators to be helpful in diagnosing maxillary sinus disease (50). In some cases, fever may be the only symptom and sign of occult sinusitis. Fineman and associates described a group of patients with AIDS with occult fevers, seven of whom were found by radionuclide scintigraphy to have clinically significant sinusitis as the cause of the fever (51).

2. Course of Disease

As discussed above, many patients have been noted to have either recurrent or chronic sinus disease when treated medically. In the majority of cases, sinus involvement tends to be both diffuse and bilateral. Patients with extensive, recurrent, or chronic disease tend to be those with severely depressed CD4 counts (6,7,17). It is noteworthy that there are few reported cases in which sinusitis has led to serious complications in this population, such as cavernous sinus thrombosis or frontal lobe abscess. Whether this paucity of description is indicative of a different disease process than in non-HIV-infected patients or whether this is simply a reporting artifact is yet to be determined.

E. Diagnosis

The diagnosis of sinusitis in this population can be difficult at times due to the high frequency of nonspecific upper airways symptoms, including rhinorrhea and nasal congestion as well as the presence of comorbid conditions. Yet, given the high frequency of sinusitis, especially among patients with advanced disease, it is imperative to retain a high index of suspicion for patients presenting with upper airways complaints, particularly if there is associated fever. In order to diagnose sinusitis properly in these patients modalities that should be considered include radiographic studies, directed otorhinolaryngologic examination, and, for selected patients with maxillary sinus disease, maxillary antral puncture.

1. Sinus Radiographs

The distribution of specific sinus involvement with disease has been addressed by several investigators. In general, diffuse, bilateral disease is a common finding. Between 75 and 85% of patients with sinusitis have unilateral or bilateral maxillary sinus involvement (6,7,22). Ethmoid involvement is next most common, 55–82%, although these percentages may not be accurate due to the difficultly in establishing the presence of ethmoid disease with certainly (6,7). Simultaneous maxillary and ethmoid disease occurs in 36–72% of patients (6,7). Sphenoid disease has been reported by one investigator to be common in this patient group (57%) (6). Because of the relative insensitivity of sinus plain films in imaging the sphenoid sinuses, it is likely that sphenoid disease is underdiagnosed in this patient group. Frontal sinus disease is least frequent, occurring in 7–37% of patients (6,7,22).

Because of both availability and relatively low cost, paranasal sinus plain films that include at least three views, Water's, Caldwell, and lateral, have been considered the traditional first-line radiographic studies to obtain when patients present with a suggestive symptom complex. Although there is a wide spectrum of opinions about their true value in diagnosing sinusitis, sinus plain films are probably useful in detecting air-fluid levels and opacification in some of the anterior sinuses such as the maxillary and frontal chambers. However, they are relatively insensitive in imaging either the ethmoid or sphenoid sinuses. In addition, the measurement of sinus mucosal thickness in all but the maxillary sinuses is often inaccurate compared with either computed tomograms (CT) or magnetic resonance imaging (MRI) studies.

Imaging the sinuses using MRI or CT clearly yields more detailed anatomy than sinus plain films. In a study of sinusitis in a non-HIV-infected population, Davidson and associates reported a lack of concordance between sinus CTs and plain films (52). In their study of 62 patients presenting to a nasal dysfunction clinic with a variety of complaints, sinus plain films and CT scans were obtained on all patients and read independently. The investigators found that plain films tended to overread the maxillary sinuses while underreading the ethmoids. Unfortunately, they included no "gold standard" on which to make an independent judgment as to the presence or absence of clinical sinusitis. They concluded that plain films were unreliable and that CTs should be considered the study of choice for evaluation of the paranasal sinuses (52).

In a study of HIV-infected patients with sinusitis, Godofsky and associates found that the sinus CT or MRI identified a higher median number of abnormal sinuses (n = 6) than did sinus plain films (n = 3). Furthermore, they noted that sphenoid disease was detected significantly more often using CT or MRI. Of their 54 patients who underwent either a CT scan or MRI, focal sinus disease was distinctly unusual, occurring in only 4% of patients (6).

Also in a study of HIV-infected patients with sinusitis, Zurlo and associates retrospectively identified all patients with radiographic evidence of sinus abnormalities from among their entire HIV-infected population. Within that group, 19 of 75 patients (33%) had no sinus symptoms despite having radiographs showing evidence of sinusitis. Although nine patients demonstrated abnormalities in multiple sinuses, 10 patients (13%) were found to have relatively mild mucosal thickening in the maxillary or ethmoid sinuses, suggesting that the MRI may have overread mucosal disease (7). No control population was available for comparison. They concluded that MRI may lack specificity in an asymptomatic population.

CT scans may also overread sinus disease. Calhoun and associates attempted to address this question in a non-HIV-infected population by comparing CT scans in two groups: one group had CTs done to evaluate sinus disease, the other for evaluation of orbital pathologic conditions. They noted that 17% of patients with no sinusitis symptoms had radiographic abnormalities in their sinuses, similar to the 13% rate reported by Zurlo using MRI (53).

In summary, despite a small percentage of apparent false-positive readings by CT or MRI in asymptomatic individuals, either of these studies should be considered superior to plain films for evaluation of the paranasal sinuses,

particularly in patients with recurrent or chronic disease in whom extensive sinus involvement is suspected. Davidson and associates have recommended a
limited CT of the sinuses using consecutive 10 mm axial cuts and 5 mm coronal
cuts. They argue that the radiation exposure and cost of this study are both acceptable given the excellent imaging provided of the sinuses, ostiomeatal complex, and other nasal structures (52).

2. Otorhinolaryngologic Assessment

For patients with an equivocal clinical presentation, an otolaryngologist experienced in the use of nasal endoscopy is an invaluable resource. Careful examination of the posterior pharynx can reveal lymphoid hypertrophy. Nasal
endoscopy is an excellent diagnostic modality since it allows the examiner to
view essential nasal structures directly, particularly the OMC. Finding purulent
material at the posterior choana or emanating from the OMC should be considered unequivocal confirmatory evidence of sinusitis.

3. Maxillary Antral Puncture

Documentation of the presence of purulent material in the sinuses with the
growth of pathogenic micro-organisms in significant quantities from aspirated
sinus fluid remains the "gold standard" for the diagnosis of sinusitis in any
population. As a practical matter, however, the maxillary sinuses are the only
sinuses from which material can easily be obtained in an office setting. In a
classic study, Evans and associates performed antral punctures in 24 healthy
adults presenting with symptomatic maxillary sinusitis (50). Several of their
observations were noteworthy. First, there was a high correlation between
fluid white cell count and quantitative bacteriologic findings: patients with
aspirates containing $> 1,000$ white cells/mm^3 almost always had bacterial
counts $\geq 10^5$/mm^3. S. pneumoniae and H. influenzae were the most common
isolates. There was a poor correlation between antral fluid cultures and cultures obtained from anterior nasal swabs. Second, there was a high correlation
between the presence of an abnormal sinus aspirate and radiographic findings
on sinus plain films. All patients with abnormal aspirates were found to have
air-fluid levels, opacification, or mucosal thickening > 7 mm. They also found
that transillumination of the sinuses was both sensitive and specific for the
diagnosis of acute sinusitis (50). Their conclusions have been corroborated
by other investigators and remain valid (54,55). It is likely, although not
proven, that their observations are applicable to HIV-infected patients with
acute maxillary sinusitis. In addition to the diagnostic utility of antral puncture,
the procedure is also therapeutic and can quickly relieve the pain and tenderness associated with acute maxillary sinus disease and hasten resolution of
infection.

F. Therapy and Management

There have been no controlled trials of medical therapy for the treatment of sinusitis in HIV-infected patients. The general principles to keep in mind are the recurrent and sometimes chronic, refractory nature of sinus disease in this population, suggesting the need for aggressive, relatively long-term therapy to treat individual episodes. This is particularly true in patients with advanced immunodeficiency, extensive sinus involvement, and/or those with a previous history of recurrent sinusitis.

1. Acute Sinusitis

Various combinations of antibacterial agents, decongestants, expectorants, and topical agents have been used by investigators and clinicians to treat acute sinusitis. The initial management decision (whether the patient can be treated as an outpatient with an oral regimen or he or she needs hospitalization for the administration of parenteral antibiotics) is based on the clinical presentation. For most patients, outpatient management is adequate. In the absence of culturable material, the antibiotic choice is empiric. We believe that agents with activity against *S. pneumoniae* and *H. influenzae* such as trimethoprim/sulfamethoxazole (TMP/SMX) or amoxicillin are first line. Given the high prevalence of beta-lactamase-producing strains of *H. influenzae* in some areas and the high incidence of TMP/SMX intolerance in this population, other excellent first-line agents include amoxicillin/clavulanic acid and cefuroxime axetil. Choice of antibiotic should take into account other antibiotics the patient may be receiving for long-term prophylaxis. For instance, for a patient receiving TMP/SMX prophylaxis for *Pneumocystis carinii* pneumonia (PCP), it probably makes little sense to use the same drug in a higher dosage as first line therapy. In such a setting, amoxicillin/clavulanic acid or cefuroxime axetil would be more appropriate.

The antibiotic(s) should be used along with a decongestant. Common practice has been to use a decongestant (pseudoephedrine or phenylpropanolamine) combined with an expectorant (guaifenesin). Topical vasoconstrictors (phenylephrine or oxymetazoline) can be effective when used for limited duration. The role of topical steroids is still undefined but we believe they may be useful due to their powerful anti-inflammatory activity. No significant toxicity has been noted in this population despite worries that long-term nasal steroid use may predispose to invasive fungal disease.

A 3 week course of treatment should be considered the minimum duration of therapy in most circumstances of acute sinusitis. Close follow-up is essential. For patients whose condition fails to respond to initial therapy, maxillary antral culture with lavage should be strongly considered to effect better drainage and allow one make a more rational decision regarding antimicrobial therapy (56,57). In practice however, it is sometimes difficult to convince patients to agree to antral puncture due to the perceived discomfort and inconvenience of the procedure. In such situations, another empiric choice of antibiotic is required. Addition of or change to another agent with activity against *P. aeruginosa* (ciprofloxacin) or anaerobes (clindamycin) is the most logical choice.

2. Recurrent Sinusitis

Even after an apparently good response to medical therapy, clinical recurrences have been reported to be common. Hadderingh and associates reported that 28 of 35 patients (80%) with acute maxillary sinusitis experienced relapse following treatment with amoxicillin and a topical vasoconstrictor (16). Lacassin reported 10 relapses in 8 of 20 patients (40%) over a 2 month period following medical therapy. Many different antibiotics were used to treat the initial episode; the mean duration of antibiotic therapy was 23 days (range, 8–51) (22).

It may be that even longer antibiotic courses are required to treat sinusitis successfully in these patients. It may also be that chronic long-term antimicrobial suppression is needed in patients who have demonstrated a high relapse rate, as has been advocated by some (58) (see section on Prophylaxis, below). A surgical drainage procedure may be needed to prevent recurrences in some patients. Hadderingh and associates performed bilateral rhinoantrostomy (nasal antral windows) in 14 patients who had a third relapse of maxillary sinusitis. No recurrences were reported over follow-up period of 4–24 months (16). More precise indications for surgery to prevent disease relapses have not been systematically determined, however.

3. Chronic Sinusitis

As some series have shown, chronic sinusitis, defined as the persistence of sinus-related symptoms along with radiographic evidence of sinus disease (mucosal thickening, typically), is the rule rather than the exception in HIV-infected patients. Godofsky and associates reported that 58% of their patient cohort with sinusitis developed chronic disease (6). Once again, data on which to develop management guidelines for this major subgroup are unavailable. In this situation, sinus CTs are likely to be helpful in defining the extent and severity of sinus disease. Long-term (4–6 weeks) medical therapy with antibiotics, decongestants, and nasal steroids should be attempted. Surgical drainage is the only remaining option for the patient whose condition fails to improve while receiving long-term medical therapy. As for recurrent sinusitis, the timing of surgery and proper surgical approach in patients with chronic sinusitis have not been well established but should be guided by the clinical course and radiographic findings.

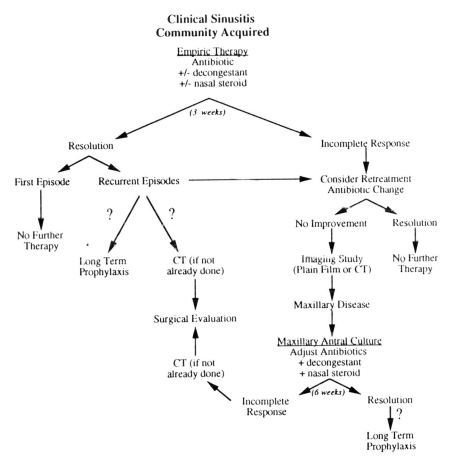

Figure 2 Algorithm for the management of sinusitis in HIV-infected patients (see text for details).

4. Prophylaxis

The use of prophylactic agents to prevent relapses in patients with a predisposition to recurrences is a promising approach that may help reduce the morbidity and, to a lesser extent, mortality of sinusitis in HIV-infected patients. A double-blinded, randomized, multicenter trial aimed at exploring prophylactic regimens is currently underway within the National Institutes of Health-sponsored AIDS Clinical Trials Group (ACTG). HIV-infected patients with low CD4 counts ($\leq 200/\text{mm}^3$) and/or with a well-documented history of recurrent sinusitis are randomized to receive one of four prophylactic regimens once their sinusitis relapse has clinically resolved. Combinations of the following agents are being studied: cefuroxime axetil, beclomethasone dipropionate aqueous nasal spray, and a decongestant/expectorant agent containing pseudoephedrine and guaifenesin. It is hoped that a superior prophylactic regimen will be defined. Other questions are also being explored in this study such as the microbiological basis of sinusitis, the clinical utility of sinus plain films compared with sinus CTs and which prognostic factors are important in predicting recurrent disease. Results of this trial will likely be forthcoming within the next few years.

IV. SUMMARY

It is apparent that there is a great information void when it comes to the subject of sinusitis in HIV-infected patients, despite the generally acknowledged fact that sinus disease is common, often difficult to treat, and has a tendency to relapse. What causative factors are involved and what pathogenic mechanisms are important are virtually unknown beyond the observation that sinusitis is associated with declining immunocompetence. The precise treatment of sinusitis and its prevention in this population have likewise not been well formulated. Therefore, at least for the time being, an empiric, common-sense approach to therapy is required that takes into account the existing literature on sinusitis in HIV-infected and noninfected patients (see algorithm, Fig. 2). Further studies are needed to clarify the relationship between sinusitis and HIV-induced immunodeficiency, to define more systematically the microbiology of disease, to determine whether any prognosticators exist that can predict which patients are and are not likely to relapse, and to establish a more precise management algorithm.

REFERENCES

1. Masur H, Michelis MA, Greene JB, et al: An outbreak of community-acquired *Pneumocystis carinii* pneumonia: initial manifestation of cellular immune dysfunction. N Engl J Med 1981; 305:1431–8.
2. Gottlieb MS, Schroff R, Schanker HM, et al: *Pneumocystis carinii* pneumonia and mucosal candidiasis in previously healthy homosexual men. N Engl J Med 1981; 305:1425–31.
3. Marcusen DC, Sooy CD. Otolaryngologic and head and neck manifestations of acquired immunodeficiency syndrome (AIDS). Laryngoscope 1985; 95:401–5.
4. Poole MD, Postma D, Cohen MS. Pyogenic otorhinologic infections in acquired immune deficiency syndrome. Arch Otolaryngol 1984; 110:130–1.
5. Lim DT, Enright T, Shetty R, Park L. Asthma, recurrent sinopulmonary disease and HIV infection. Ann Allergy 1988; 61:175–6.
6. Godofsky EW, Zinreich J, Armstrong M, Leslie JM, Weikel CS. Sinusitis in HIV-infected patients: a clinical and radiographic review. Am J Med 1992; 93:163–70.
7. Zurlo JJ, Feuerstein IM, Lebovics R, Lane HC. Sinusitis in HIV-1 infection. Am J Med 1992; 93:157–62.

8. Greene WC. The molecular biology of human immunodeficiency virus type 1 infection. N Engl J Med 1991; 324:308–17.

9. Haseltine WA. Molecular biology of the human immunodeficiency virus type 1. FASEB J 1991; 5:2349–60.

10. Rosenberg ZF, Fauci AS. The immunopathogenesis of HIV infection. Adv Immunol 1989; 47:377–431.

11. Barin F, M'Boup S, Denis F, et al. Serological evidence for virus related to simian T-lymphotropic retrovirus III in residents of West Africa. Lancet 1985; 2:1387–9.

12. Rosenberg ZF, Fauci AS. Induction of expression of HIV in latently or chronically infected cells. AIDS Res Hum Retroviruses 1989; 5:1–4.

13. Lane HC, Masur H, Edgar LC, et al: Abnormalities of B-cell activation and immunoregulation in patients with the acquired immunodeficiency syndrome. N Engl J Med 1983, 309:453–8

14. Ammann AJ, Schiffman G, Abrams D, Volberding P, Ziegler J, Conant M. B-cell immunodeficiency in acquired immune deficiency syndrome. JAMA 1984; 251:1447–9.

15. Pahwa SG, Quilop MTJ, Lange M, Pahwa RN, Grieco MH. Defective B-lymphocyte function in homosexual men in relation to the acquired immunodeficiency syndrome. Ann Intern Med 1984; 101:757–63.

16. Hadderingh RJ. Recurrent maxillary sinusitis in AIDS patients [abstract M.B.P.203]. Proceedings of the Vth International Conference on AIDS. Montreal, Canada, 1989:255.

17. Simpson G, Martin M, Cox P, Beck K, Beall G. Bacterial ear and sinopulmonary infections in HIV infected persons [abstract] 2044]. Proceedings of the VIth International Conference on AIDS, San Francisco, California, 1990:365.

18. Spech TJ, Rahm SJ, Longworth DL, Keys TF, McHenry MC. Frequency of sinusitis in AIDS patients [abstract 7088]. Proceedings of the IVth International Conference on AIDS. Stockholm, Sweden, 1988:399.

19. Lamprecht J, Wiedbrauck C. Sinusitis und andere typische Erkrankungen im HNO-bereich im rahmen des erworbenen immundefekt-syndroms (AIDS). HNO 1988; 36:489–92.

20. Sample S, Lenahan GA, Serwonska MH, et al. Allergic diseases and sinusitis in acquired immune deficiency syndrome (AIDS). J Allergy Clin Immunol 1989; 83:190.

21. Pon C, Don C, Conway B, Garber G, Walters D, Cameron DW. Sinusitis in HIV infection and immune disease [abstract M.B.2422]. Proceedings of the VIIth International Conference on AIDS, Florence, Italy, 1991:287.

22. Lacassin F, Leport C, Gehanno P, et al. Bacterial sinusitis in HIV infected patients [abstract F.B.528]. Proceedings of the VIth International Conference on AIDS, San Francisco, California, 1990:210.

23. Polsky B, Gold JWM, Whimbey E, et al. Bacterial pneumonia in patients with the acquired immunodeficiency syndrome. Ann Intern Med 1986; 104:38–41.

24. Witt DJ, Craven DE, McCabe WR. Bacterial infections in adult patients with the acquired immune deficiency syndrome (AIDS) and AIDS-related complex. Am J Med 1987; 82:900–6.

25. Whimbey E, Gold JWM, Polsky B, et al. Bacteremia and fungemia in patients with acquired immunodeficiency syndrome. Ann Intern Med 1986; 104:511–4.
26. Aucouturier P, Couderc LJ, Gouet D, et al. Serum immunoglobulin G subclass dysbalances in the lymphadenopathy syndrome and acquired immune deficiency syndrome. Clin Exp Immunol 1986; 63:234–40.
27. Kekow J, Hobusch G, Gross WL. Predominance of the IgG_1 subclass in the hypergammaglobulinemia observed in pre-AIDS and AIDS. Cancer Treat Prev 1988; 12:211–6.
28. Parkin JM, Helbert M, Hughes CL, Pinching AJ. Immunoglobulin G subclass deficiency and susceptibility to pyogenic infections in patients with AIDS-related complex and AIDS. AIDS 1989; 3:37–9.
29. Siber GR, Schur PH, Aisenberg AC, Weitzman SA, Schiffman G. Correlation between serum IgG-2 concentrations and the antibody response to bacterial polysaccharide antigens. N Engl J Med 1980; 303:178–82.
30. Freijd A, Hammarstrom L, Persson MAA, et al. Plasma anti-pneumococcal antibody activity of the IgG class and subclasses in otitis prone children. Clin Exp Immunol 1984; 56:233–8.
31. Matter L, Wilhelm JA, Angehrn W, Skvaril F, Schopfer K. Selective antibody deficiency and recurrent pneumococcal bacteremia in a patient with Sjogren's syndrome, hypergammaglobulinemia G, and deficiencies of IgG_2 and IgG_4. N Engl J Med 1985; 312:1039–42.
32. Janoff EN, Douglas JM, Gabriel M, et al. Class-specific antibody response to pneumococcal capsular polysaccharides in men infected with human immunodeficiency virus type 1. J Infect Dis 1988; 158:983–90.
33. Klein RS, Selwyn PA, Maude D, Pollard C, Freeman K, Schiffman G. Response to pneumococcal vaccine among asymptomatic heterosexual partners of persons with AIDS and intravenous drug users infected with human immunodeficiency virus. J Infect Dis 1989; 160:826–31.
34. Simberkoff MS, El Sadr WE, Schiffman G, Rahal JJ. *Streptococcus pneumoniae* infections and bacteremia in patients with acquired immunodeficiency syndrome with report of a pneumococcal vaccine failure. Am Rev Respir Dis 1984; 130:1174–6.
35. Nelson KE, Clements ML, Miotti P, Cohn S, Polk BF. The influence of human immunodeficiency virus (HIV) infection on antibody responses to influenza vaccines. Ann Intern Med 1988; 109:383–8.
36. The National Institute of Child Health and Human Development Intravenous Immunoglobulin Study Group. Intravenous immune globulin for the prevention of bacterial infections in children with symptomatic human immunodeficiency virus infection. N Engl J Med 1991; 325:73–80.
37. Cooperative Group for the Study of Immunoglobulin in Chronic Lymphocytic Leukemia. Intravenous immunoglobulin for the prevention of infection in chronic lymphocytic leukemia. N Engl J Med 1988; 319:902–7.
38. Wright DN, Nelson RP, Ledford DK, Fernandez-Caldas E, Trudeau WL, Lockey RF. Serum IgE and human immunodeficiency virus (HIV) infection. J Allergy Clin Immunol 1990; 85:445–52.

39. Parkin JM, Eales L-J, Galazka, AR, Pinching AJ. Atopic manifestations in the acquired immune deficiency syndrome: response to recombinant interferon gamma. Br Med J 1987; 294:1185–6.

40. Greenspan JS, Greenspan D, Winkler JR. Diagnosis and management of the oral manifestations of HIV infection and AIDS. Infect Dis Clin North Am 1988; 2:373–85.

41. Sooy CD. The impact of AIDS in otolaryngology–head and neck surgery. Adv Otolaryngol Head Neck Surg 1987; 1:1–27.

42. Mendelson MH, Szabo S, Gurtman AC, et al. *Pseudomonas aeruginosa* bacteremia in AIDS patients [abstract M.B.2411]. Proceedings of the VIIth International Conference on AIDS, Florence, Italy, 1991:284.

43. Schlanger G, Lutwick LI, Kurzman M, Hoch B, Chandler FW. Sinusitis caused by *Legionella pneumophila* in a patient with the acquired immune deficiency syndrome. Am J Med 1984; 77:957–60.

44. Wiest PM, Wiese K, Jacobs MR, et al. *Alternaria* infection in a patient with acquired immunodeficiency syndrome: case report and review of invasive *Alternaria* infections. Rev Infect Dis 1987; 9:799–803.

45. Choi SS, Lawson W, Buttone EJ, et al. Cryptococcal sinusitis: A case report and review of literature. Otolaryngol Head Neck Surg 1988; 99:414–418.

46. Gonzalez MM, Gould E, Dickinson G, et al. Acquired immunodeficiency syndrome associated with *Acanthamoeba* infection and other opportunistic organisms. Arch Pathol Lab Med 1986; 110:749–51.

47. Brillhart T, Gathe J, Piot D, et al. Symptomatic cytomegalovirus rhinosinusitis in patients with AIDS [abstract M.B.2182]. Proceedings of the VIIth International Conference on AIDS, Florence, Italy 1991:227.

48. Zurlo JJ, O'Neill D, Polis M, et al. Relationship between CMV culture positivity and circulating CD4 counts in patients with HIV infection [abstract Th.B431]. Proceedings of the VIth International Conference on AIDS, San Francisco, California, 1990:229.

49. Millar AB, Patou G, Miller RF, et al. Cytomegalovirus in the lungs of patients with AIDS: Respiratory pathogen or passenger. Am Rev Respir Dis 1990; 141:1474–7.

50. Evans FO, Sydnor JB, Moore WEC, et al. Sinusitis of the maxillary antrum. N Engl J Med 1975; 293:735–9.

51. Fineman DS, Palestro CJ, Kim CK, et al. Detection of abnormalities in febrile AIDS patients with In-111-labeled leukocyte and Ga-67 scintigraphy. Radiology 1989; 170:677–80.

52. Davidson TM, Brahme FJ, Gallagher ME. Radiographic evaluation for nasal dysfunction: Computed tomography versus plain films. Head Neck 1989; 11:405–9.

53. Calhoun KH, Waggenspack GA, Simpson CB, Hokanson JA, Bailey BJ. CT evaluation of the paranasal sinuses in symptomatic and asymptomatic populations. Otolaryngol Head Neck Surg 1991; 104:480–3.

54. Berg O, Bergstedt H, Carenfelt C, Lind MG, Perols O. Discrimination of purulent from nonpurulent maxillary sinusitis: Clinical and radiographic diagnosis. Ann Otol Rhinol Laryngol 1981; 90:272–5.

55. Hamory BH, Sande MA, Sydnor A, Seale DL, Gwaltney JM. Etiology and antimicrobial therapy of acute maxillary sinusitis. J Infect Dis 1979; 139:197–202.
56. Meiteles LZ, Lucente FE. Sinus and nasal manifestations of the acquired immunodeficiency syndrome. Ear Nose Throat J 1990; 69:454–9.
57. Rubin JS, Honigberg R. Sinusitis in patients with the acquired immunodeficiency syndrome. Ear Nose Throat J 1990; 69:460–3.
58. Schrager LK. Bacterial infections in AIDS patients. AIDS 1988; 2(Suppl.1): S183–9.

13

Chronic Fungal Sinusitis in the Nonimmunocompromised Host

RONALD G. WASHBURN
Wake Forest University Medical Center
Winston-Salem, North Carolina

I. HISTORY AND DEFINITION

Chronic fungal sinusitis in apparently normal hosts is being recognized and reported with increasing frequency worldwide (1–12). The first case of possible fungal sinusitis was reported by Plaignaud in 1791 (13). In 1885, a specific diagnosis of noninvasive aspergillosis of the paranasal sinus was established (14). The first carefully documented case of invasive fungal sinusitis was reported by Oppe in 1897 (15); in that patient, *Aspergillus* infection extended through the walls of the sphenoid sinus into the cerebrum. Invasive fungal sinusitis was again reported in 1927 by Wright, who documented two cases with extension into the orbit (16).

Currently, three different types of fungal sinusitis are recognized: chronic noninvasive disease (2,4,10,11,17–29), invasive disease that may have either an acute (24,30–43) or chronic presentation (3,5,11,12,24,36,39,44–72) depending on host factors, and the most recently described form, allergic fungal sinusitis (6,7,9,73–85).

Chronic noninvasive fungal sinusitis is defined as the presence of a mycelial mass in the sinus cavity for months or years without tissue invasion. A local inflammatory response may be seen, but the integrity of anatomical architecture is preserved. In contrast, invasive fungal sinusitis does not respect anatomical barriers and the fungi penetrate across mucosa, submucosa, and bone, as well as neighboring structures such as the orbit and brain. The acute fulminant form of the disease, which is found in patients with poorly controlled diabetes and patients with prolonged neutropenia, has been described elsewhere and will not be discussed further here. The central attention of this chapter will be on the chronic forms of fungal sinusitis.

The most recently described form of chronic fungal sinusitis is allergic fungal sinusitis. Patients with this form of sinusitis usually have a long-standing history of atopy, peripheral blood eosinophilia, and elevated serum concentrations of total IgE. The hallmark of allergic fungal sinusitis is the presence of "allergic mucin," which contains eosinophils, Charcot-Leyden crystals, and fungal hyphae. Rearrangement of bony walls may be seen in these patients, but hyphae do not actually invade tissue, judged by histopathologic examination. The suggestion has been made that the fungi might serve as allergens that are crucial in the disease process, based on the fact that patients with allergic fungal sinusitis often exhibit positive immediate-type hypersensitivity skin testing responses to antigens from their fungal isolates and that specific antifungal IgE or IgG can be found in patients' sera.

II. CAUSES

Many different species of fungi can cause chronic fungal sinusitis (Table 1). It is important to note that hyphal organisms, as opposed to yeast, are responsible for the vast majority of cases. Most of the species listed in Table 1 are ubiquitous in the environment and therefore their recovery from superficial swab specimens of the nares or sinus mucosa ordinarily should be considered to represent saprophytic colonization unless the clinical presentation, histopathologic evidence, and anatomical studies in a given case indicate that the fungus is likely to be playing a causative role.

In Table 1, the hyphal organisms are subdivided according to their appearance in tissue. Listed first are the fungi with broad nonseptate hyphae. These include the agents of mucormycosis, such as the *Rhizopus* species. The organisms most commonly responsible for chronic fungal sinusitis in nonimmunocompromised hosts possess narrower septate hyphae. The genus accounting for the majority of cases, *Aspergillus*, is not pigmented in tissue. Several different fungal species such as *Pseudallescheria boydii* are indistinguishable morphologically from *Aspergillus* in tissue, and therefore cultures are required for definitive identification. This is an important distinction because the choice of antifungal chemotherapy is guided in part by the fungal species isolated (see section on Chronic Invasive Fungal Sinusitis, Therapy and Prognosis).

In contrast to the nonpigmented fungi, the dematiaceous fungi (e.g., *Bipolaris* spp.) produce brownish pigment on synthetic media and often *in vivo* as well. Thus, the finding of brownish hyphae in sinus biopsy material can

Table 1   Agents of Chronic Fungal Sinusitis: Appearance in Tissue

Current name	Other names	References
Broad nonseptate hyphae		
Rhizopus oryzae	*Rhizopus arrhizus*	30,33,37,40,86–88
Rhizomucor pusillus	*Mucor pusillus*	
Rhizopus microsporus	*Rhizopus rhizopodiformis*	
var. *rhizopodiformis*		
Cunninghamella bertholletiae		89
Conidiobolus coronatus	*Entomophthora coronata*	90
Basidiobolus haptosporus	*Basidiobolus ranarum*	91
Absidia corymbifera		92
Narrower septate hyphae		
Nonpigmented fungi		
Aspergillus spp.		2,4,5,6,9–11,19,20, 22,24,27,43,48,50, 53,55,56,59,65,69, 70,72,73,77,81–83, 93–99
Pseudallescheria boydii	*Allescheria boydii*	11,39,55,64,68, 100–102
	Petriellidium boydii	
Scedosporium apiospermum	*Monosporium apiospermum*	17
Penicillum spp.		103
Fusarium spp.		104
Paecilomyces spp.		23,29,105,106
Schizophyllum commune		18,107,108
Dematiaceous fungi		
Bipolaris spp.	*Drechslera*	1,7,11,12,28,44,54, 57,60,61,63,67,71, 75,76,81,109
	Helminthosporium	
Drechslera biseptata		11
Exserohilum rostratum	*Drechslera rostrata*	1,11,12,45,75,81, 96,109
Curvularia spp.		11,12,21,46,57,58,62, 73,74,80,81,84,110
Alternaria spp.		1,3,12,39,51,52, 66,74,81,110,111
Cladosporium spp.		4,47,75
Rounded Forms		
Candida sp.		112
Sporothrix schenckii		39
Rhinosporidium seeberi		8

Source: From ref. 11.

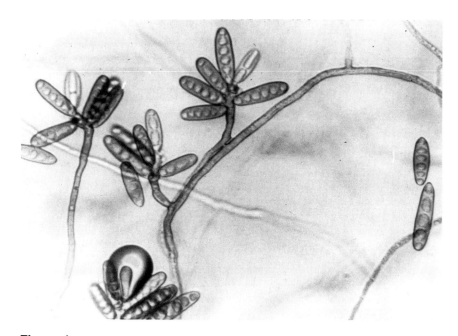

Figure 1 *Bipolaris hawaiiensis* conidia, with four to five septa (400X).

sometimes provide an early clue that the responsible agent may be a dematiaceous mold. Final identification is based chiefly on morphologic analysis of conidia from *in vitro* growth of the organism (Fig. 1). These ubiquitous pigmented fungi are of special interest because they account for an increasing number of published reports of chronic fungal sinusitis (1,7,11,12,45,46,49,52,57,58,60–62,80).

In the cases of allergic fungal sinusitis originally reported by Katzenstein et al., *Aspergillus* was thought to be the responsible organism (78,79,85), and several subsequent papers have also implicated *Aspergillus* (6,9,73,77,81–83), but a number of additional species have been reported recently, including the dematiaceous molds *Alternaria alternata* (74,81), *Bipolaris hawaiiensis* (7), *B. spicifera* (76,81), *Curvularia lunata* (73,74,80,81,84), *C. senegalensis* (84), and *Exserohilum rostratum* (75,81). Patients with allergic fungal sinusitis may rarely also have concomitant allergic bronchopulmonary disease caused by the same fungus (9,82–84).

III. NONINVASIVE FUNGAL SINUSITIS

A. Clinical Features

Noninvasive fungal sinusitis is a relatively benign entity. The symptoms that lead to surgery are chronic nasal congestion, postnasal drip, and pain localizing to a single sinus, usually a maxillary sinus (1,4,10,11,17–19,21,22,24,26,28, 107,113). The clinical course may be punctuated by exacerbations of pain and fever during episodes of superimposed acute bacterial sinusitis. The mechanism by which the mycelial mass predisposes to the intermittent episodes of bacterial sinusitis is probably obstruction of the sinus ostium.

B. Immunologic Studies

In a study of 25 patients with noninvasive *Aspergillus* masses, Loidolt et al. found that lymphocyte proliferative responses to the mitogens concanavalin A and phytohemagglutinin were depressed, compared to responses in patients with nonfungal sinusitis (97). Patients with noninvasive hyphal masses also exhibited an enhanced frequency of CD 25-positive cells (interleukin 2-receptor-bearing cells). However, the authors recognized that the study was limited by the fact that the immunologic findings could have represented effects of the fungal sinusitis rather than factors that actually predisposed to the disease.

C. Radiographic Findings

Computed tomography (CT scanning) is the single most helpful radiologic technique for differentiating between noninvasive and invasive fungal sinusitis. Noninvasive mycelial masses usually appear as an increased soft tissue density confined to one sinus. The maxillary sinus is the most commonly involved, but solitary noninvasive fungal masses of the sphenoid sinus (25,29,99) or frontal sinus (27) have also been reported. Very dense opacities can be observed due to calcium phosphate deposition in *Aspergillus* masses (4,10).

When soft tissue densities are found in more than one sinus, the presence of invasive disease is strongly suggested, because normal structures constitute natural barriers to spread of noninvasive fungal disease between sinuses.

D. Surgical Findings and Pathologic Appearance

In the sinus cavity, the surgeon encounters a thick friable, cheeselike, gritty, rubbery, or greasy mass that can easily be separated from mucosa. The mass may be one of several different colors including black, dark reddish-brown, brownish-yellow, or brownish-green and it may have a foul odor (3,11,18,21–23,26,29). The mucosa itself may appear either completely normal or hypertrophic or polypoid, and mucosal biopsy often shows submucosal edema and lymphocytic infiltration. However, underlying bony structures are intact, and hyphae are never found in mucosa, submucosa, or bone. The hyphal mass itself usually appears as a mass of entangled mycelia on routine hematoxylin and eosin stain, but the fungal structures can be more easily visualized with properly prepared silver stains. Sporulation may be seen at the periphery of the mycelial mass, a feature that can provide an early clue to the causative species before culture results become available (2,10,11,19,64,95).

E. Differential Diagnosis

On gross inspection, masses of fungi embedded in mucin may be confused with mucin impactions (114), mucoceles, inclusion cysts, or Pindborg tumors. Silver stains or periodic acid–Schiff stains readily demonstrate the fungi, leading to the correct diagnosis.

F. Therapy and Prognosis

Restoration of adequate sinus drainage by complete removal of the mycelial mass is generally curative, and recurrence is unusual. Thus, it is not necessary to use antifungal chemotherapy in the treatment of noninvasive fungal sinusitis (1,2,4,10,11,18–22,24,26,27,29,67,113).

IV. CHRONIC INVASIVE FUNGAL SINUSITIS

A. Clinical Features

Patients with chronic invasive fungal sinusitis typically have a long-standing history of upper respiratory allergies, nasal polyposis, and chronic sinusitis punctuated by repeated sinus surgeries (11,12,45,49,57,58,60,61,64,68); peripheral blood eosinophilia may be seen (11,46). Rearrangement of normal sinus architecture impairs drainage and can lead to superimposed bacterial sinusitis (11). Chronic fungal sinusitis usually progresses relentlessly over months or years, eroding through anatomical barriers that separate the paranasal sinuses from each other (11,55,63,66,71) and from contiguous structures such as the orbit (11,24,36,47,48,53,55–58,60,64,68,70,72), brain (5,11,36,39,45,53,54,65, 69,98,109), or pituitary gland (36,50,94). Therefore, the clinical manifestations of chronic invasive fungal sinusitis can be understood on the basis of its insidious violation of the normal anatomy of the paranasal sinuses and neighboring structures. Lesions reported to arise from extension through walls of sinuses into contiguous structures are listed in Table 2. For example, a common presentation of chronic invasive disease is unilateral proptosis based on erosion of disease superiorly through the roof of the maxillary sinus (5,11,36,56,65,69,72). By the same token, disease may penetrate inferiorly through the floor of the maxillary sinus into the hard palate (51,52,66), laterally into the nasal turbinates and ethmoid sinuses, or posteriorly through the pterygopalatine fossa (11).

Invasion of ethmoid sinus disease laterally through the lamina papyracea (Fig. 2a) may produce proptosis or hypertelorism (11,24,98). In a similar vein, superior invasion through the roof of the ethmoid sinus has caused frontal lobe abscess (98) or cerebritis (Fig. 2b; 11), lesions that may present with chronic headaches, lateralizing neurologic findings, seizures, altered sensorium, or urinary incontinence. Ethmoidal sinusitis may also extend directly along mucosal

Table 2 Structures that May be Involved by Contiguous Extension of Fungal Sinusitis

Paranasal sinus	Adjacent structure
Maxillary	Maxillary bone, skin of cheek
	Orbit, orbital floor, infraorbital vessels and nerve
	Lateral wall of nose, including turbinates
	Ethmoid sinus
	Hard palate
	Pterygopalatine space
Ethmoid	Cribriform plate, olfactory bulb
	Orbital plate of frontal bone, frontal lobe of brain
	Frontal sinus
	Sphenoid sinus
	Lamina papyracea, orbit, and skin near inner canthus
	Maxillary sinus
Sphenoid	Frontal lobe of brain
	Dorsum sella, pituitary gland
	Clivus, brainstem
	Optic nerve, cranial nerves III, IV, V, and VI
	Sphenopalatine canal, artery, nerve, and ganglion
	Internal carotid artery, cavernous sinus
	Ethmoid sinus
Frontal	Frontal lobe of brain
	Ethmoid sinus
	Orbit
	Skin of forehead

Source: From ref. 11.

surfaces into either the sphenoid sinus posteriorly or into the hiatus semilunaris, middle meatus, and nares inferiorly.

Chronic invasive fungal infection of the sphenoid sinus has produced particularly serious consequences, including lateral extension into the cavernous sinus (36,50,70) or compression of the optic nerve (11,48). Thus, visual impairment may overshadow sinus discomfort early in the course of disease. Peripheral extension along the optic nerve can likewise produce orbital apex syndrome, superior orbital fissure syndrome, or orbital abscess. Finally, infection may erode superiorly into the sella turcica or frontal lobe of the brain, or posteriorly through the clivus and brainstem.

Frontal lobe abscess and fungal meningitis have resulted from extension of fungal infection across the posterior wall of the frontal sinus (36,44,47). Chronic fungal meningitis caused by hyphal organisms such as *Aspergillus* is

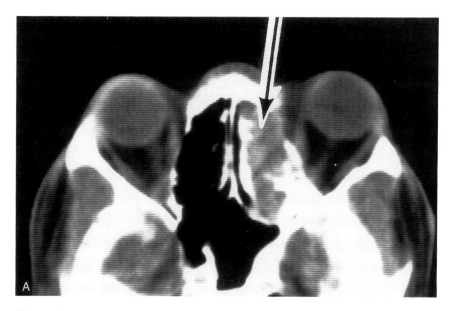

Figure 2   A. Sagittal view of CT scan shows soft tissue mass in ethmoid sinus and nasal cavity in patient with chronic invasive disease caused by *Exserohilum rostratum*. B. The MRI outlines bilateral frontal lobe cerebritis in the same patient (from ref. 11).

difficult to control despite prolonged courses of antifungal chemotherapy with intravenous amphotericin B.

B. Immunologic Studies

A number of different tests of immunologic function have been performed to assess for abnormalities associated with chronic invasive fungal sinusitis, but the studies to date have failed to identify any consistent defects. The list of normal studies includes absolute neutrophil counts and monocyte counts, the percentage of mononuclear cells with positive staining for nonspecific esterase and myeloperoxidase, the phagocytic and fungicidal activity of peripheral blood monocytes against conidia, and such additional phagocyte functions as superoxide generation, chemiluminescence, nitroblue tetrazolium reduction, and chemotaxis (11,46,49).

Berry et al. found a transient decrease in numbers of circulating T-lymphocytes associated with invasive fungal sinusitis (46); but in general, lymphocyte subpopulations, total lymphocyte counts, and natural killer cell activity have been shown to be normal (1,11,49,52,63). Delayed-type hypersensitivity skin testing revealed anergy in at least one case (11), but most patients tested

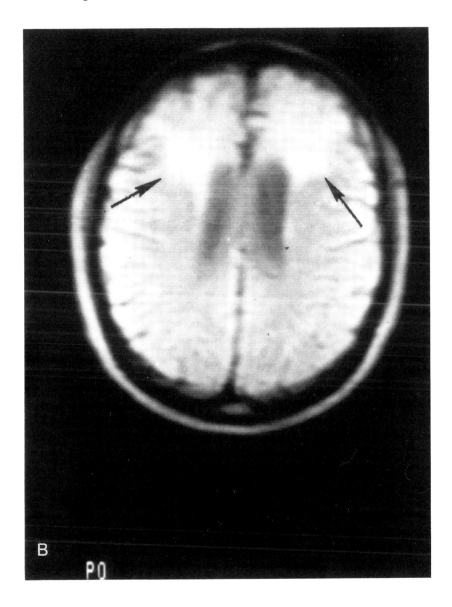

have exhibited normal reactivity to control antigens (1,11,46,49,51,54,60, 63,66). In a single case, specific immunologic tolerance to the causative organism was reported (52), but further studies are needed to ascertain whether the defect can be found in additional patients.

Serum concentrations of immunoglobulin classes G, A, and M were normal (11,49,54,63,66) as were complement studies (46,49,54,63,66), but total serum concentration of IgE may be elevated (49). Tests for human immunodeficiency virus (HIV) yielded negative results in several patients (11,45,60,68), but one patient with chronic sinusitis caused by *Schizophyllum commune* had acquired immunodeficiency syndrome (AIDS) (108).

Since these studies have not been uniformly applied in all cases, no firm conclusion can be reached concerning the immunologic integrity of patients with chronic invasive fungal sinusitis. However, in general, the collective published studies seem to suggest that most patients with chronic invasive fungal sinusitis probably possess intact immunologic function.

C. Radiographic Findings

Among the available radiologic techniques, CT scanning is the most useful for differentiating between noninvasive and invasive fungal sinusitis (1,4,11,50,54, 63,98,109). Extension of abnormal soft tissue density into contiguous structures such as orbit, brain, or sella turcica indicates the presence of invasive disease. CT examination often shows foci of increased attenuation in soft tissue masses of patients with chronic invasive fungal sinusitis (12,57,64,115). Magnetic resonance imaging (MRI) T1- and T2-weighted images can be very useful for resolving soft tissue structures. An especially valuable clinical feature of MRI is that it can provide crucial information to determine if intracranial masses are intradural or extradural (Fig. 3). However, the inability of MRI to reveal bony details has prevented that modality from replacing CT scanning for diagnostic imaging of fungal sinusitis. T2-weighted images of patients with chronic fungal sinusitis showed hypointense signal characteristics; in patients with bacterial sinusitis, high T2 signal intensity occurred (12,57,115). Evidence from furnace atomic absorption spectrometry suggested that the low T2 signal in patients with chronic fungal sinusitis may be due to high concentrations of iron, manganese, and calcium in the fungal lesions (115).

D. Surgical Findings

Invasion may be strongly suspected on the basis of bony erosion detected by CT scanning and crossing of bony barriers by soft tissue densities seen with either CT or MRI. However, the gold standard for documenting tissue invasion continues to be the surgeon's description of soft tissue and bone, combined with thorough histopathologic examination of excised tissue. The surgeon usually sees hypertrophic or polypoid mucosa (1,3,11,28,51,54,57,58,63,71,109,113), and in some cases the sinus cavity may appear to contain a mucocele (11,45,99). As with noninvasive mycelial masses, one may find tenacious rubbery or putty-

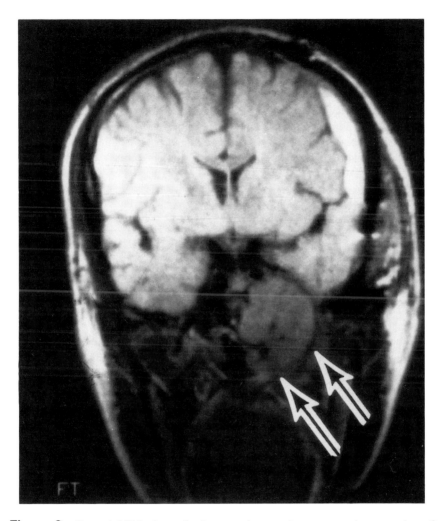

Figure 3 Coronal MRI view of subtemporal mass due to posterior extension of chronic invasive *Aspergillus* sinusitis (from ref. 11).

like material or greasy mucus in the sinus cavity (11,12,24,45,58,67,70,99). The material is usually brown or green and may be so thick and inspissated as to require curettage. It often has a foul odor, which may help to explain the cacosmia described by many patients (11). The surgeon may also find loss of bony integrity of the sinus wall, with softening detected by probing or friable bone noted during curettage.

E. Pathologic Findings

Careful examination of excised tissue shows invasion of mucosa, submucosa, bone, or contiguous structures by hyphal fragments (Fig. 4; 1,3,11,12,39, 51,53,54,59,60,65,66,69,71,72,99,109), The organisms may be present in large numbers in excised mucus, but the key diagnostic feature is to find the organisms actually invading tissue. The number of invasive organisms may be extremely low, requiring prolonged searching through numerous tissue sections stained with methenamine silver or periodic acid–Schiff before the hyphae can be located. The inflammatory response is usually granulomatous with Langhans' giant cells (5,11,24,36,51–53,56,60,65,66,69,94), but other responses that may be seen with some frequency include eosinophils (1,5,11,12,36,65,69, 71,109) mixed with collagenous scar tissue, and palisading histiocytes (5,94), plasmacytes (11,65,71,94,99,109), and mast cells (49).

F. Differential Diagnosis

As noted above, pathologic examination of excised tissue is usually diagnostic, and fungal cultures yield specific identifications of causative fungi. However, it is important to caution that cultures without histopathologic examination are not very helpful because almost all the pathogens listed in Table 1 can also be found as airborne contaminants. Heavy growth of fungus from a sinus aspirate would be suggestive, but should prompt the surgeon to obtain diagnostic material including mucosa and, if clinically indicated, bone for special stains.

The problem of most consequence in the differential diagnosis is failure to consider the possibility of fungal sinusitis in a patient with chronic destructive lesions of the paranasal sinus, orbit, or brain. For example, failure to obtain silver stains in a case with prominent granulomatous inflammation could potentially lead to a mistaken diagnosis of Wegener's granulomatosis; chronic lymphocytic inflammation may raise the possibility of lymphoma or malignant plasmacytoma (11). Use of silver stains would prevent this confusion. Additional diseases that cause bony erosion in the paranasal sinuses are squamous cell carcinomas, inverting papillomas, meningiomas, schwannomas, and malignant melanomas.

G. Therapy and Prognosis

The eventual outcome of patients with invasive fungal sinusitis is less certain than that of patients with noninvasive hyphal masses. Some reports have suggested that cure might be achieved with surgical debridement alone (5,65,67), or perhaps followed by a short course of antifungal therapy (45,48,50,55,71). However, follow-up in several of those reports was too brief to allow a confident assessment of the likelihood of relapse.

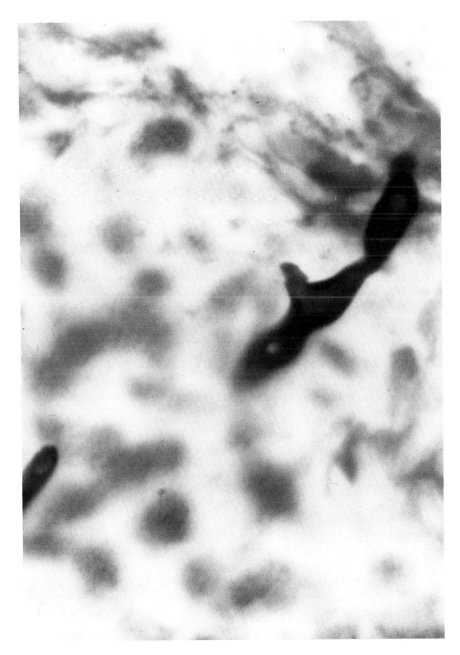

Figure 4 Irregular septate hyphae of *Bipolaris hawaiiensis* in sinus tissue (silver stain, 1000X).

The surgery should include thorough excision of diseased soft tissue, but of course it is important at the same time to preserve essential anatomical barriers such as dura and orbital periosteum. Several reported cases with careful long-term follow-up have relapsed even after surgical debridement and prolonged courses of antifungal chemotherapy (11,24,36,51,53,56,66,72,111). These cases provide compelling evidence that a prolonged course of amphotericin B exceeding 2 g for adults should be administered after surgery (11,12,24,60,64, 70,72). Treatment with an imidazole agent would be preferable for patients with sinusitis caused by *Pseudallescheria boydii* (55,64,68).

The high risk of relapse has prompted many clinicians to follow the initial intensive period of antifungal chemotherapy with a prolonged course of oral therapy with an agent such as ketoconazole or itraconazole (11,49,57,60). The long-term stability of several reported patients treated in this manner supports this approach (11).

Patients with far advanced disease, (e.g., some patients with intracranial extension) may not be curable, but palliation is certainly a realistic goal in such cases (11,60). In those more fortunate patients whose diseased tissue can be completely or almost completely surgically extirpated, and who receive a prolonged course of antifungal chemotherapy, CT scan should be obtained approximately 1 month after surgery. The study should then be repeated every 3 or 4 months to look for early evidence of recurrence such as new abnormal soft tissue densities or loss of normal bony architecture. That recommendation is based on the impression that early intervention against a small mass of recurrent disease is more effective than later treatment of more extensive disease.

V. ALLERGIC FUNGAL SINUSITIS

A. Clinical Features and Immunologic Studies

Patients with allergic fungal sinusitis usually have a history of atopy with long-standing allergic rhinitis, nasal congestion, nasal polyposis, headaches, and sometimes visual disturbances (7,73–76,78,81,85). The chronic sinusitis often leads to repeated sinus surgery over a period of months or years, and patients may have peripheral blood eosinophilia. These historical features are not specific because of considerable overlap with the clinical presentation of chronic invasive fungal sinusitis (11,12). Therefore, in a given allergic patient with fungi in the nares or paranasal sinuses, several additional criteria should be met before the diagnosis of allergic fungal sinusitis is seriously considered. The first of these is the presence of "allergic mucin," which contains eosinophils, Charcot-Leyden crystals, and hyphae (78). Patients usually have elevated serum concentrations of total IgE, and may exhibit immediate-type hypersensitivity skin testing responses to antigens from their fungal isolates, as well as circulating specific antifungal IgE and IgG antibodies (7,73,74,76,78,83–85). The suggestion has therefore been made that the disease may be mediated by both type I hypersensitivity (IgE-mediated) and type III antibody–antigen reactions to specific fungal antigens (74). In contrast, immunologic tests proven to be normal in patients with allergic fungal sinusitis include delayed-type hypersensitivity skin testing, total numbers of circulating T-lymphocytes and B-lymphocytes, T-lymphocyte subsets, serum concentrations of IgG (and IgG subclasses), IgA, and IgM, absolute neutrophil counts, and total hemolytic complement (7,74,76).

Due to the expansile nature of the disease, bony remodeling is commonly observed (73–75,78,80,81,85) and may produce clinical presentations similar to those seen in patients with chronic invasive fungal sinusitis, including proptosis, hypertelorism, and periorbital swelling. However, despite these sometimes destructive clinical presentations, it is important to emphasize that actual tissue invasion by hyphae is never a feature of allergic fungal sinusitis.

B. Radiographic Findings

Soft tissue masses usually occupy more than one sinus (80) and most reports describe pansinusitis (73,76,78,81,85). As noted above, rearrangement of bony barriers has been described in several case reports, but histopathologic examination does not reveal tissue invasion, so the bony changes are thought to reflect pressure remodeling, as may be seen with expansile mucoceles.

C. Surgical and Pathologic Findings

The surgeon finds abundant inspissated mucus that is red-gray to green-brown (75) and may be either gelatinous or peanut-butter-like in consistency (76,80). Excised mucosa is pinkish-tan (75). In addition to eosinophils, Charcot-Leyden crystals, and hyphae, the "allergic mucin" may contain neutrophils, plasma cells, histiocytes, and lymphocytes (6,75). Prominent eosinophilic infiltration is usually also found in the edematous submucosa, along with mast cells and lymphocytes (7,73,80). However, it is important to caution that a high proportion of patients with chronic invasive fungal sinusitis also exhibit eosinophilic infiltration of the submucosa, and Zieske et al. even found "allergic mucin" in several patients with documented invasive disease (12). Thus, it is imperative to exclude invasive disease in patients with "allergic mucin" or with submucosal eosinophilia through painstaking examination of silver-stained mucosa, submucosa, and, if clinically indicated, bone. The distinction between the two different diagnoses is critical because the recommended treatments are different. Therapy for allergic fungal sinusitis is directed primarily at relieving the allergic response, whereas successful therapy for invasive disease mandates intensive antifungal chemotherapy.

D. Differential Diagnosis

As noted in the section on clinical features, specific immune responses to the fungal isolates can often be demonstrated, but there still remains considerable controversy over the issue of whether the allergic sinusitis is driven by fungal products or nonfungal antigens. It is certainly possible that the presence of fungi in some of these patients could represent saprophytic colonization of inspissated mucus in situations in which the allergic response is triggered by nonfungal antigens.

E. Therapy and Prognosis

The first step is to restore normal sinus drainage by thoroughly extirpating abnormal soft tissue masses. Another goal of the surgery is to reduce the burden of fungal antigens. The suggestion has been made that some patients will be cured with surgery alone (74–77), but most authors recommend that therapy should also include an attempt to ameliorate the allergic response with steroid therapy (7,73,74,78,81,85). Dissenters advocate postoperative antifungal chemotherapy (80).

It is important to caution that steroid therapy can be confidently recommended only when vital structures such as the orbit and brain are not threatened, and when careful histopathologic examination excludes the presence of tissue invasion. Long-term topical nasal corticosteroids are a commonly employed treatment, but relapses during therapy have prompted some authors to recommend a tapering course of systemic steroids early in the postoperative period. One regimen that has met with therapeutic success is prednisone 0.5 mg/kg for 2 weeks, followed by tapering dosages on an every other day schedule for 3 months (73). However, a controlled study of steroid therapy remains to be performed. Patients should be evaluated closely during steroid therapy because there is a theoretical concern that even topical steroids could increase the likelihood of fungal invasion. The role of immunotherapy has not been defined (9,74,75).

VI. SUMMARY

A number of different fungal species can cause noninvasive sinusitis, chronic invasive sinusitis, or allergic fungal sinusitis. The diagnosis of invasive disease is based on the presence of hyphae in mucosa, submucosa, bone, and deeper adjacent structures. Computerized tomography and magnetic resonance imaging can help to differentiate among the three forms of chronic fungal sinusitis by outlining soft tissue masses, bone, and contiguous structures.

The three forms of fungal sinusitis require different therapeutic approaches. Patients with noninvasive hyphal masses require only surgical removal of fungi and restoration of normal sinus drainage for a successful result. In contrast, patients with chronic invasive fungal sinusitis not only require thorough surgical extirpation of infected tissues but most also need a prolonged course of antifungal chemotherapy. The high risk of relapse renders prolonged suppressive oral antifungal therapy an attractive option for many patients with this infection. Patients with allergic fungal sinusitis seem to have the best results when surgery is followed by treatment with topical corticosteroids and/or a tapering course of systemic steroids.

REFERENCES

1. Adam RD, Paquin MI, Petersen FA, Saubolle MA, Rinaldi MG, Corcoran JG, Galgiani JN, Sobonya RE. Phaeohyphomycosis caused by the fungal genera *Bipolaris* and *Exserohilum*. Medicine 1986; 65:203–17.
2. Axelsson H, Carlsii B, Weibring J, Winblad B. Aspergillosis of the maxillary sinus. Acta Otolaryngol 1978; 86:303–8.
3. Bassiouny A, Maher A, Bucci TJ, Moawad MK, Hendawy DS. Noninvasive antromycosis. J Laryngol Otol 1982; 96:215–28.
4. Kopp W, Fotter R, Steiner H, Beaufort F, Stammberger H. Aspergillosis of the paranasal sinuses. Radiology 1985; 156:715–6.
5. Milosev B, Mahgoub ES, Aal OA, El Hassan AM. Primary aspergilloma of paranasal sinuses in the Sudan. Br J Surg 1969; 56:132–7.
6. Philip G, Keen CE. Allergic fungal sinusitis. Histopathology 1989; 14:222–4.
7. Robson JMB, Hogan PG, Benn RAV, Gatenby PA. Allergic fungal sinusitis presenting as a paranasal sinus tumor. Aust NZ J Med 1989; 19:351–3.
8. Satyanarayana C. Rhinosporidiosis. Acta Otolaryngol 1960; 51:348–66.
9. Shah A, Khan ZU, Chaturvedi S, Malik GB, Randhawa HS. Concomitant allergic *Aspergillus* sinusitis and allergic bronchopulmonary aspergillosis associated with familial occurrence of allergic bronchopulmonary aspergillosis. Ann Allergy 1990; 64:507–12.
10. Stammberger H, Jakse R, Beaufort F. Aspergillosis of the paranasal sinuses. Ann Otol Rhinol Laryngol 1984; 93:251–6.
11. Washburn RG, Kennedy DW, Begley MG, Henderson DK, Bennett JE. Chronic fungal sinusitis in apparently normal hosts. Medicine 1988; 67:231–47.
12. Zieske LA, Kopke RD, Hamill R. Dematiaceous fungal sinusitis. Otolaryngol Head Neck Surg 1991; 105:567–77.
13. Plaignaud M. Observation sur un fongus du sinus maxillaire. J Chir (Paris) 1791; 1:111–6.
14. Schubert P. Zur Casuistik der Aspergillusmykosen. Dtsch Arch Klin Med 1885; 36:162–79.
15. Oppe W. Zur Kentniss der Schimmelmykosen bei den Menschen. Zbl Allg Path 1897; 8:301–6.
16. Wright RE. Two cases of granuloma invading orbit due to aspergillosis. Br J Ophthalmol 1927; 11:545–59.

17. Bloom SM, Warner RR, Weitzman I. Maxillary sinusitis: isolation of *Scedo-sporium* (*Monosporium*) *apiospermum*, anamorph of *Petriellidium* (*Allescheria*) boydi. Mt Sinai J Med 1982; 49:492–4.

18. Catalano P, Lawson W, Bottone E, Lebenger J. Basidiomycetous (mushroom) in-fection of the maxillary sinus. Otolaryngol Head Neck Surg 1990; 102:183–5.

19. Levine PA, Yanagisawa E. Aspergillosis of the maxillary sinus. Arch Otolaryngol 1977; 103:560–3.

20. McGinnis MR, Buck DL, Katz B. Paranasal aspergilloma caused by an albino vari-ant of *Aspergillus fumigatus*. South Med J 1977; 70:886–8.

21. Nishioka G, Schwartz JG, Rinaldi MG, Aufdemorte TB, Mackie E. Fungal max-illary sinusitis caused by *Curvularia lunata*. Arch Otolaryngol Head Neck Surg 1987; 113:665–6.

22. Peña CE. Aspergillus intranasal fungus ball. Am J Clin Pathol 1975; 64:343–4.

23. Rockhill RC, Klein MD. *Paecilomyces lilacinus* as the cause of chronic maxillary sinusitis. J Clin Microbiol 1980; 11:737–9.

24. Rommet JL, Newman RK. Aspergillosis of the nose and paranasal sinuses. Laryn-goscope 1982; 92:764–6.

25. Simmons BP, Johnson G, Abar RC. Fungus ball of the sphenoidal sinus in an im-munocompetent host. South Med J 1982; 75:762–4.

26. Stammberger H. Endoscopic surgery for mycotic and chronic recurring sinusitis. Ann Otol Rhinol Laryngol 1985; 94 (Suppl. 119):1–11.

27. Stevens MH. Aspergillosis of the frontal sinuses. Arch Otolaryngol 1978; 104:153–6.

28. Stutman HR, Clark KF, Sexton DJ, Guruswamy A, Marks MI. Human infections caused by *Drechslera* (*Bipolaris*) (abstract). 86th Annual Meeting of the American Society of Microbiology, Washington, DC, March 1986.

29. Thompson RF, Bode RB, Rhodes JC, Gluckman JL. *Paecilomyces variotii*. An un-usual cause of isolated sphenoid sinusitis. Arch Otolaryngol Head Neck Surg 1988; 114:567–9.

30. Baker RD. Mucormycosis (opportunistic phycomycosis). In: Baker RD, ed. The Pathologic Anatomy of Mycoses, Human Infection with Fungi, Actinomycetes, and Algae, New York: Springer-Verlag, 1971; 832–918.

31. Bodey GP. Fungal infections complicating acute leukemia. J Chron Dis 1966; 19:667–87.

32. Colman MF. Invasive *Aspergillus* of the head and neck. Laryngoscope 1986; 95:898–9.

33. Gass JDM. Ocular manifestations of acute mucormycosis. Arch Ophthalmol 1961; 65:226–37.

34. Kavanagh KT, Parham DM, Hughes WT, Chanin LR. Fungal sinusitis in immuno-compromised children with neoplasms. Ann Otol Rhinol Laryngol 1991; 100:331–6.

35. McGill TJ, Simpson G, Healy GB. Fulminant aspergillosis of the nose and para-nasal sinuses: a new clinical entity. Laryngoscope 1980; 90:748–54.

36. McGill TJI. Mycotic infection of the temporal bone. Arch Otolaryngol 1978; 104:140–4.

37. Sugar AM. Agents of mucormycosis and related species. In: Mandell GL, Douglas RG Jr, Bennett JE, eds. Principles and Practice of Infectious Diseases. New York: Churchill Livingstone, 1990; 1962–72.

38. Meyer RD, Young LS, Armstrong D, Yu B. Aspergillosis complicating neoplastic disease. Am J Med 1973; 54:6–15.
39. Morgan MA, Wilson WR, Neel B, Roberts GD. Fungal sinusitis in healthy and immunocompromised individuals. Am J Clin Pathol 1984; 82;597–601.
40. Parfrey NA. Improved diagnosis and prognosis of mucormycosis. Medicine 1986; 65:113–23.
41. Swerdlow B, Deresinski S. Development of aspergillus sinusitis in a patient receiving amphotericin B. Am J Med 1984; 76:162–6.
42. Talbot GH, Huang A, Provencher M. Invasive Aspergillus rhinosinusitis in patients with acute leukemia. Rev Infect Dis 1991; 13:219–32.
43. Young RC, Bennett JE, Vogel CL, Carbone PP, DeVita VT. Aspergillosis: The spectrum of the disease in 98 patients. Medicine 1970; 49:147–73.
44. Ahuja GK, Jain N, Vijayaraghovan M, Roy S. Cerebral mycotic aneurysm of fungal origin. J Neurosurg 1978; 49:107–10.
45. Aviv JE, Lawson W, Bottone EJ, Sachdov VP, Som PM, Biller HF. Multiple intracranial mucoceles associated with phaeohyphomycosis of the paranasal sinuses. Arch Otolaryngol Head Neck Surg 1990; 116:1210–3.
46. Berry AJ, Kerkering TM, Giordano AM, Chiancone J. Phaeohyphomycotic sinusitis. Pediatr Infect Dis 1984; 3:150–2.
47. Brown JW, Nadell J, Sanders CV, Sardenga L. Brain abscess caused by *Cladosporium trichoides (Bantianum)*: a case with paranasal sinus involvement. South Med J 1976; 69:1519–21.
48. Crivelli G, Riviera LC. Unilateral blindness from aspergilloma at the right optic foramen. J Neurosurg 1970; 33:207–11.
49. Frenkel L, Kuhls TL, Nitta K, Clancy M, Howard DH, Ward P, Cherry JD. Recurrent *Bipolaris* sinusitis following surgical and antifungal therapy. Pediatr Infect Dis J 1987; 6:1130–2.
50. Fuchs HA, Evans RM, Gregg CR. Invasive aspergillosis of the sphenoid sinus manifested as a pituitary tumor. South Med J 1985; 78:1365–7.
51. Garau J, Diamond RD, Lagrotteria LB, Kabins SA. *Alternaria* osteomyelitis. Ann Intern Med 1977; 86:747–8.
52. Goodpasture HC, Carlson T, Ellis B, Randall G. *Alternaria* osteomyelitis. Arch Pathol Lab Med 1983; 107:528–30.
53. Green WR, Font RL, Zimmerman LE. Aspergillosis of the orbit. Arch Ophthalmol 1969; 82:302–13.
54. Harpster WH, Gonzalez C, Opal SM. Pansinusitis caused by the fungus *Drechslera*. Otolaryngol Head Neck Surg 1985; 93:683–5.
55. Holt GR, Standefer JA, Brown WE, Gates GA. Infectious diseases of the sphenoid sinus. Laryngoscope 1984; 94:330–5.
56. Hora JF. Primary aspergillosis of the paranasal sinuses and associated areas. Laryngoscope 1965; 75:768–73.
57. Jay WM, Bradsher RW, LeMay B, Snyderman N, Angtuaco EJ. Ocular involvement in mycotic sinusitis caused by *Bipolaris*. Am J Ophthalmol 1988; 105:366–70.
58. Killingsworth SM, Wetmore SJ. *Curvularia/Drechslera* sinusitis. Laryngoscope 1990; 100:932–7.
59. Lew D, Southwick FS, Montgomery WW, Weber AL, Baker AS. Sphenoid sinusitis. A review of 30 cases. N Engl J Med 1983; 309:1149–54.

60. Maskin SL, Fetchick RJ, Leone CR Jr, Sharkey PK, Rinaldi MG. *Bipolaris hawaiiensis*-caused phaeohyphomycotic orbitopathy. Ophthalmology 1989; 96:175–9.

61. Pingree TF, Holt R, Otto RA, Rinaldi MG. *Bipolaris*-caused fungal sinusitis. Otolaryngol Head Neck Surg 1992; 106:302–5.

62. Rinaldi MG, Phillips P, Schwartz JG, Winn RE, Holt GR, Shagets FW, Elrod J, Nishioka G, Aufdemorte TB. Human *Curvularia* infections: report of five cases and review of the literature. Diagn Microbiol Infect Dis 1987; 6:27–39.

63. Rolston KVI, Hopfer RL, Larson DL. Infections caused by *Drechslera* species. Case report and review of the literature. Rev Infect Dis 1985; 7:525–9.

64. Salitan ML, Lawson W, Som PM, Bottone EJ, Biller HF. Pseudallescheria sinusitis with intracranial extension in a nonimmunocompromised host. Otolaryngol Head Neck Surgery 1990; 102:745–50.

65. Sandison AT, Gentles JC, Davidson CM, Branko M. Aspergilloma of paranasal sinuses and orbit in northern Sudanese. Sabouraudia 1969; 6:57–69.

66. Shugar MA, Montgomery WW, Hyslop NE. *Alternaria* sinusitis. Ann Otol Rhinol Laryngol 1981; 90:251–4.

67. Sobol SM, Love RG, Stutman HR, Pysher TJ. Phaeohyphomycosis of the maxillo-ethmoid sinus caused by *Drechslera spicifera*: a new fungal pathogen. Laryngoscope 1984; 94:620–7.

68. Stamm MA, Frable MA. Invasive sinusitis due to *Pseudallescheria boydii* in an immunocompetent host. South Med J 1992; 85:439–41.

69. Veress B, Malik OA, El Tayeb AA, El Daoud S, El Mahgoub S, El Hassan AM. Further observations on the primary paranasal aspergillus granuloma in the Sudan. Am J Trop Med Hyg 1973; 22:765–72.

70. Weinstein M, Theron J, Newton TH. Aspergillosis involving the sphenoid sinus. Neuroradiology 1976; 11:137–9.

71. Young CN, Swart JG, Ackermann D, Davidge-Pitts K. Nasal obstruction and bone erosion caused by *Drechslera hawaiiensis*. J Laryngol Otol 1978; 92:137–43.

72. Zinneman HH. Sino-orbital aspergillosis. Minn Med 1972; 55:661–4.

73. Allphin AL, Strauss M, Abdul-Karim FW. Allergic fungal sinusitis: problems in diagnosis and treatment. Laryngoscope 1991; 101:815–20.

74. Bartynski JM, McCaffrey TV, Frigas E. Allergic fungal sinusitis secondary to dematiaceous fungi—*Curvularia lunata* and *Altrenaria*. Otolaryngol Head Neck Surg 1990; 103:32–9.

75. Friedman GC, Hartwick RWJ, Ro JY, Saleh GY, Tarrand JJ, Ayola AG. Allergic fungal sinusitis. Report of three cases associated with dematiaceous fungi. Am J Clin Pathol 1991; 96:368–72.

76. Gourley DS, Whisman BA, Jorgensen NL, Martin ME, Reid MJ. Allergic *Bipolaris* sinusitis: clinical and immunopathologic characteristics. J Allergy Clin Immunol 1990; 85:583–91.

77. Jonathan D, Lund V, Milroy C. Allergic aspergillus sinusitis—an overlooked diagnosis? J Laryngol Otol 1989; 103:1181–3.

78. Katzenstein A-L A, Sale SR, Greenberger PA. Allergic Aspergillus sinusitis: a newly-recognized form of sinusitis. J Allerg Clin Immunol 1983; 72:89–93.

79. Katzenstein A-L A, Sale SR, Greenberger PA. Pathologic findings in allergic aspergillus sinusitis. Am J Surg Pathol 1983; 7:439–43.
80. MacMillan RH III, Cooper PH, Body BA, Mills AS. Allergic fungal sinusitis due to *Curvularia lunata*. Hum Pathol 1987; 18:960–4.
81. Manning SC, Schaefer SD, Close LG, Vuitch F. Culture-positive allergic fungal sinusitis. Arch Otolaryngol Head Neck Surg 1991; 117:174–8.
82. Safirstein B. Allergic bronchopulmonary aspergillosis with obstruction of the upper respiratory tract. Chest 1976; 70:788.
83. Sher TH, Schwartz HJ. Allergic *Aspergillus* sinusitis with concurrent allergic bronchopulmonary *Aspergillus*: report of a case. J Allergy Clin Immunol 1988; 81:844–6.
84. Travis WD, Kwon-Chung KJ, Kleiner DE, Geber A, Lawson W, Pass HI, Henderson D. Unusual aspects of allergic bronchopulmonary fungal disease: report of two cases due to *Curvularia* organisms associated with allergic fungal sinusitis. Hum Pathol 1991; 22:1240–8.
85. Waxman JE, Spector JG, Sale SR, Katzenstein A-LA. Allergic aspergillus sinusitis: Concepts in diagnosis and treatment. Laryngoscopy 1987; 97:261–6.
86. Ferstenfeld JE, Cohen SH, Rose HD, Rytel MW. Chronic rhinocerebral phycomycosis in association with diabetes. Postgrad Med J 1977; 53:337–42.
87. Finn DC, Farmer JC Jr. Chronic mucormycosis. Laryngoscope 1982; 92:761–6.
88. Helderman JH, Cooper HS, Mann J. Chronic phycomycosis in a controlled diabetic. Ann Intern Med 1974; 80:419.
89. Brennan RO, Crain BJ, Proctor AM, Durack DT. *Cunninghamella*: a newly recognized cause of rhinocerebral mucormycosis. Am J Clin Pathol 1983; 80:98–102.
90. Clark BM, Edington GM. Subcutaneous phycomycosis and rhinoentomophthoromycosis. In: Baker RD, ed. Human Infection with Fungi, Actinomycetes, and Algae. New York: Springer-Verlag 1971; 684–90.
91. Dworzack DL, Pollock AS, Hodges GR, Barnes WG, Ajello L, Padhye A. Zygomycosis of the maxillary sinus and palate caused by *Basidiobolus haptosporus*. Arch Intern Med 1978; 138:1274–6.
92. Ryan RM, Warren RE. Rhinocerebral mucormycosis due to *Absidia corymbifera*. Infection 1987; 15:120–1.
93. Feely M, Steinberg M. Aspergillus infection complicating trans-sphenoidal yttrium-90 pituitary implant. J Neurosurg 1977; 46:530–2.
94. Goldhammer Y, Smith JL, Yates BM. Mycotic intrasellar abscess. Trans Am Ophthalmol Soc 1974; 72:65–78.
95. Gonty AA, Page LR. Aspergillosis of the maxillary sinus. Oral Surg Med Pathol 1977; 43:350–6.
96. Hartwick RW, Batsakis JG. Sinus aspergillosis and allergic fungal sinusitis. Ann Otol Rhinol Laryngol 1991; 100:427–30.
97. Loidolt D, Mangge H, Wilders-Truschnig M, Beaufort F, Schauenstein K. In vivo and in vitro suppression of lymphocyte function in Aspergillus sinusitis. Arch Otorhinolaryngol 1989; 246:321–3.
98. Lowe J, Bradley J. Cerebral and orbital *Aspergillus* infection due to invasive aspergillosis of ethmoid sinus. J Clin Pathol 1986; 39:774–8.

99. Miglets AW, Saunders WH, Ayers L. Aspergillosis of the sphenoid sinus. Arch Otolaryngol 1978; 104:47–50.

100. Bryan CS, DiSalvo AF, Kaufman L, Kaplan W, Brill AH, Abbott DC. *Petriellidium boydii* infection of the sphenoid sinus. Am J Clin Pathol 1980; 74:846–51.

101. Schiess RJ, Coscia MF, McClellan GA. *Petriellidium boydii* pachymeningitis treated with miconazole and ketoconazole. Neurosurgery 1984; 14:220–4.

102. Winn RE, Ramsey PD, McDonald JC, Dunlop KJ. Maxillary sinusitis from *Pseudallescheria boydii*: Efficacy of surgical therapy. Arch Otolaryngol 1983: 109:123–5.

103. Morriss FH, Spock A. Intracranial aneurysm secondary to mycotic orbital and sinus infection. Am J Dis Child 1970; 119:357–62.

104. Valenstein P, Schell WA. Primary intranasal *Fusarium* infection. Arch Pathol Lab Med 1986; 110:751–4.

105. Otcenasek M, Jirousek Z, Nozicka Z, Mencl K. Paecilomycosis of the maxillary sinus. Mykosen 1984; 27:242–51.

106. Rowley SD, Strom CG. Paecilomyces fungus infection of the maxillary sinus. Laryngoscope 1982; 92:332–4.

107. Kern ME, Uecker FA. Maxillary sinus infection caused by the homobasidiomycetous fungus *Schizophyllum commune*. J Clin Micro 1986; 23:1001–5.

108. Rosenthal J, Katz R, DuBois DB, Morrissey A, Machicao A. Chronic maxillary sinusitis associated with the mushroom *Schizophyllum commune* in a patient with AIDS. Clin Infect Dis 1992; 14:46–8.

109. Padhye AA, Ajello L, Wieden MA, Steinbronn KK. Phaeohyphomycosis of the nasal sinuses caused by a new species of *Exserohilum*. J Clin Microbiol 1986; 24:245–9.

110. Loveless MO, Winn RE, Campbell M, Jones SR. Mixed invasive infection with *Alternaria* species and *Curvularia* species. Am J Clin Pathol 1981; 76:491–3.

111. Murtagh J, Smith JW, Mackowiak PA. Case report: *Alternaria* osteomyelitis: eight years of recurring disease requiring cyclic courses of amphotericin B for cure. Am J Med Sci 1987; 293:399–402.

112. Iwamoto H, Katsura M, Fujimaki T. Mycosis of the maxillary sinuses. Laryngoscope 1972; 82:903–9.

113. Chapnik JS, Bach MC. Bacterial and fungal infections of the maxillary sinus. Otolaryngol Clin North Am 1976; 9:43–54.

114. Wenig BL, Sciubba JJ, Zielinski BZ, Stegnjajic A, Abramson AL. Mucin impaction tumor of the paranasal sinuses: a new clinical entity? Laryngoscopy 1983; 93:621–6.

115. Zinreich SJ, Kennedy DW, Malat J, Curtin HD, Epstein JI, Huff LC, Kuman AJ, Johns ME, Rosenbaum AE. Fungal sinusitis: diagnosis with CT and MR imaging. Radiology 1988; 169:439–44.

14

Tetrad of Nasal Polyps, Aspirin Sensitivity, Asthma, and Rhinosinusitis

GUY A. SETTIPANE
*Brown University School of Medicine
and Rhode Island Hospital
Providence, Rhode Island*

RUSSELL A. SETTIPANE
*Rhode Island Hospital
Providence, Rhode Island*

Widal in 1922 (1,2) first described the triad of nasal polyps, asthma, and aspirin intolerance. Another entity should be added to this triad: chronic rhinosinusitis. Very frequently nasal polyps are associated with chronic rhinosinusitis for at least three reasons. First, polyps may disrupt or entirely block the ostiomeatal complex leading to chronic sinusitis on a mechanical basis. Second, the eosinophilia associated with most polyps is toxic to the ciliated membranes, producing a decrease in mucus flow and this stasis could result in sinusitis (3). This mechanism is thought to be through the toxic effect of the major basic protein associated with eosinophilia. Third, polyps can occur within the paranasal sinus causing a mechanical and toxic obstruction (eosinophilia) from within the sinus. Also, pressure on the intrasinus membranes and bone can actually cause destruction of bone, Woakes' disease, or midfacial expansion. Facial deformation occurring with juvenile nasal polyposis is well described (frog face). The tetrad of nasal polyps, asthma, aspirin intolerance, and rhinosinusitis is a more realistic grouping of this pattern of classic symptoms.

227

Nasal polyps also are associated with other systemic diseases: cystic fibrosis, Kartagener's syndrome (chronic dyskinetic cilia syndrome), Young's syndrome (sinopulmonary disease, azoospermia), Churg-Strauss syndrome (allergic vasculitis), and allergic fungal sinusitis. In some cases, nasal polyps may be visualized only with the use of the rhinoscope. In many situations, the nasal polyp may present as a minor symptom but in reality may represent the "tip of the iceberg" with the major associated syndromes often being severe manifestations of systemic disorders. In this chapter, nasal polyps will be evaluated on the basis of their history, epidemiology, anatomy, histopathologic appearance, differential diagnosis, in association with systemic diseases, chemical mediators, pathogenesis, relationship to atopy, relationship to aspirin intolerance, and treatment.

I. HISTORY

Nasal polyps were known as far back as 1000 B.C. Vancil (5) has presented an excellent historical survey of treatment for nasal polyps. In about 400 B.C. Hippocrates developed two surgical methods for nasal polypectomy: extraction by pulling a sponge through the nasal canal and cauterization. Cato the Censor (234–149 B.C.) developed the first known medical management of nasal polyps using the local application of herbs. Other authors who have written about nasal polyps through the centuries include Celsus (42 B.C.–37 A.D.), Paulus of Aegina (625–690 A.D.), Avicenna (980–1037 A.D.), Saliceto (1210–1270 A.D.), Fallopius (1523–1562 A.D.), Petros Forestus (1522–1597 A.D.), Fabricius ab Acquapendente (1537–1619 A.D.), Aranzi (1530–1589 A.D.), and Juncker, who in 1721 wrote: "According as the moon fills or wanes, the polypi of the nose increase or decrease in size. . . ." an excellent clinical observation of remissions and exacerbations of polyps but certainly a faulty lunar correlation. Thus, it appears that nasal polyps have been a medical problem as far back as we can remember.

II. EPIDEMIOLOGY

Nasal polyps are most commonly found in nonatopic asthmatic patients over 40 years of age, especially in those patients with severe, steroid-dependent asthma. The overall frequency of nasal polyps in asthmatic patients between the ages of 10 and 50 years is 7% (Table 1). In a subgroup of asthmatic patients over 40 years old with negative skin tests, the frequency ranges from 10 to 15% (Table 2) (6). In patients with aspirin intolerance, the frequency of nasal polyps may be as high as 36% (7,8). Slavin's group (9) reported on 33 patients with severe asthma and sinusitis. Fifteen of these patients were receiving corticosteroids: 10 who received continuous corticosteroids and 5 who required intermittent bursts. Of these 33 patients, 30 (90%) had a diagnosis of nasal polyps and 17 (52%) had

Table 1 Frequency of Nasal Polyps in Various Conditions

Diagnosis	Frequency (%)
Aspirin intolerance	36
Adult asthma	7
Intrinsic asthma	13
Atopic asthma	5
Chronic rhinosinusitis	2
Nonallergic rhinitis	5
Allergic rhinitis	1.5
Childhood asthma/rhinitis	0.1
Cystic fibrosis	20
Churg-Strauss syndrome	50
Allergic fungal sinusitis (49)	85
Kartagener's syndrome	?
Young's syndrome	?

Source: Reprinted with permission from ref. 42.

aspirin intolerance. These data demonstrate that the nasal polyps as well as aspirin intolerance found in asthmatic patients usually indicate the presence of a
severe asthmatic state. In children, the frequency of nasal polyposis is extremely
low, about 0.1% (6,10). Any child 16 years or younger with nasal polyps should
be evaluated for cystic fibrosis.

Table 2 Frequency of Nasal Polyps in Various Age Groups of Asthmatic Patients

Age when first seen (yrs)	No. with asthma		No. with nasal polyps		%		p
10–19	491		9		1.8		
20–29	465	1,374	18	43	3.9	3.1	
30–39	418		16		3.8		<0.01[a]
40–49	410		41		10.0		
50 and over	444	854	65	106	14.6	12.4	
Total	2,228		149		6.7		

[a]The difference between the 10–39-year-old group (43/1,374) (3.1%) compared to the 40-year-old
and over group (106/854) (12.4%) is statistically significant.
Source: Reprinted with permission from ref. 42.

III. ANATOMY

Nasal polyps are frequently bilateral and multiple and have a characteristic appearance. They are glistening, semitranslucent, pale gray, smooth, soft, freely movable, attached by a pedicle, and arise from the surfaces of the middle turbinates, the hiatus semilunaris, or ostia of the ethmoid and maxillary sinuses. Most commonly they are found in the middle meatus, extending to the nasal cavity, filling the nose, and finally protruding from the anterior nares. If the polyp projects posteriorly into the nasopharynx, it is called a choanal polyp and may not be seen by routine examination through the anterior nares. Choanal polyps may be single, usually occur during the first two decades of life, and are classified in three groups: antrochoanal polyps arising from the antrum; polyps arising from other sinuses; or polyps that are the posterior part of multiple ethmoidal polyps (11). Polyps are one of the most common types of mass found in the nasal passage.

IV. HISTOPATHOLOGIC CHARACTERISTICS

Nasal polyps have pseudostratified columnar epithelium and cellular constituents of normal nasal mucosa (Fig. 1). Polyps from patients who do not have cystic fibrosis have extensive thickening of the epithelial basement membranes with extension into the submucosa as an irregular hyaline membrane, high stromal eosinophil count, and mainly neutral mucin in mucous glands, cysts, and mucous blanket (12). Glands are few and denervated. Polyp tissue is essentially free of nerve endings, except for nerve terminals in the base of the polyps associated with blood vessels. In most cases, the cells consist of a mixture of lymphocytes, plasma cells, and eosinophils (Fig. 2). Occasionally, neutrophils are numerous. Nasal smears from these patients usually reveal "sheets" of eosinophils. In contrast, polyps from patients with cystic fibrosis have a delicate, barely visible basement membrane of surface epithelium without submucosal hyalinization, lack of extensive infiltration of eosinophils, and a preponderance of acid mucin in glands, cysts, and surface mucous blanket. Polyps from patients with Kartagener's and Young's syndromes usually lack an eosinophilic component and have neutrophils as the predominant cell.

As to polyps not in cystic fibrosis, one report (13) demonstrated that all polyps showed evidence of epithelial damage, either ulceration or marked desquamatization. In another study (14), a small proportion of polyps showed a focal dysplastic change of the surface lining of the mucosa with no related changes in the immediately underlying stroma. On follow-up, in none of these patients did an invasive feature supersede, and these changes appear to constitute a local reaction to recurrent irritation.

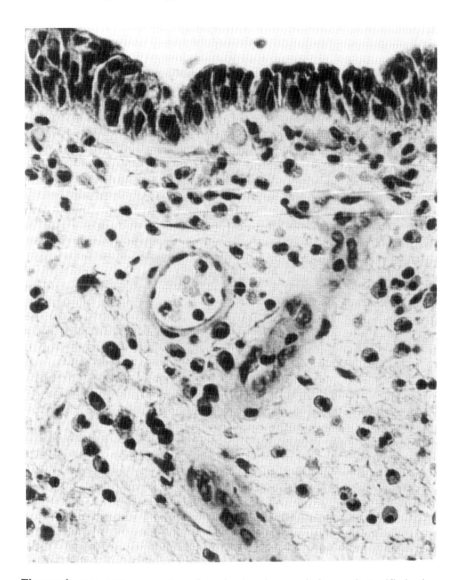

Figure 1 This high-power view of nasal polyp shows orderly pseudostratified colum-nar epithelium overlying an intact basement membrane. The stroma is edematous, vas-cular, and contains eosinophils (hematoxylin and eosin; 400×; from ref. 42).

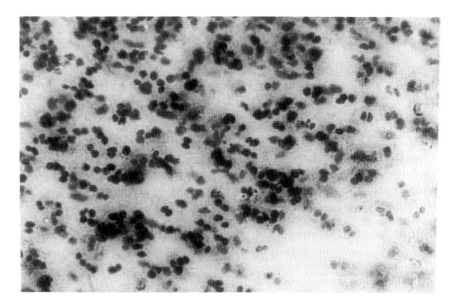

Figure 2 Smear of nasal secretions from a patient with nasal polyps reveals eosinophils (from ref. 42).

V. DIFFERENTIAL DIAGNOSIS

The differential diagnosis of nasal polyps includes chordoma, chemodectoma, neurofibroma, angiofibroma, inverting papilloma, squamous cell carcinoma, sarcoma, and encephaloceles or meningoceles. Most of these lesions present as unilateral lesions. Meningoceles enter the nasal cavity via the cribriform plate. They increase in size with straining, lifting, or crying and may have a pulsating characteristic. The other lesions included in this differential diagnosis are immobile, bleed easily, and may be sensitive to manipulation. Nasal polyps are characteristically mobile, rarely bleed, are not sensitive to manipulation, and are frequently bilateral and multiple. Malignant tumors frequently are associated with bony, destructive changes. In rare cases, benign paranasal sinus cysts or polyps may also produce bone destruction (Woakes' disease) (4). Diagnostic procedures for the differential diagnosis include angiography, tomographic x-rays, computer tomographic scan, magnetic resonance imaging, and biopsy.

VI. ASSOCIATION WITH SYSTEMIC DISEASES

The most common systemic disease associated with nasal polyps is nonallergic asthma, followed by aspirin intolerance. The tetrad of nasal polyps, asthma, aspirin intolerance, and rhinosinusitis will be discussed in a separate category later. Patients with cystic fibrosis have a high frequency of nasal polyps (20%). Children age 16 or younger who have nasal polyps should be evaluated for cystic fibrosis. As in cystic fibrosis, the polyps associated with the chronic dyskinetic cilia syndrome and Young's syndrome have the neutrophil as the predominant cell. Primary ciliary dyskinesia is classically manifested in Kartagener's syndrome, which is an uncommon genetic condition with an estimated incidence of 1:20,000 births (15,16). It appears to be inherited as an autosomal recessive trait and is characterized by bronchiectasis, chronic sinusitis, and situs inversus (complete reversal of internal organs with heart on the right, liver on the left, etc.). The ciliary abnormality in these cases usually involves the entire body including the respiratory tract and sperm cells. The disorder is in the cilia itself in which the dynein arms are missing and the cilia remains completely immotile. Situs inversus is found in only 50% of patients with this syndrome. Infections caused by *Pseudomonas aeruginosa* are often found in patients with Kartagener's syndrome or cystic fibrosis (17).

Young's syndrome consists of recurrent respiratory diseases, azoospermia, and nasal polyposis. The respiratory disease consists of severe chronic sinusitis that may be associated with bronchiectasis (18,19). These patients have normal sweat chloride values and pancreatic function and, therefore, do not have a variant of cystic fibrosis. Cilia structures are normal in sperm tails taken from testicular biopsy specimens and in the cilia from tracheal biopsy specimens and, therefore, these patients do not have a chronic form of immotile cilia syndrome. The azoospermia in Young's syndrome is due to a block in the epididymis that can be differentiated from the defect in the vas deferens associated with cystic fibrosis. However, spermatogenesis is normal. The prevalence of Young's syndrome is considerably higher than that of cystic fibrosis or Kartagener's syndrome. It is responsible for 7.4% of cases of male infertility. In Churg-Strauss syndrome (allergic vasculitis), 50% of patients have nasal polyps. Thus, it is apparent that the presence of nasal polyps may be a sign that a basic generalized disease may be present. The systemic diseases associated with nasal polyps are listed in Table 3 in order of frequency found in the general population.

VII. CHEMICAL MEDIATORS

Chemical mediators found in nasal polyps are histamine, serotonin, leukotrienes (slow reactive substance of anaphylaxis [SRS-A], LTC4, LTD4, LTE4, LTB4), eosinophilic chemotactic factor of anaphylaxis (ECF-A), norepinephrine, kinins, TAME-esterase, and possibly prostaglandin (PGD) (20,21.) Kaliner et al. (22) reported that the release of chemical mediators in nasal polyps is modulated by agents affecting the intracellular concentrations of cyclic nucleotides. These authors also stated that the quantity of SRS-A released in relation to the amount of

Table 3 Nasal Polyps Associated with Systemic Diseases[a]

Asthma (nonallergic)
Aspirin intolerance (bronchospastic type)
Tetrad of asthma, aspirin intolerance, nasal polyps and rhinosinusitis
Allergic fungal sinusitis (49)
Churg-Strauss syndrome (vasculitis)
Young's syndrome (sinopulmonary disease, azoospermia, nasal polyps)
Cystic fibrosis
Kartagener's syndrome (bronchiectasis, chronic sinusitis, and situs inversus)

[a]The first five diseases are associated with tissue eosinophilia, while in the latter group of diseases the predominant cell is the neutrophil.
Source: Reprinted with permission from ref. 42.

histamine released from nasal polyps is considerably less than that released from the human lung. Bumsted et al. (21) reported that there is more histamine in nasal polyps than in normal nasal mucosa and that norepinephrine is present in greater concentration in the base of nasal polyps than in normal nasal mucosa. However, there is no difference in serotonin levels in nasal polyps and normal nasal mucosa. In addition, there is no difference in levels of histamine, serotonin, and norepinephrine in nasal polyps from groups of patients with or without inhalant allergies or asthma.

An interesting finding is that patients with aspirin intolerance have levels of histamine in nasal polyps much lower than all other types of patients with nasal polyps, approximating the histamine levels found in normal mucosa. Chandra and Abrol (23) reported that polyp fluid contains albumin and immunoglobulins (IgA, IgE, IgG, IgM, and macroglobulins). The concentrations of IgA and IgE and, in some cases, IgG and IgM were greater in the polyp fluid than in the serum. Using the Prausnitz-Kustner procedure, Berdal (24) in 1952 reported that skin sensitivity antibody in polyp fluid was many times more concentrated than that found in sera. An explanation for these increased concentrations of serum components found in polyp fluid may be that the polyp acts as a dialyzing membrane with water evaporating through the mucosa. This causes an increased concentration of large substances in the polyp sac.

VIII. PATHOGENESIS

A current theory on the pathogenesis of polyps has been presented by Bumsted et al. (21). Their theory is based on data that norepinephrine is present in greater concentration in the base of nasal polyps than in normal mucosa. They stated that this norepinephrine at the base of the polyp could produce excessive adrenergic receptor-mediated vasoconstriction that might lead to rebound mucosal congestion and edema, potentiating the effects of histamine and kinins. Norepinephrine, through adrenergic receptor activation, would lower the effects of cyclic adenosine monophosphate, which would enhance the release of histamine, SRS-A, and ECF-A. These mediators would cause an increased vascular permeability, edema, and the leakage of macromolecules out of the vascular system, eventually causing the polyp formation. They explain the lower levels of histamine found in polyps of aspirin-intolerant patients by stating that these patients have an increased sensitivity to histamines.

Mygind (25) believes that polyp formation is related to denervation of blood vessels and degranulation of mast cells in the nasal mucosa. This process leads to increased vascular permeability, edema, and finally polyp formation. IIc lists causative factors for denervation to be infection, cystic fibrosis, and aspirin intolerance. He lists contributing factors to be mast cell degeneration and IgE-dependent reactions.

An old theory (26) on polyp formation starts with Bernoulli's theorem that gases or fluid passing through a constrictor results in an area of negative pressure in its vicinity. Weakened, denervated tissue such as polyps may theoretically be sucked out by this negative pressure, leading to edema and enlargement of the polyp.

Other theories of polyp formation have been postulated. Tos and Mogensen's (27) theory is based on rupture of the epithelium with protrusion of the subepithelial tissue through the epithelial defect and the epithelization of the prolapsed tissue.

A new theory from Bernstein et al. (28) is that a greater rate of transepithelial ion transport occurs in nasal polyps. They suggest that this increased rate may have an effect on the movement of water into the cell and interstitial tissue, causing edema and formation of nasal polyps. They base their theory on the transepithelial bioelectric potential difference and resistance of nasal polyps and turbinate epithelial cells.

None of these theories appears to be adequate to account for all of the known facts involving nasal polyps. However, the theory of Bumsted et al. (21) is more closely related to biochemical events and, perhaps with some modification, may be more plausible. The fact that nasal polyps are frequently associated with systemic diseases indicates that the underlying cause of polyposis may be related to a basic generalized biochemical disorder. At the present time, the pathogenesis of polyp formation is unknown.

IX. RELATIONSHIP TO ATOPY

Nasal polyps are more found frequently in patients with asthma/rhinitis who have negative skin tests than those with positive skin tests (6–8). There is a relationship to asthma: more than 70% of patients with nasal polyps have associated

Table 4 Nasal Polyps (211 Cases): Characteristics

Clinical categories	No.	%
Males	106	50.2
Females	105	49.8
Asthma	149	70.6
Rhinitis (alone)	62	29.4
Positive allergy skin tests	117	55.5
Total aspirin intolerance	30	14.2
Subtypes of aspirin intolerance		
Bronchospasm	21	70.0
Urticaria	4	13.3
Both bronchospasm and urticaria	2	6.7
Rhinitis	3	10.0

Source: Reprinted with permission from ref. 42.

asthma (Table 4) (6). Some patients with nasal polyps not only have no history of asthma but also have negative methacholine challenge tests (29,30). Therefore, not all patients with nasal polyps have an associated lower respiratory disease (31,32). Whiteside et al. (33) reported that in five of six cases of nasal polyps in nonatopic patients, no IgE-bearing lymphocytes were detected in the polyp tissue. However, in atopic patients, IgE-bearing lymphocytes in nasal polyps correlated well with serum IgE levels.

We reviewed (34) 167 patients with nasal polyps, 143 (86%) of whom had undergone polypectomies (Table 5). A number of these patients had a verified history of two, three, four, or even five or more polypectomies. Our data suggest that patients with positive allergy skin tests (pollen, animal dander, or molds) have a progressively higher rate of repeated polypectomies (Table 6).

Table 5 Data on 167 Patients with Verified Polyps and Polypectomies

Total patients	No. of polypectomies	No. of patients	%
167	1 or more	143	86
143	2 or more	57	40
143	3 or more	34	24
143	4 or more	22	15
143	5 or more	17	12
143	6 or more	11	8

Source: Reprinted with permission from ref. 42.

Table 6   Frequency of Polypectomies in Patients with Positive Allergy Skin Tests

No. of polypectomies	Total patients[a]	No. with positive allergy skin tests	%
None	24	12	50
One or more	143	81	57
Two or more	57	33	53
Three or more	34	20	59
Four or more	22	15	68
Five or more	17	12	71
Six or more	11	8	73

[a]Total patients = 167: one patient did not have a skin test
Source: Reprinted with permission from ref. 42.

The frequency of one or more possible allergy skin tests (pollens, danders, or molds) in our patient population with nasal polyps is 56% (6). However, this population was obtained from an allergy-biased practice, both in private practice and in the allergy clinic at Rhode Island Hospital, where the overall frequency of one or more positive allergy skin tests was 77% (6). Therefore, the 56% positive allergy skin tests in patients with nasal polyps is lower than that found in our allergy practice and is not directly related to polyp formation.

It appears that atopy or IgE-mediated disease is not a cause of nasal polyps, but once polyp formation occurs, atopy or IgE-mediated disease may aggravate and increase the risk of nasal polyp formation. Acute upper respiratory infections are also known to cause an exacerbation or enlargement of nasal polyps (32).

X. RELATIONSHIP TO ASPIRIN INTOLERANCE

The full-blown tetrad of asthma, aspirin intolerance, chronic sinusitis, and nasal polyps usually is associated with a severe type of asthma that is frequently steroid-dependent. The type of aspirin intolerance associated with nasal polyps is the bronchospastic type, not the urticaria/angioedema type. In many cases, only two components of the tetrad are present, asthma and aspirin intolerance, which usually have onset within 1 year of each other. However, nasal polyps may occur about 10 years later (34). The mean age of onset of the asthma and aspirin intolerance part of the tetrad is about 31 years (35). However, the cumulative frequency increases with age so that in asthmatic patients older than 40, the frequency of nasal polyps is 10% and above (Table 2).

Other characteristics of this tetrad are listed in Table 7. It is most commonly associated with nonallergic or negative skin test asthma and with a normal

Table 7   Characteristics of the Bronchospastic Type of Aspirin Intolerance

Found in asthmatic patients
Correlated with nasal polyposis
Similar age of onset to asthma
Severe rhinorrhea with reactions to aspirin
Increased frequency in older age groups
Familiar occurrence
Eosinophil in nasal smear
Elevated total (blood) eosinophil count
Nonsteroidal anti-inflammatory drug cross-reaction
No specific IgE (antiaspiryl)
Normal total IgE
Desensitization possible to aspirin
Pathogenic mechanism: prostaglandins

Source: Reprinted with permission from ref. 42.

serum IgE level. Specific IgE against aspirin has not been found. During acute bronchospasm produced by aspirin challenge, histamine levels, neutrophil chemotactic activity, and complement activation were not found to be significantly different from baseline levels (36). Elevated blood eosinophils and a marked eosinophilia in the nasal secretions are also characteristic of this syndrome. There is a hereditary disposition of aspirin intolerance: clusters of this syndrome are found in certain families (35). The frequency of aspirin intolerance increases with age, especially over 40. However, it is the bronchospastic type of aspirin intolerance not the urticaria/angioedema type that increases with age.

It is apparent that there are many similarities between aspirin intolerance and nasal polyps. Besides being associated together in the triad of asthma, aspirin intolerance (bronchospastic type), and nasal polyps, both are associated with chronic sinusitis and nasal eosinophilia. Both conditions increase in frequency with age, both are commonly associated with negative skin test or nonallergic asthma, and both conditions are associated with a high frequency of steroid-dependent asthma as stated.

It is important to remember that nonsteroidal anti-inflammatory drugs (NSAID) cross-react with aspirin and cause a similar acute bronchospasm in aspirin-intolerant asthmatic persons. These drugs are cyclooxygenase inhibitors. Some of these NSAID, such as indomethacin and ibuprofen, cross-react with aspirin in intolerant individuals about 100% of the time. Other NSAID cross-react with aspirin in intolerant individuals at a somewhat decreased rate, depending on the dosage used and degree of inhibition of cyclo-oxygenase.

The pathologic mechanism of aspirin intolerance is unknown. One theory is based on the association between prostaglandin and SRS-A. It is possible that in certain individuals inhibition of the cyclooxygenase pathway may cause a shunting toward the lipoxygenase pathway resulting in increased production of leukotrienes LTC4, LTD4, and LTE4 (SRS-A), which will produce bronchospasm. In addition, products of the lipoxygenase system such as 5-HPETE, 5-HETE, and LTB4 are chemotactic for eosinophils. Both aspirin intolerance and nasal polyps are associated with eosinophils. A similar mechanism including arachidonic acid and prostaglandins for the formation of nasal polyps has not been developed at this time, but further research is needed in this area.

XI. TREATMENT

A. Nasal Polyps

Polypectomy is not the treatment of choice for routine nasal polyposis. We reviewed 167 patients with verified nasal polyps (Table 5). Eighty-six percent (143) had undergone polypectomies. Of these 143, 57 (40%) required 2 or more polypectomies, 34 (24%) required 3 or more polypectomies, 22 (15%) required 4 or more polypectomies, 17 (12%) had 5 or more polypectomies, and 11 (8%) had 6 or more polypectomies. Three of our patients had a history of 20 or more polypectomies. Therefore, nasal polyposis frequently is a recurrent problem in more than 40% of cases. Other studies (23) have found a recurrence rate of more than 31%. Also, polyps in patients with aspirin intolerance appear to have a greater recurrence rate than in aspirin-tolerant patients.

It is apparent that surgical polypectomy does not permanently eliminate this disease. However, in certain selected cases, especially in those in whom corticosteroids are not effective or are contraindicated, surgical polypectomy may be considered. Steroid injection of nasal polyps has been used with some success in the hands of expert otolaryngologists (38). However, injection of steroids in the nasal turbinates and polyps has resulted in 10 instances of visual loss, 5 of which were permanent as of 1981. Steroid emboli were demonstrated in the retinal vessels in six cases. This type of treatment for nasal polyps should certainly be reserved for the very skilled otolaryngologist if it is used at all.

At the present time, I believe that the treatment of choice is a 10-day course of systemic corticosteroid therapy beginning with about 60 mg of prednisone orally and decreasing by 5 mg daily. This short burst of corticosteroids should not cause a clinically significant suppression of the pituitary–adrenal axis. Patients may occasionally need a second burst of steroids a few weeks later if symptoms do not improve with the first course of corticosteroid treatment (40).

Afterwards, patients may be maintained on topical beclomethasone or flunisolide, but one must realize that long-term use of these topical medications may result in questionable suppression of the pituitary–adrenal axis, which may not be clinically significant. Newer products, such as topical fluocortin butyl and fluticasone, may help to prevent these complications since these have not been found to have a significant pituitary–adrenal effect. Fluocortin butyl is still undergoing clinical investigation and has not been released to the practicing physician in the United States yet.

Even with systemic and topical corticosteroid therapy, nasal polyps frequently may still be a recurrent disease and periodic bursts of systemic corticosteroids may have to be administered. When treatment with systemic corticosteroids has no effect, or is contraindicated, a surgical procedure may be contemplated.

Our recent investigation (41) has shown that surgical polypectomy may delay the recurrence rate of polyps compared to those treated with corticosteroids, but certainly the trauma and morbidity are much worse with surgery.

Contrary to previous opinion, the surgical removal of nasal polyps does not cause or aggravate asthma. In our laboratory, 10 patients with nasal polyps and no history of asthma were studied. Results of methacholine challenge tests done before and about 5 months after polypectomy were similar (29). In a report by Miles-Lawrence et al. (30), similar data were obtained. They performed methacholine challenge tests 1 month prior to polypectomy and up to 1 year following polypectomy. They found essentially no change in methacholine sensitivity, confirming our conclusion that polypectomy does not cause or worsen asthma. However, the occurrence rate for nasal polyps following polypectomy is notoriously high and may be aggravated by many nonspecific factors such as upper respiratory infection and allergies to pollens, danders, and molds (when the chance occurrence of these diseases coexists) (34,37).

To extend these laboratory findings to clinically relevant data, we evaluated pulmonary function tests just prior to polypectomy and up to 5 months following polypectomy. There was no significant change in pulmonary function tests (34).

We also evaluated seven steroid-dependent asthmatic patients for steroid requirements before and approximately 6 months following polypectomy (Table 8). The steroid requirements were essentially unchanged in five patients and decreased in two, possibly because of less stimulation through the rhinosinobronchial reflex. Thus, our initial data with methacholine sensitivity have been confirmed with subsequent clinical information.

Patients with nasal polyps deserve an allergic evaluation despite the fact that a large percentage of them are nonatopic. If clinically relevant IgE-mediated disease is found in these patients, a course of hyposensitization may be given, especially in those with recurrent polyposis. IgE-mediated disease is not the cause of nasal polyps, but it may contribute to episodes of exacerbations (41,42).

B. Aspirin Sensitivity

The most important treatment for aspirin intolerance is avoidance of aspirin and nonsteroidal anti-inflammatory drugs (43). Nonsteroidal anti-inflammatory

Table 8   Effect of Polypectomy on Steroid-Dependent Asthma (6 Month Interval)

| | | Prednisone Dosage | | |
Patient	Age (yr)	Preoperative	Postoperative (6 mo)	Change in asthma
1	48	10 mg alt days	10 mg alt days	Same
2	25	10 mg alt days	10 mg alt days[a]	Same
3	66	10 mg alt days	2.5 mg daily	Better
4	66	5 mg daily	10 mg alt days	Better
5	42	10 mg alt days	10 mg alt days	Same
6	58	10 mg daily	10 mg daily	Same
7	76	10 mg alt days	10 mg alt days	Same

[a]Data collected at 9 months.
Source: Reprinted with permission from ref. 42.

drugs that inhibit cyclo-oxygenase cross-react with aspirin in aspirin-intolerant patients (Table 1). The cyclo-oxygenase inhibitors listed in Table 9 cross-react with aspirin in intolerant patients almost 100% of the time. Weak inhibitors of cyclo-oxygenase such as nonacetylated salicylates and acetaminophen are less likely to cross-react. However, an occasional case report has noted a cross-reactivity resulting in adverse reactions with the use of high dosages (44). Hundreds of over-the-counter drugs contain aspirin, and sensitive patients should be familiar with them.

Non-cyclo-oxygenase inhibitors such as the yellow dye tartrazine occasionally have been reported to cross-react with aspirin in intolerant individuals. More recent studies have not been able to confirm tartrazine cross-reactivity (45).

Table 9   Nonsteroidal Anti-Inflammatory Drugs: *Cyclo-Oxygenase Inhibitors*

Aminophenazone	Indomethacin
Aspirin	Mefenamic acid
Benzydamine	Naproxen
Diftalone	Nictindole
Ditazole	Noramidopyrine
Fenoprofen	Piroxicam
Flumizole	Sulindac
Ibuprofen	Tolmetin

Source: Reprinted with permission Settipane GA. Aspirin sensitivity and allergy. Biomed Pharmacother 1988;42:493–8.

Acute reactions after the accidental ingestion of aspirin or nonsteroidal anti-inflammatory drugs usually constitute a medical emergency. These reactions may begin with severe rhinorrhea followed rapidly by acute bronchospasm and even shock; an occasional patient may have acute urticarial and/or angioedema with or without respiratory distress. Severe reactions involving shock should be treated promptly with epinephrine 1/1000, 0.1–0.5 ml, which could be repeated in 20 min. Bronchospastic reactions may be treated with aerosolized beta-agonists such as albuterol or metaproterenol in repeated dosages. If symptoms persist, aminophylline in intravenous dosages sufficient to achieve or maintain therapeutic blood levels may be used. Cyanosis should be treated immediately with oxygen (2–5 liters/min via nasal catheter or 34% by Venturi mask). Hypotension should be treated with intravenous fluid administration, volume expanders, dopamine hydrochloride, or norepinephrine bitartrate. In prolonged reactions, the intravenous administration of methylprednisolone, 125 mg, or hydrocortisone sodium succinate (Solu-Cortef), 100–200 mg, may prevent status asthmaticus.

The chronic treatment of asthma in aspirin-intolerant patients frequently requires glucocorticoids for the control of respiratory symptoms in addition to the initiation of oral doses of theophylline and aerosolized beta-agonist medication.

Since these patients frequently have associated chronic rhinosinusitis or nasal polyps, treatment also should be directed to the upper airway. Through the rhinosinobronchial reflex, acute or chronic sinusitis and nasal polyps can aggravate asthma, and successful treatment of the upper airway disease may decrease the asthma. Sinusitis should be treated vigorously with antibiotics, topical glucocorticoids, and oral and nasal administration of decongestants.

Desensitization with aspirin followed by long-term daily aspirin treatment has recently been demonstrated to result in improvement of both upper and lower airway symptoms in aspirin-sensitive asthmatic patients (46–48). Selected patients with aspirin intolerance and resistant arthritis or cardiovascular disease may also be candidates for desensitization. These arthritic symptoms should be severe enough to warrant the inherent risk associated with desensitization procedures, as outlined by Stevenson and his colleagues. Desensitization is initiated immediately following aspirin challenge studies. The 1 day challenge procedure is useful when aspirin sensitivity is not suspected and the patient has limited time (Table 10).

The usual procedure in the patient with a history of aspirin intolerance is the 3-day aspirin challenge, (Table 11). It is important to remember that one must start with a 3 mg aspirin dose in patients with a history of severe reactions. If aspirin is continued over the ensuing days, the patient will continue to be desensitized to aspirin. However, in rare cases the aspirin reaction may again break through even though the desensitized patient is taking aspirin daily. The refractory period after a positive aspirin challenge usually is 2–4 days if aspirin ad-

Table 10   1 Day Acetylsalicylic (ASA) Acid Challenge

Time	ASA dosage (mg)	Cumulative dosage (mg)
8 AM	30	30
10 AM	60	90
12 PM	100	190
2 PM	325	515
4 PM	650	1,165
6 PM	End[a]	

[a]If a reaction does not occur, patient is not ASA sensitive. If forced expiratory volume in 1 sec is reduced ≥25%, 7 or more days later carry out placebo challenge to confirm specificity. One-day challenge is useful when ASA sensitivity is not suspected and patient has a limited amount of time.
Source: From ref. 45.

ministration is not maintained daily. Desensitization to aspirin also desensitizes the patient to other nonsteroidal anti-inflammatory drugs. The use of nonacetylated salicylic acid in desensitizing procedures is being investigated.

XII. SUMMARY

The association of the tetrad symptoms of nasal polyps, asthma, aspirin intolerance, and chronic rhinosinusitis are described in detail. Nasal polyps frequently are associated with aspirin intolerance, intrinsic asthma, chronic sinusitis, Young's syndrome, cystic fibrosis, Kartagener's syndrome, and Churg-Strauss syndrome. Children 16 years or younger with nasal polyps should be evaluated for cystic fibrosis. Nasal polyps are frequently bilateral, multiple, freely movable, pale-gray and arise from the middle meatus of the nose.

Table 11   3 Day Acetylsalicylic Acid (ASA) Challenge

Time	Days		
	1	2	3
8 AM	Placebo	ASA 30(3) mg	ASA 150 mg
11 AM	Placebo	ASA 60 mg	ASA 325 mg
2 PM	Placebo	ASA 100 mg	ASA 650 mg

Protocol: 1. Discontinue antihistamines; cromolyn and sympathomimetics; 2. Increase glucocorticoids for 3 days before challenge to produce forced expiratory volume in 1 sec >70% or a value of 1.5 liters per minute; 3. History of severe reactions: start challenge at 3 mg of ASA (20% of time).
Source: Reprinted with permission from Ref. 45.

On histologic examination, they classically have pseudostratified ciliated co-lumnar epithelium, thickening of the epithelial basement membrane, high stro-mal eosinophil count, mucin with neutral pH, few glands, and essentially no nerve endings. Cells consists of a mixture of lymphocytes, plasma cells, and eosinophils. Polyps from patients with Young's syndrome, Kartagener's syn-drome, and cystic fibrosis have predominantly neutrophils with insignificant eosinophils. Chemical mediators found in nasal polyps are as follows: histamine, serotonin, leukotrienes (SRS-A or LTC4, LTD4, LTE4, LTB4), ECF-A, nor-epinephrine, kinins, TAME-esterase, and possibly PGD2. There is more hista-mine in nasal polyps than in normal nasal mucosa, and norepinephrine is present in greater concentration in the base of nasal polyps than in normal nasal mucosa. The concentrations of IgA and IgE and, in some case, IgG and IgM are greater in polyp fluid than in serum. IgE-mediated disease is not the cause of nasal pol-yps but, when present, may contribute to episodes of exacerbation. At the present time, the pathogenesis of polyp formation is unknown. Despite medical or surgical management, a significant number of nasal polyps are recurrent es-pecially in patients with aspirin intolerance. For treatment, systemic corticos-steroids should be tried before surgical polypectomy. Polypectomy does not increase the risk of developing asthma or making asthma worse.

REFERENCES

1. Widal, MF, Abram P, Lermoyez J. Anaphylaxie et idiosyndraise. Presse Med 1922;22:191.
2. Settipane GA. Landmark commentary: history of aspirin intolerance. Allergy Proc 1990;11:251–2.
3. Davidson AE, Miller DS, Settipane RJ, Ricci AR, Klein DE, Settipane GA. De-layed nasal mucociliary clearance in patients with nonallergic rhinitis and nasal eosinophilia. Allergy Proc 1991;12(6): 402.
4. Wentges RTR. Edward Woakes: the history of an eponym. J Laryngol Otol 1972;86:501–12.
5. Vancil ME. A historical survey of treatments for nasal polyposis. Laryngoscope 1969;79:435–45.
6. Settipane GA, Chafee FH. Nasal polyps in asthma and rhinitis: a review of 6,037 patients. J Allergy Clin Immunol 1977;59:17–21.
7. Chafee FH, Settipane GA. Aspirin intolerance: I. Frequency in an allergic popu-lation. J Allergy Clin Immunol 1974;53:193–9.
8. Settipane GA, Chafee FH, Klein DE. Aspirin intolerance: II. A prospective study in an atopic and normal population. J Allergy Clin Immunol 1974;53:200–4.
9. Slavin RG, Linford P, Friedman WH. Sinusitis and bronchial asthma. J Allergy Clin Immunol 1982;69(Part 2): 102.
10. Lanoff G, Daddono A, Johnson E. Nasal polyps in children: a ten-year study. Ann Allergy 1973;31:551–4.

11. Ballantyne J., Groves J., eds. The nose. In: Grooves, ed. *Scott Brown's Diseases of the Ear, Nose and Throat, ed 3*. Philadelphia: JB Lippincott, 1971:179.
12. Oppenheimer EH, Rosenstein BJ. Differential pathology of nasal polyps in cystic fibrosis and atopy. Lab Invest 1979;40:445–9.
13. Wladislavosky-Wasserman P, Kern EB, Holley KE, Gleich GJ. Epithelial damage is commonly seen in nasal polyps. J Allergy Clin Immunol 1982;69(part 2): 148.
14. Busuttil A. Dysplastic epithelial changes in nasal polyps. Ann Otol Rhinol Laryngol 1978;87:416–20.
15. Atzelius BA. Disorders of ciliary motility. Hosp Pract 1986;21:73–80.
16. Rossman CM, Lee RM, Forrest JB, Newhouse MT. Nasal ciliary ultrastructure and function in patients with primary ciliary dyskinesia compared with that in normal subjects and in subjects with various respiratory diseases. Am Rev Respir Dis 1984;129:161–7.
17. MacKay DN. Antibiotic treatment of rhinitis and sinusitis. Am J Rhinol 1987;1:83–5.
18. Schanker HM, Rajfer J, Saxon A. Recurrent respiratory disease, azoospermia, and nasal polyposis. Arch Intern Med 1985;145:2201–3.
19. Handelsman DJ, Conway AJ, Boylan LM, Turtle JR. Young's syndrome. Obstructive azoospermia and chronic sinopulmonary infections. N Engl J Med 1984;310:3–9.
20. Pelletier G, Hebert J, Bedard PM, Salari H, Borgeat P. Profile of leukotrienes and histamine from human nasal polyps. J Allergy Clin Immunol 1986;77(part 2): 177, (abstr).
21. Bumsted RM, El-Ackad T, Smith JM, Brody MJ. Histamine, norepinephrine and serotonin content of nasal polyps. Laryngoscope 1979;89:832–43.
22. Kaliner M, Wasserman SI, Austen KF. Immunologic release of chemical mediators from human nasal polyps. N Engl J Med 1973;289:277–81.
23. Chandra RK, Abrol BM. Immunopathology of nasal polypi. J Laryngol Otol 1974;88:1019–24.
24. Berdal P. Serologic investigations on the edema fluid from nasal polyps. J Allergy 1952;23:11–14.
25. Mygind N, ed. Nasal polyps. In: *Nasal Allergy, ed 2*. Oxford/London: Blackwell Scientific Publications, 1979:233–8.
26. Gray L. Deviated nasal septum. III. Its influence on the physiology and disease of the nose and ear. J Laryngol 1967;81:953–86.
27. Tos M, Mogensen C. Density of mucous glands in normal adult nasal septum. Arch Otorhinolaryngol 1977;215:101.
28. Bernstein JM, Cropp JA, Nathanson I, Yankaskas J. Bioelectric properties of cultured human nasal polypi and turbinate epithelial cells. Am J Rhinol 1990; 4(2): 45–9.
29. Downing ET, Braman S, Settipane GA. Bronchial reactivity in patients with nasal polyps before and after polypectomy. J Allergy Clin Immunol 1982;69(part 2): 102.
30. Miles-Lawrence R, Kaplan M, Chang K. Methacholine sensitivity in nasal polyposis and the effects of polypectomy. J Allergy Clin Immunol 1982;69(part 2): 102.
31. Connell JT. Nasal disease. N Engl Soc Allergy Proc 1982;3:389–96.

32. Settipane GA. Aspirin intolerance presenting as chronic rhinitis. RI Med J 1980;63:63–5.
33. Whiteside TL, Rabin BS, Zetterberg J, Criep L. The presence of IgE on the surface of lymphocytes in nasal polyps. J Allergy Clin Immunol 1975;55:186–94.
34. Settipane GA, Klein DE, Lekas MD. Asthma and nasal polyps. In: Myers E, ed. New Dimensions in Otorhinolaryngology, Head and Neck Surgery. Amsterdam: Excerpta Medica, 1987:499–500.
35. Settipane GA, Pudupakkam RK. Aspirin intolerance. III. Subtypes, familial occurrence and cross-reactivity with tartrazine. J Allergy Clin Immunol 1975; 56:215–21.
36. Simon R, Pleskow W, Kaliner M, Wasserman S. Plasma mediator studies in aspirin sensitive asthma. J Allergy Clin Immunol 1983;71(part 2): 146.
37. Settipane GA. Nasal polyposis. N Engl Soc Allergy Proc 1982;3:497–504.
38. McCleve D, Gatos L, Goldstein J, Silvers S. Corticosteroid injections of the nasal turbinates: past experience and precautions. ORL J Otorhinolaryngol Rel Spec 1978;86:851–7.
39. Mabry RL. Visual loss after intranasal corticosteroid injection. Arch Otolaryngol 1981;107:484–6.
40. Settipane GA. Nasal polyps: epidemiology, pathology, immunology and treatment. Am J Rhinol 1987;1:119–26.
41. Settipane GA, Klein DE, Settipane RJ. Nasal polyps, state of the art. Rhinology 1991;11:33–6.
42. Settipane GA, ed. Nasal polyps. In: *Rhinitis*, 2nd ed. Providence: Oceanside Publications, 1991:178.
43. Samter M, Beers RF. Concerning the nature of intolerance to aspirin. J Allergy 1967;40:281.
44. Settipane RA, Stevenson DD. Cross sensitivity with acetaminophen in aspirin-sensitive subjects with asthma. J Allergy Clin Immunol 1989;84:26–33.
45. Stevenson DD. Oral challenge: aspirin, NSAID, tartrazine and sulfites. N Engl Reg Allergy Proc 1984;5:111.
46. Zeiss CR, Lockey RF. Refractory period to aspirin in a patient with aspirin-induced asthma. J Allergy Clin Immunol 1976;57:440.
47. Stevenson DD, Pleskow WW, Simon RA, et al. Aspirin sensitive rhino-sinusitis asthma: a double-blind crossover study of treatment with aspirin. J Allergy Clin Immunol 1984;73:500.
48. Sweet JM, Stevenson DD, Simon RA, Mathison DA. Long-term effects of aspirin desensitization-treatment of aspirin-sensitive rhinosinusitis-asthma. J Allergy Clin Immunol 1990;85:59–65.
49. Schwietz LA, Gourley DS. Allergic fungal sinusitis. Allergy Proc 1992;13:3–6.

15

Sinusitis and Nasal Polyposis in Cystic Fibrosis

RICHARD B. MOSS
Stanford University School of Medicine
Stanford, California

I. BASIC SCIENCE ASPECTS OF CYSTIC FIBROSIS

Cystic fibrosis (CF) is an inherited disease of electrolyte and fluid transport primarily affecting secretory and absorptive mucosal epithelia, including the respiratory and gastrointestinal tracts. It is inherited in mendelian autosomal recessive fashion, indicating that inheritance of two mutated alleles at the *CF* locus in the human genome is necessary for manifestation of clinical pathologic change. Recognized as a distinct clinical entity in the late 1930s, it is only within the last few years that the underlying cellular pathophysiology has been defined and the genetic basis of the disease identified at the molecular level. The clinical presentation of the disease always includes respiratory signs and symptoms due to luminal obstruction and mucosal infection, as well as clinical pancreatic insufficiency in ~90% of cases. With improved treatment due to better medical and nutritional intervention, the median survival is now approaching 30 years, resulting in emergence of previously neglected or ignored problems as new foci of clinical concern. Prominent among these are the upper respiratory tract problems of chronic pansinusitis and nasal polyposis. In addition, advances in cell culture and relative ease of access to the nasal mucosa have made the upper respiratory surface a major source of tissue for basic and clinical research in cystic fibrosis. This section provides a brief summary of scientific understanding of cystic fibrosis, reviews the upper respiratory tract manifestations of CF with particular attention to sinusitis and polyposis, and suggests future directions for treatment.

A. CF Gene and Its Product

The CF gene was cloned and sequenced in 1989 by molecular geneticists Lap-Chee Tsui, Francis Collins, and colleagues after a major international effort (1). The CF gene is large (250,000 base pairs); only ~5% of it (mRNA transcript ~6.5 kb) codes for a 1480 amino acid protein termed the cystic fibrosis transmembrane conductance regulator (CFTR) of molecular weight ~170 kD when fully glycosylated in the Golgi after translation in the endoplasmic reticulum. CFTR is expressed in most differentiated secretory epithelial cells. CFTR consists of two homologous structural units each consisting of a transmembrane domain and a nucleotide-binding fold, which are connected by a unique central R (regulatory) domain. The predicted tertiary structure suggests a cell membrane transport function (2).

The major mutation in CFTR, which is responsible for ~70% of mutant alleles and therefore most clinical cases of CF, is due to a deletion of a 3 base pair coding for the amino acid phenylalanine at position 508 of CFTR (ΔF508); this ΔF508 mutation is associated with pancreatic insufficiency (3). More than 200 other mutations in the CFTR gene have been identified, but the most common handful account for nearly 90% of CF cases in white subjects (4). Specific oligonucleotide probes are available for polymerase chain reaction diagnosis of these most common mutations using peripheral blood mononuclear cells, amniotic cells, or chorionic villous cells as source material. Prenatal diagnosis and carrier detection are thus clinically available, but there are many unresolved medical, socioeconomic, and ethical issues (5-8).

B. Molecular Pathophysiological Characteristics

The first major insights into the basic cellular pathophysiology of CF occurred in the early 1980s with demonstration of altered Cl^- transport across sweat gland and respiratory epithelial cell membranes (9-11). Technical advances in epithelial cell culture in the mid-1980s facilitated biochemical and physiological studies that focused on distal steps in the regulatory pathways for Cl^- transport (12-19). The pathologic basis of Cl^- transport always involves a failure of Cl^- secretion via a pathway involving β-adrenergic agonists, adenylate cyclase, cAMP, a cAMP-dependent protein kinase, and a Cl^- ion channel in the cell membrane. In CF all steps in this pathway are normal except the Cl^- channel itself. Transcellular Cl^- reabsorption is also blocked, presumably due to the same defective Cl^- channel (see below). In some tissues defective cholinergic, GMP-, and/or Ca^{2+}-mediated Cl^- secretory pathways, excessive Na^+ reabsorption, and increased sulfation of mucus glycoproteins have also been found (20,21).

Current trials of drug therapy aimed at correcting the pathologic defects in ion exchange are underway. One of these involves using the Na^+ channel blocker amiloride administered by aerosol to reduce excessive luminal Na^+ absorption in the airways of patients with CF (22). Another involves bypassing the defective Cl^- channel by utilizing alternative intracellular pathways to Cl^- secretion with regulatory extracellular triphosphate nucleotides (23). It is also possible to modulate directly the function of the defective CFTR protein pharmacologically, opening the possibility of direct effective drug therapy at the molecular level (24,25). Molecular biologists have also succeeded in correcting Cl^- transport defects in vitro by transfecting CF cells with normal CFTR gene delivered by viral vectors (26-28). (In most cases of CF, due to inheritance of $\Delta F508$ mutations in both CFTR gene alleles, the defective CFTR protein is incompletely processed in the endoplasmic reticulum and is not properly inserted into the cell's apical membrane) (29). This in vitro gene therapy has dramatically raised hopes for eventual clinical treatment of CF by transfection and induction of normal CFTR genes into airway cells in patients with CF, a feat accomplished in vivo in the airways of rats in late 1991 (30). The road to human gene therapy with CFTR is thus open, but remains long and potentially rocky. One of the interesting approaches to future drug and gene therapy in CF is to capitalize on the involvement of the nasal and sinus mucosa and the relative ease of access to this tissue, as discussed below.

C. CFTR Function: Cl^- Channel, and More?

The physiological studies outlined above suggest that the defect in CF resides in the Cl^- channel itself. However, a molecular model of CFTR structure–function relationships, based upon sequence and domain organization in other proteins of a homologous gene superfamily of ATPase transport proteins, was proposed soon after the CFTR gene was cloned (31). In this model, CFTR functions as a *pump*, transporting some solute in or out of cells. CFTR in this model must *regulate* Cl^- channels either directly by physical association (making them sensitive to cAMP-mediated phosphorylation) or indirectly via activity of the solute pumped by CFTR (perhaps by pumping a Cl^- channel inhibitory factor out of the cell or pumping in a factor needed to make Cl^- channels sensitive to cAMP). Support for the pump hypothesis came from studies with synthetic peptides derived from the critical nucleotide-binding folds of CFTR where the most common mutations occur, in which a variety of adenine nucleotides were in fact bound (32). However, compelling evidence for the hypothesis that CFTR is *itself* a Cl^- channel comes from studies in which cell types that do not normally express a Cl^- transport function (and are thus intrinsically incapable of responding to kinase with Cl^- secretion) do so after transfection with normal CFTR gene (33,34). Even more persuasive are studies in which specific mutations introduced into CFTR alter the anion transport properties of cells into which they are introduced (35,36). In this model, potential nucleotide-binding fold pump features might be related to channel activity by an interaction with the R domain, which seems to serve as a movable "ball and chain" occluder of the ion pore (1,36). The case for CFTR as a Cl⁻ channel seems clinched by in vitro reconstitution of Cl⁻ channel activity in a lipid bilayer with purified CFTR (37).

It remains entirely possible that CFTR could be *both* a Cl⁻ channel and a pump/regulator. Another member of the ATPase transport gene superfamily, P-glycoprotein (which, when sufficiently expressed, is responsible for multiple-drug resistance by pumping chemotherapeutic drugs out of cancer cells) appears to also function as a Cl⁻ channel (38). Moreover, acidification of intracellular organelles, which is involved in secretion of macromolecules, also appears to be partly determined by CFTR, although the mechanism is obscure (39). Cellular endocytosis and exocytosis of a variety of molecules appear to be somehow regulated by CFTR (40). Thus, the mysteries of what CFTR does, and how the genetic defects of CF affect the biological function of CFTR at the cellular level and result in the clinical pathology of CF, are far from solved.

D. Respiratory Mucosal Infection

The basic clinical presentation of CF is inspissation of mucus-containing secretions and chronic sinopulmonary infection with a restricted spectrum of microbial pathogens. In particular, *Pseudomonas aeruginosa* is a driving force in the natural history of progressive lung disease (41,42). Chronic endobronchial infection with *P. aeruginosa* in CF is a complex process encompassing many aspects of bacterial and host factors, their interactions, and their mutual modulation (43). In addition, the roles of other bacteria (especially *Staphylococcus aureus* and unencapsulated *Haemophilus influenzae*) and respiratory viruses remain largely unknown (44,45). It remains unclear whether the goal of antimicrobial therapy should be to eliminate *S. aureus* and *H. influenzae* or, conversely, to allow their persistence as a hedge against the more intransigent *P. aeruginosa*. Nor is it known if respiratory viruses are a critical bridge between the uninfected CF respiratory mucosa and chronic bacterial colonization (45). The relative role of bacteria and viruses in clinical exacerbations of CF respiratory disease has not been defined (46). The importance of fungal colonization with *Aspergillus fumigatus* is becoming more widely recognized but is still largely unknown (47). Finally, and perhaps most importantly, it is not clear how selective viruses, bacteria, fungi, and perhaps other microbial pathogens appear to utilize changes in the local microenvironment arising from the genetic defect of CF to colonize the respiratory mucosal surface.

With respect to the upper respiratory tract, we shall see below that our knowledge of which microbial pathogens colonize the mucosal epithelium is incomplete. We do not know what the relation is between upper and lower respiratory tract colonization. We do not know what the role of microbial colonization is in initiating or sustaining chronic pansinusitis and nasal polyposis, nor why the middle ear is clinically spared. Finally, although we know about control of symptoms and quality of life, we do not know what effective therapy of sinusitis in CF would mean in terms of overall prognosis.

E. Should We Be Aggressive?

Interest in aggressive management of sinusitis has recently emerged as an important element in the care of patients at our CF Center at Stanford. In this approach, the entire respiratory epithelium is conceptualized as a contiguous and relatively uniform mucosal surface vulnerable to infection and inflammation, but also amenable to treatment. The availability of fiberoptic rhinosinuscopy, selective coronal sinus computed tomographic CT imaging, endoscopic sinus surgery, and use of antimicrobial lavage via indwelling antral catheters placed in the maxillary antra, has substantially changed the management of respiratory disease in CF, particularly in adults. The impact of such care upon the course of pulmonary disease remains to be determined.

II. UPPER RESPIRATORY TRACT DISEASE IN CF: SINUSITIS AND POLYPOSIS

A. Nasal Polyps in CF

Although first mentioned in a survey of pathologic conditions associated with CF published in 1952 (48), upper respiratory tract disease in CF received scant attention before the 1960s. In 1956 Claude Pennington, an otolaryngologist at Columbia's Babies' Hospital in New York, pointed out the frequency of nasal suppuration and obstruction in children with CF. He showed examples of maxillary sinus pathologic involvement, emphasizing glandular dilatation and hyperplasia, and mentioned radiographic maxillary sinus opacification in two cases (49). He speculated, prophetically, that glandular malfunction led to chronic infection, that the sinuses were likely reservoirs for bronchopulmonary infection, that the goal of therapy was to reduce infection to a minimum, and that the study of nasal mucosa "may prove to be an excellent means of recording the interval pathologic changes." The past quarter century has borne out much of what Pennington wrote. In 1959, Lurie first reported the occurrence of nasal polyposis in CF patients, remarking on their appearance as early as age 5 (50).

The first major investigation, still widely cited, was Shwachman et al.'s encyclopedic description of nasal polyposis among 742 patients with CF evaluated at the Children's Hospital Medical Center in Boston, published in 1962

Table 1 Prevalence of Nasal Polyposis in Patients with CF

Reference	Site	Year	Patients	Prevalence (%)	
Shwachman et al. (51)	Boston	1962	742	6.7	
				10	>3 yrs old
Rulon and Brown (52)	Mayo	1963	26	28	
Magid et al. (55)	Salt Lake	1967	34	6	
Neely et al. (59)	Houston	1972	93	24	
Taylor et al. (60)	London	1974	50	20	
Cunningham et al. (61)	Chicago	1975	26	27	
			19	36	>5 yrs old
Moler & Thomsem (82)	Copenhagen	1978	161	32	
Bak-Pedersen and Larsen (62)	Copenhagen	1979	111	32	
DiSant'Agnese and Davis (110)	Bethesda	1979	75	48	Adults
Ledesma-Medina et al. (75)	Pittsburgh	1980	187	10	
Stern et al. (87)	Cleveland	1982	605	26	
Lee and Pitcher-Wilmott (89)	London	1982	117	19	
Cepero et al. (64)	Houston	1987	450	10	

(51). In this paper, an incidence of polyposis of 6.7% over a 4 year period was found, with most patients presenting between ages 4 and 13 years (Table 1). No correlation of polyposis and atopy was found, a finding since confirmed repeatedly. The first microbiological results are also to be found in this report: of 45 patients with nasopharyngeal cultures performed, 30 had *S. aureus* and 15 had *P. aeruginosa* identified, with other bacteria found much less often. The first systematic description of results of therapeutic intervention was given, with recurrence of polyps noted in 13 of 31 patients following polypectomy during the study period (Table 2). The pathologic findings of Pennington were confirmed and extended: comparison to polyps from an allergic individual suggested that in CF some changes might be distinct, particularly a lesser degree of epithelial basement membrane thickening and stromal eosinophilia. Sinus radiographs in patients with polyps showed universal opacification (Table 3). This report defined the terrain for subsequent clinical descriptions of upper respiratory tract involvement in CF.

In the decade following the study of Shwachman et al., a series of reports did not add a great deal to the information previously provided (52-58). Mendelsohn and Cohen first reported the use of antral irrigation as a treatment modality in CF, but provided no data on its efficacy (53). They also first reported the ocurrence of a mucocele (a secretory, enlarging cyst lined by epithelium) in a patient with CF who presented with unilateral ocular displacement. Of some interest was their observation that maxillary secretions obtained with antral irrigation in CF were grossly different from that seen in other patients with sinusitis: the CF

Table 2 Recurrence of Nasal Polyposis after Surgery in Patients with CF

Reference	Year	N	Recurrence (%)	Comments
Shwachman et al. (51)	1962	31	40	After polypectomy (P), as early as 3 wks
Jaffe et al. (85)	1977	23	87	2 mos–8 yr after P
		9	45	1–5 yr after P + ethmoidectomy (E)
		10	60	1–5 yr after P + E + nasoantral windows
		5	0	One yr after P + Caldwell-Luc (CL) procedure
Schram and Effron (111)	1980	35	40	Less recurrence with more extensive surgery
Stern et al. (87)	1982	95	67	31% spontaneous disappearance if not operated upon (? duration)
Reilly et al. (76)	1985	39	59	Average 2.1 procedures/patient (range, 1–12)
Cepero et al. (64)	1987	22	61	Less recurrence with more extensive surgery
Crockett et al. (86)	1987	92	78	P alone within 18 months (most at 7–12 mo)
			89	P along with 8 year follow-up
			3	P + E ± CL within 18 months
			35	P + E ± CL with 8 year follow-up
Cuyler (80)	1992	10	20	2-3 years after endoscopic surgery (P + antrostomy + partial E)

N = patients, except for in Crockett et al., where n = procedures

Table 3 Prevalence of Radiographic Sinusitis in Patients with CF[a]

Reference	Site	Year	Patients	Prevalence (%)
Shwachman et al. (51)	Boston	1962	50	93
Gharib et al. (54)	Denver	1964	53	92
Magid et al. (55)	Salt Lake City	1967	28	100
Neely et al. (59)	Houston	1972	81	100
Cunningham et al. (61)	Chicago	1975	26	100
Ledesma-Medina et al. (75)	Pittsburgh	1980	187	99
Reilly et al. (76)	Pittsburgh	1985	35	100
Cepero et al. (64)	Houston	1987	50	100
Cuyler and Monaghan (78)	Edmonton	1989	10	100

[a]All imaging by plain films except for Cuyler and Munaghan's coronal sinus CT study.

secretions were described as "characteristic grayish-green pasty putty-like material with a musty odor" (53). Gharib et al. conducted the first systemic radiographic investigation of CF sinuses, finding that 49 of 53 patients had asymptomatic radiographic abnormalities, most commonly bilateral maxillary and ethmoid opacification (Table 3) (54). Magid et al. observed normal ciliary motility in excised CF nasal polyp epithelium under phase contrast microscopy (55).

B. The Middle Ear in CF

In 1972 Neely et al. reported on 93 patients with CF evaluated at Baylor in Houston (59). This study is of interest for a number of reasons. The first systemic results of otologic and audiometric studies in CF were reported. These were uniformly normal. Neely et al. raised the intriguing and still unanswered question of why, given the presence of an epithelium morphologically similar to that in the rest of the respiratory tract, the middle ear is clinically spared in CF. Second, Neely et al. briefly described a novel treatment program in two patients consisting of surgical placement of nasoantral windows followed by temporary placement of indwelling antral catheters for maxillary irrigation. Details of this treatment and its outcome were not mentioned. Third, Neely et al.'s study was the first to suggest that mucocele formation may be a common and important complication of sinusitis in CF: 17 patients were thought to have mucocele development. (The basis for this judgment was, however, not described.) Finally, a histopathologic differentiation of CF from non-CF polyps was suggested on the basis of general lack of basement membrane thickening and eosinophilic stromal infiltrates in CF, in agreement with Shwachman et al.

The relative lack of middle ear disease in CF, an impression widely shared by clinicians and established by Neely et al., has been confirmed in subsequent studies (60-65). Direct clinical otologic and audiometric observations recently received interesting indirect objective substantiation in a study of the degree of temporal bone pneumatization by computed tomographic imaging. Patients with CF had significantly greater pneumatization volume than normal controls, an indication of a reduced incidence and/or severity of otitis media (65).

Taylor et al. speculated that the frequent use of antibiotics is more effective in preventing otitis media than sinusitis or bronchitis in patients with CF (60). This seems to beg the question of why such a differential therapeutic effect should be observed. The density of mucus-secreting glands does not appear to be the basis of the effect either, since gland density is highest in nasal mucosa and lowest in sinus mucosa, yet chronic sinusitis is essentially inherent to CF (66).

Another possibility that holds some promise of shedding light on the pathogenesis of CF respiratory tract disease has to do with the function of mucus-secreting goblet cells. The nose, sinuses, and bronchi have a relatively uniform distribution of goblet cells in their epithelium (66). In contrast, the eustachian tube and middle ear cavity, according to one quantitative study, have lower numbers of goblet cells relative to ciliated epithelial cells and other cell types in normal individuals (67). Although mucosal cell types have not been quantitated in the upper respiratory tract of patients with CF, it seems unlikely that gross alterations in distribution will be found given generally comparable epithelial morphology of CF and atopic polyps or neonatal CF and normal bronchial epithelium. However, if goblet cells are an important cell type for CFTR expression and function, a lesser role in normal middle ear function, resulting from diminished proportional numbers, could manifest itself in lesser disease involvement clinically in patients with CF. At present, the distribution of CFTR expression and function among the various cell types of the respiratory epithelium is under study.

C. Histopathologic Appearance of CF Polyps

Nonsystematic comparisons of CF and non-CF (usually atopic) polyps such as those cited above suggested possible differentiating morphologic differences (51,59). A lesser degree of basement membrane thickening and stromal eosinophilic infiltrate has been reported, but most earlier studies were essentially anecdotal and impressionistic (49,51-52,55,59). CF polyps have been found by some investigators to have a greater number of mucus-secreting glands, often filled with inspissated secretions. Tos et al. performed the first careful quantitative comparison of mucus glands from CF and non-CF polyps in 1977. In this study, gland density, number, distribution, and architecture were all comparable in the two groups. Even though almost all CF polyps lacked eosinophilic infiltration in the stroma, a majority (59%) of non-CF polyps also lacked eosinophilia, and in both groups stromal infiltration by lymphocytes and plasmacytes was present in most specimens. In short, blinded review of polyps by light microscopy could not reliably differentiate CF from non-CF specimens (69). In contrast, Oppenheimer and Rosenstein identified three distinguishing histologic features of CF polyps. (70). First, CF polyps were found, as previously suggested, to have thinner epithelial basement membranes. Second, CF polyps lacked extensive eosinophilic infiltration on Giemsa stains (prior studies used hematoxylin–eosin, a less specific stain for eosinophils). Third, although CF polyps did not consistently display more mucous glands, the mucin contained in them and on the epithelial surface of the polyp was more acidic in CF specimens with Alcian blue–periodic acid–Schiff staining. However, Oppenheimer and Rosenstein did not apply their criteria to a blinded analysis of specimens (70).

The increased acidity of CF mucins in nasal polyps is consistent with other reports of increased acidity of mucins from lower respiratory tract secretions in CF. This observation has been attributed to the effect of infection and inflammation, which results in a more highly sulfated and acidic mucinous secretory product in diseases such as asthma and chronic bronchitis, as well as in CF. Therefore, this finding appeared secondary and thus seemed to shed little light on the pathogenesis of CF.

However, in 1974 Boat et al. described increased sulfation of mucinous glycoproteins secreted by CF nasal polyp epithelium maintained in an explant organ culture system, raising at least the possibility that increased mucin sulfation could be a primary manifestation of CF (71). Of note, these explants contained few glands, and it seems likely the mucins analyzed were mostly derived from epithelial goblet cells. This line of investigation recently received powerful support from similar results obtained under long-term cell culture conditions, in which secondary effects of infection and inflammation appear to be excluded (72). It remains unclear how oversulfation of CF mucins is related to CFTR function. As in the case of the spared middle ear, however, there is a hint that the goblet cell may play an important role in this aspect of CF pathophysiology. The only published electron microscopic analysis of CF nasal polyps appears to support this role by suggesting pathologic mucus formation in goblet cells (73). In fact, this study, published in 1977 by Jahnke and Theopold in Munich, is impressive for their conclusion, based on morphologic analysis alone, that "a disturbance of membrane transport or in the dilution of the secretions must be assumed," an analysis supported by current CF research.

Recent electron micrographic studies comparing CF and non-CF polyps by Beju et al. have further contributed to our understanding of the cellular pathologic basis (74). Both CF and non-CF polyps possess a pseudostratified colum-

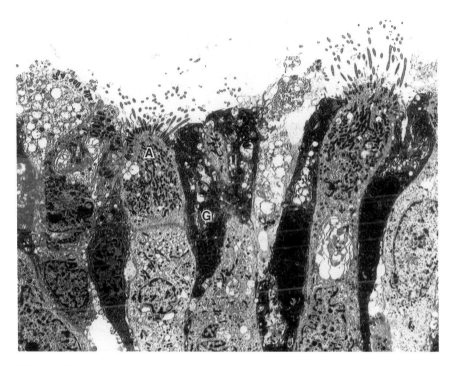

Figure 1 Electron micrograph (3500 ×) of nasal polyp epithelium from patient with CF shows pseudostratified columnar epithelium with ciliated cell (A) and emptied goblet cell (G) (courtesy of D. Beju, Saint Francis Hospital of Tulsa Medical Research Institute).

nar epithelium generously endowed with secreting goblet cells (Fig. 1). Additional ultrastructural characteristics common to CF and non-CF include the following:

1. Intraepithelial edema (Fig. 2)
2. Squamous metaplasia (Fig. 3)
3. Neutrophilic or eosinophilic mucosal and submucosal infiltration (Fig. 4)
4. Varying degrees of stromal fibrosis (Fig. 4)
5. Occasional hyperplastic mucous glands
6. Aberrant cilia (Fig. 5)

In addition, CF polyps exhibit several distinct features at the ultrastructural level when compared to non-CF polyps:

1. Relative epithelial integrity, whereas non-CF epithelium is often eroded (Fig. 6)

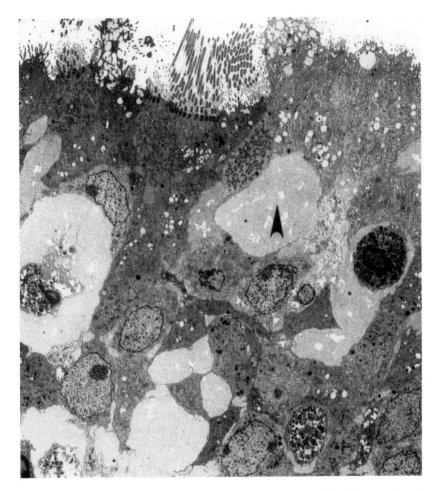

Figure 2   Electron micrograph (2428 ×) of nasal polyp epithelium from patient with CF shows intraepithelial edema (arrowhead) (courtesy of D. Beju, Saint Francis Hospital of Tulsa Medical Research Institute).

2. A predominantly plasmacytic and mast cell mucosal and submucosal infiltrate (Fig. 7), with a high incidence of metabolically active plasmacytes (indicated by extensive and distended rough endoplasmic reticulum) and mast cells (indicated by degranulation) (Fig. 8)
3. Extensive focal inflammation in the stroma
4. A higher incidence of small blood vessels
5. Occasional unmyelinated nerve endings near mucous glands and vessels

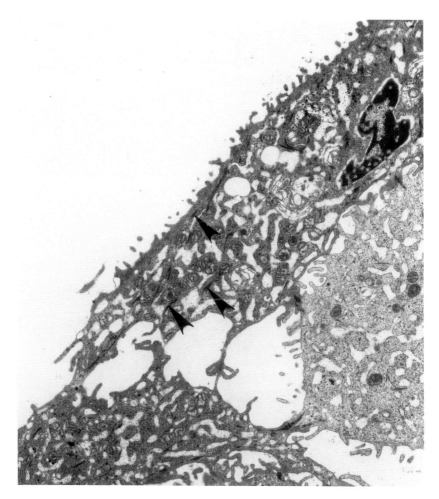

Figure 3   Electron micrograph (8640 ×) of nasal polyp epithelium from patient with CF shows squamous metaplasia with flattened epithelial cell (A) that shows loss of polarity and intracytoplasmic tonofilaments (arrow) (courtesy of D. Beju, Saint Francis Hospital of Tulsa Medical Research Institute).

6.   Intraluminal accumulation of a dense secretory product in mucous glands

The apparently unique profile of infiltrating inflammatory cell types in CF polyps seems to suggest that products of plasmacytes (i.e., antibodies or non specific immunoglobulin) and/or mast cells (i.e., mediators of allergic inflammation such as histamine and leukotrienes) may play a role in the pathogenesis

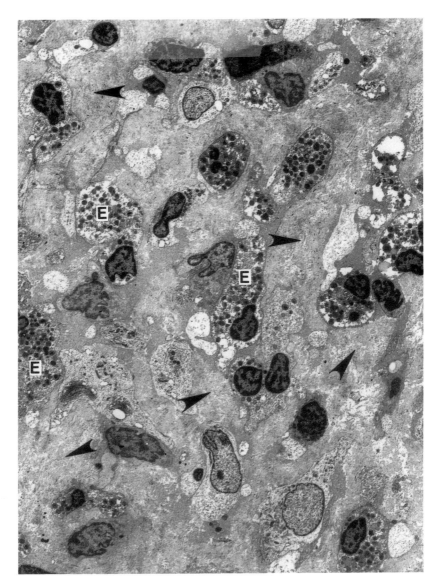

Figure 4   Electron micrograph (2124 ×) of nasal polyp stroma from patient with CF
shows focal eosinophilic infiltration of the submucosa (E) and fibrosis (arrow) (courtesy
of D. Beju, Saint Francis Hospital of Tulsa Medical Research Institute).

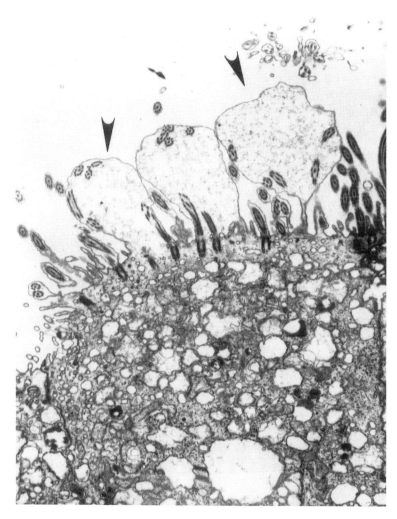

Figure 5   Electron micrograph (9400 ×) of nasal polyp epithelium from patient with CF shows aberrant compound cilia (arrowheads) (courtesy of D. Beju, Saint Francis Hospital of Tulsa Medical Research Institute).

of these lesions. However, direct measurements of these or other soluble proinflammatory molecules have not been made.

D. Sinusitis in CF

As summarized earlier, the observation of sinusitis in association with CF goes back at least to 1956, and radiographic surveys have indicated that sinusitis is

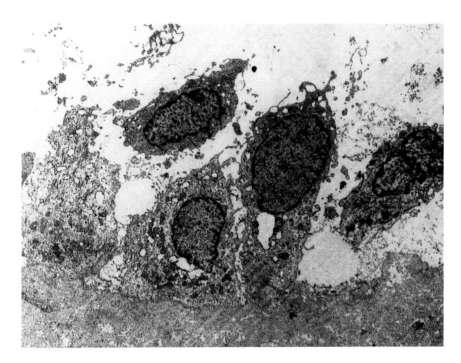

Figure 6   Electron micrograph (5100 ×) of nasal polyp epithelium from control subject without CF shows focal erosion (courtesy of D. Beju, Saint Francis Hospital of Tulsa Medical Research Institute).

very nearly universal in CF, with a prevalence of 92–100% (Table 3) (51,54-55,,59,61,64,75,76). The few cases in the literature in which plain films did not demonstrate sinusitis must be questioned in light of evidence from coronal computed tomography (CT) that plain sinus films can miss significant sinus disease, especially ostiomeatal and anterior ethmoid pathologic involvement (77). Indeed, recent studies employing sinus CT in selected patients with CF have found universal occurrence of sinusitis by this sensitive imaging technique (78-80).

One of the difficulties in assessing the problem of sinusitis in patients with CF is the impression of many clinicians that this is often an asymptomatic phenomenon, and therefore of questionable clinical importance. Moreover, given the life-threatening nature of pulmonary and gastrointestinal involvment, it is often regarded as no more than a trivial nuisance. Perhaps because of this attitude, systematic attempts to quantify incidence or severity of symptoms referable to nasal or sinus disease in CF are virtually nonexistent in the literature. Neely et al. described ''severe'' nasal symptoms in 20% of their 93 patients (i.e., continuous nasal congestion, purulent postnasal drip, frequent morning

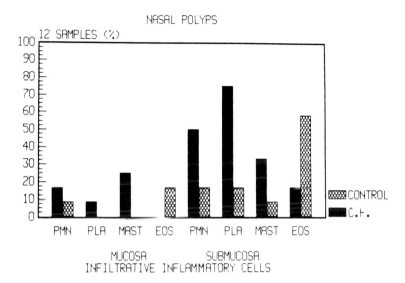

Figure 7   Differential distribution of inflammatory cell types in nasal polyp mucosa (*left*) and submucosa (*right*) from CF and non-CF and control subjects. PMN, neutrophils; PLA, plasmacytes; MAST, mast cells; EOS, eosinophils (data courtesy of D. Beju, Saint Francis Hospital of Tulsa Medical Research Institute).

coughing or gagging), and "mild" symptoms in all but 6 of the remainder (i.e., nasal congestion, postnasal drip, and rhinorrhea). No symptoms specifically referable to sinusitis were described except for one severe case with mucocele formation displacing the eyes (59). Taylor found a "history of sinusitis" (no details given) in 8 of 50 patients (16%) (60). Cepero et al. diagnosed clinical sinusitis based on physical findings of tenderness, fever, pain, and postnasal discharge in 50 of 450 cases (11%) (64). Thus, one could easily conclude that patients with CF are not seriously troubled by their virtually universal sinus opacification and frequent polyposis.

However, there are sound reasons to doubt this downgrading of the upper respiratory problems of patients with CF. In fact, this disregard could in part be a result of the attention given by patient, family, and physician to other more immediately concerning manifestations of CF. Second, given the lack of effective therapeutic interventions until recently (see below), the patient as well as the physician has a difficult time knowing how to place nasal or sinus symptoms in perspective. Could not anosmia, congestion, intermittent headache, postnasal drip, and other symptoms just be regarded as essentially trivial "facts of life" in CF? Third, it is clear that pain as an index of disease cannot be relied upon when approaching sinusitis, since chronic inflammation may well cause little pain

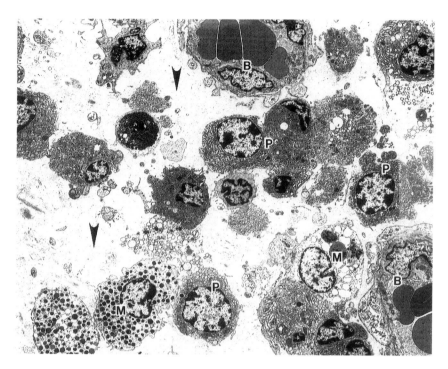

Figure 8   Electron micrograph (2700 ×) of nasal polyp submucosa from patient with CF shows focal accumulation of plasmacytes (P) and mast cells (M). Blood vessels (B) and collagen fibrils (arrowheads) are also visible. Note metabolic activity of plasmacytes (indicated by profusion of endoplasmic reticulum, *center*) and mast cells (indicated by degranulation, *lower right*) (data courtesy of D. Beju, Saint Francis Hospital of Tulsa Medical Research Institute).

(often no pain), and is to be contrasted with the sometimes excruciating pain of acute sinusitis associated with rapid changes in ostiomeatal patency and mucosal swelling (81).

It is also clear that untreated sinusitis in patients with CF can lead to complications. The most common of these appears to be mucocele formation, first reported in 1964 (53). Neely et al. reported an incidence of 18%, but the criteria for diagnosis were not specified (59). Bony destruction and compromise of the orbit usually lead to the diagnosis (82). Mucocele may be the presenting sign of CF and may occur as early as early infancy (83,84).

E. Therapy of Sinusitis and Polyposis in CF

Early attempts at surgical treatment by simple polypectomy, described above, led to an appreciation of the high likelihood of recurrence and a search for alternative treatment methods. Recurrences of polyps after conventional sinus surgery, summarized in Table 2, indicate that more extensive sinus surgery decreases the likelihood of recurrence. Jaffe et al., summarizing the experience at Boston Children's Hospital to the mid-1970s, found that addition of ethmoidectomy with or without nasoantral window formation decreased recurrence of polyps from 87% to 45–60%, and also suggested that the most radical procedure, the Caldwell-Luc operation, might further diminish recurrences (85). This experience appears to be confirmed by subsequent experience at the same institution, where Crockett et al. reported in 1987 that addition of ethmoidectomy and (in some cases) Caldwell-Luc operation reduced recurrences by over 50% (86). In general, nasal surgery in patients with CF can be performed safely if careful attention to general care is maintained (64,76).

Enthusiasm for extensive sinus surgery must, however, be tempered by at least two major developments in the therapy of sinusitis. Before discussing them, it is also necessary to account for the data of Stern et al., who reported an astonishing 31% rate of spontaneous disappearance of polyps in patients with CF in Cleveland (87). This study seems to me to be seriously, if not fatally, flawed by its methodology. Data were obtained by retrospective chart review and patient/family interview. In this study, there is no objective verification if polyps were in fact definitively identified, or how their "disappearance" was verified. There is no evidence that physical examinations were performed. There is no corroborating evidence elsewhere in the literature that polyps of patients with CF spontaneously regress or disappear.

The advent of effective and nontoxic intranasal steroid sprays such as beclomethasone dipropionate offers some hope for nonsurgical management of polyposis in at least some cases (68). Only one systematic attempt to treat nasal symptoms with topical steroids has been reported (88). In this study, 100 μ beclomethasone per nostril twice daily produced improvement in nasal symptoms in 11 of 14 patients without polyps and disappearance or regression of polyps in 10 of 16 patients. However, duration of follow-up was either unreported or short-term (3 months). Based on these preliminary data, a trial of intranasal steroids seems advisable as initial therapy of nasal symptoms with or without polyps in patients with CF. There are no systemic data on other medical therapy including antibiotics, decongestants, antihistamines, or mucoevacuants. Although specific allergic management should be part of the therapeutic plan for atopic patients, there is no evidence that patients with CF with polyps are more likely to be allergic than patients with CF without polyps (89).

With the development of functional endoscopic sinus surgery (FESS) in the mid-1980s, new hopes arose for more successful and less invasive surgical treatment of nasal–sinus disease in CF (78,90,92). FESS offers theoretical advantages of safety, decreased postoperative morbidity, preservation of physiological mucosal function, and, perhaps most importantly, intervention at the critical site of disease pathogenesis in otherwise healthy individuals (92). Cuyler and

Monaghan reported on the safety of FESS in seven patients with CF (ages 3–19 years) (78). Unfortunately, a recent follow-up report showed recurrence or persistence of sinusitis in all seven patients when studied by CT 2–3 years later, despite variable improvement in symptoms (80).

A unique approach was developed at Stanford in the late 1980s that combines the theoretical benefits of FESS with other modalities (79). Our efforts have been spurred by the success of an aggressive approach to sinusitis in CF in controlling symptoms of reactive airways disease, prednisone use, and hospitalization rates in selected patients with CF (93). This approach has also reduced the incidence of pneumonia in patients with CF following double lung or heart–lung transplantation. (94).

This approach combines the use of FESS with other interventions mentioned in the literature but never systematically applied, namely use of antral lavage and indwelling antral catheters (Fig. 9) (56,59). After preoperative evaluation by rhinoscopy and coronal CT imaging, FESS is performed with endoscopic ethmoidectomy, transnasal antrostomy (Fig. 10) and, if necessary, partial inferior turbinectomy. Indwelling catheters are placed into the maxillary antra and a 7–10 day course of lavage with antibiotics is performed in concert with treatment of lower respiratory tract infection. The external appearance after catheter placement is illustrated in Figure 11, and an endoscopic view of catheter lavage via the antrostomy is shown in Figure 12. At surgery, highly inspissated purulent secretions adherent to the inflamed mucosa are removed from the maxillary antra under direct endoscopic visualization (Figs. 13, 14). After removal of secretions, severe mucosal hyperplasia can often be easily seen (Fig. 15).

For the typical patient with aminoglycoside-sensitive *P. aeruginosa* growing in sinus secretions obtained at surgery, tobramycin is instilled into each maxillary antrum at a dosage of 40 mg three times daily during the initial postoperative treatment course. After removal of the catheters the patient is evaluated closely. Most patients require subsequent outpatient single-dose bilateral lavage via temporarily placed catheters with antibiotics at 2–4 week intervals to maintain control of symptoms and prevent recurrence of antral opacification. With this regimen both subjective and objective control of upper respiratory tract disease can be maintained for months to years (95). Figure 16 shows the CT appearance of the sinuses before and 10 months after institution of this treatment regimen in one of our patients who had resolution of symptoms of congestion, rhinorrhea, postnasal drip, headache, and paroxysmal morning cough. The effect of this treatment program on pulmonary manifestations and respiratory bacteriologic results is being investigated. Since institution of this program, the recurrence rate for polyposis has fallen to below 10%; comparable figures for recurrence of sinusitis are not available since follow-up CT has not been routinely performed.

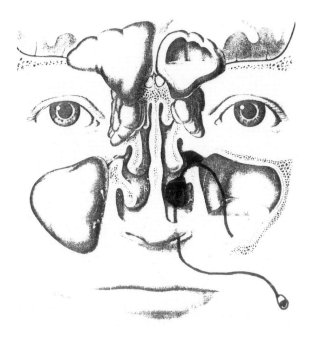

Figure 9   Illustration of use of indwelling antral catheters for topical therapy of maxillary sinusitis following functional endoscopic transnasal antrostomy (courtesy of Jeffrey Wine, Stanford University).

F. Infection and Sinusitis in CF

Despite the acknowledged importance of endobronchial infection in the pathogenesis of CF lung disease, there is surprisingly sparse information available on the nature and role of infection in the sinusitis of patients with CF. The first study to report results of bacterial cultures obtained directly from the maxillary antrum, acquired during sinus surgery, was that of Jaffe et al. (85). They reported that of 13 patients studied, normal oral flora was grown from 4 despite grossly purulent appearance of the secretions, and they attributed this to concurrent antibiotic therapy. Pathogens included *P. aeruginosa* (2), *E. coli* (2), alpha *Streptococcus* (2), nonencapsulated *H. influenzae* (1), diphtheroids (1), and *Streptococcus faecalis* (1). They also stated that there was no correlation between sinus and throat, sputum, or bronchial cultures, but provided no data.

Shapiro et al. studied 20 patients using quantitative aerobic and anaerobic bacterial cultures of samples obtained via transantral aspiration, 14 of these being bilateral punctures (96). In contrast to Jaffe et al., these investigators found pathogens at densities suggestive of pathogenicity for infection ($\geq 10^4$

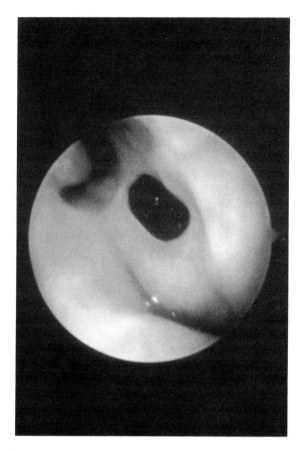

Figure 10 Endoscopic appearance of transnasal antrostomy (courtesy of Victoria King, Stanford University).

colony-forming units/ml) in 95% of patients, with *P. aeruginosa* being the most common organism (13 aspirates), followed by *H. influenzae* (10), streptococci (5), and anaerobes (5). In addition, 9 of 10 patients were taking antibiotics to which the organism was sensitive in vitro prior to the procedure, indicating the ineffectiveness of systemic antibiotics in penetrating the maxillary cavity adequately. The majority of aspirates contained only one pathogen, although 21% contained two organisms.

An important corollary conclusion of Shapiro et al. was that there was no association between the bacterial species recovered from the sinus and the predominant bacterial species in routine nasopharyngeal, throat, or sputum cultures "interpreted semiquantitatively" (96).

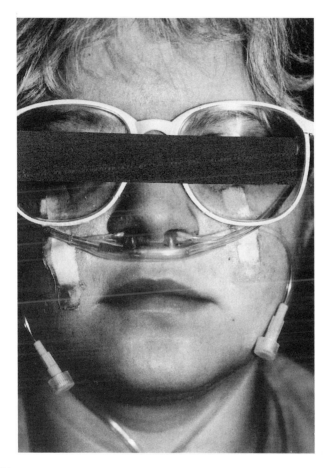

Figure 11   External appearance of indwelling maxillary catheters in patient with CF following functional endoscopic sinus surgery. Patient is also receiving supplemental oxygen via nasal cannula for chronic obstructive lung disease (courtesy of Victoria King, Stanford University).

This conclusion deserves close scrutiny because, as in the study of Jaffe et al., it suggests that microbial colonization of the sinuses and the remainder of the respiratory tract is dichotomous rather than uniform in patients with CF. Such a finding would imply differences in mucosal properties in these sites that seem important in understanding the pathogenesis of cystic fibrosis respiratory disease. For example, Plotkowski et al. have recently shown that *P. aeruginosa* does not adhere differentially to nasal polyp cells in primary culture from CF and non-CF sources, but that mucin secretion by CF cells may be increased

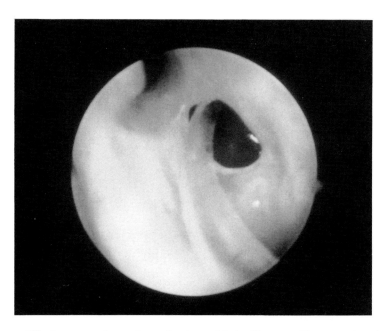

Figure 12 Intraoperative endoscopic view of indwelling maxillary antral cathether following placement through antrostomy in patient with CF (courtesy of Victoria King, Stanford University).

compared to normal, and could result in increased aggregation of *P. aeruginosa*, favoring successful mucosal colonization (97). The clinical significance of these findings depends in no small degree upon the extent to which they reflect a general property of respiratory epithelium, or only represent a regional phenomenon. Shapiro et al. base their conclusion on the fact that organisms grown from the sinus were "predominant" in nasopharyngeal, throat, or sputum cultures in only three patients (16%). However, they were "present but not predominant" in 13 other patients (68%) and absent in only 3 patients' cultures (16%). Adding the first two categories would give a concordance of 84%, which would yield a conclusion opposite to that of the authors. The problem lies in the assumption in this study that the routine cultures from nasopharyngeal, throat, and sputum sites "interpreted semiquantitatively" are comparable or equivalent to quantitative cultures from sinus aspirates. This is an erroneous assumption, since it is known that "semiquantitative" cultures such as those used in this study to characterize nasopharyngeal, throat, and sputum flora do *not* correlate with quantitative cultures using selective media, which yield an accurate picture of the

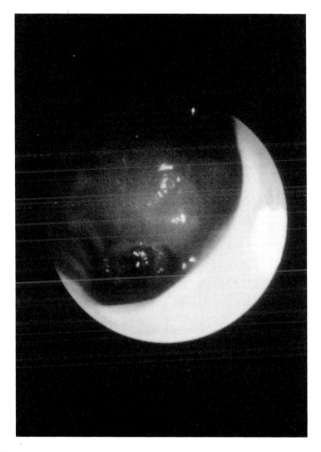

Figure 13 Intraoperative endoscopic appearance of maxillary secretions in patient with CF show highly viscid dark adherent secretions on lower lateral maxillary mucosa (courtesy of Victoria King, Stanford University).

actual bacterial ecology (98). In our own studies employing similar culture methodology of sinus aspirates obtained at endoscopic surgery and sputum, a high concordance of colonization with *P. aeruginosa* (>80%) has been found (95). Our results also contrast with the frequent inability to grow organisms from sputum as well as sinus aspirates in a recent study of 10 patients from London (99). Ultimately, genotyping ("DNA fingerprinting") of *P. aeruginosa* from sinus aspirates, throat, and sputum will be necessary to resolve the issue of whether the CF upper and lower respiratory tracts are homogeneous with respect to colonization properties or not (100).

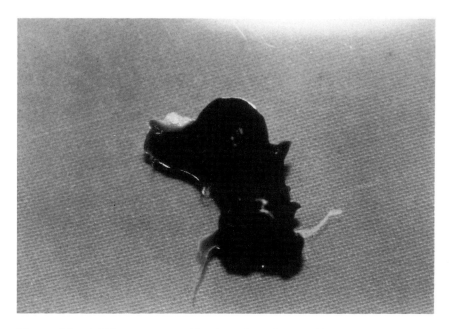

Figure 14   Gel-like appearance of inspissated purulent maxillary secretions from patient with CF after removal during functional endoscopic sinus surgery. Cultures grew mucoid *P. aeruginosa*, as did sputum culture (courtesy of Victoria King, Stanford University).

III. CF RESEARCH AND THE UPPER RESPIRATORY TRACT

We have seen that the nose and sinuses are deeply involved by clinical manifestations of CF. It seems only fitting, therefore, to note the great importance this tissue has played in both in vitro and in vivo studies of CF molecular and cellular pathophysiology. Most of the important work demonstrating in vivo electrophysiological differences differentiating CF from non-CF epithelia was obtained from measurements made on ciliated pseudostratified epithelium of the inferior nasal turbinate by Michael Knowles, Richard Boucher, and colleagues at the University of North Carolina (UNC) (9,11,101). These studies, along with in vitro studies of isolated sweat glands, established the electrophysiological basis of CF in an abnormally low Cl⁻ permeability of the apical membrane of surface epithelial cells.

Better understanding of pathogenesis is dependent upon laboratory-based methodologies. Rudimentary efforts at in vitro studies of CF nasal epithelium using short-term organ explant cultures were described in the 1960s and 1970s (51,71). In the last several years successful cell culture systems for differenti-

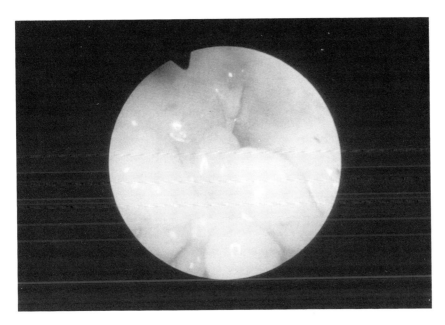

Figure 15 Intraoperative endoscopic appearance of maxillary antral mucosa in patient with CF after lavage and removal of adherent inspissated purulent secretions. Note gross mucosal inflammation and hypertrophy with possible early mucocele formation (courtesy of Victoria King, Stanford University).

ated dissociated nasal epithelial cells derived from excised polyps have been achieved by the UNC group and others (102,103). The Cl⁻ transport abnormalities observed in vivo are retained in vitro by nasal epithelial cells cultured on collagen matrix supports, in plastic tissue culture dishes, or in heterologous grafts (104-106). These studies established that the defects were intrinsic to the epithelium and not due to circulating or local soluble factors or secondary effects of disease.

Clinical applicability of transepithelial nasal potential difference measurements was recently independently confirmed, although the technical difficulties involved are considerable (107). In selected cases, nasal potential difference may be a useful adjunct to the standard pilocarpine iontophoresis sweat test in the diagnosis of CF. Such cases could include individuals in whom the sweat test is nondiagnostic, and in neonates in whom sweat is difficult to obtain (108). The recent explosion of genetic knowledge of CFTR mutations also raises interesting possibilities for genotype–phenotype studies. Finally, the possibility of exploiting the accessibility of the nasal and sinus epithelium for studies of novel

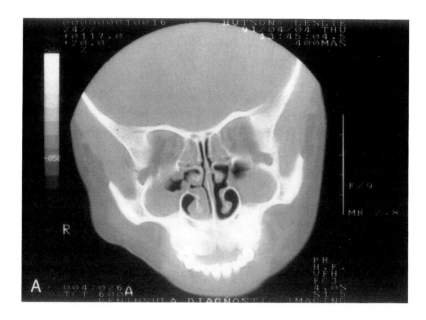

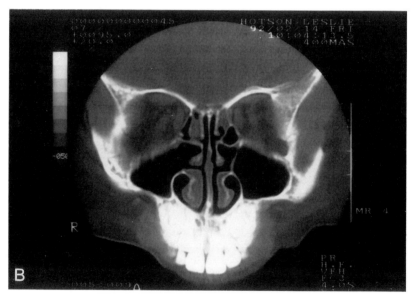

Figure 16   Coronal computed tomographic view of sinuses before (A) and 10 months after (B) institution of treatment regimen consisting of initial functional endoscopic sinus surgery, 1 week course of sinus lavage three times daily with tobramycin via indwelling antral catheters, and monthly maintenance outpatient lavages in patient with CF whose sinus aspirate culture grew mucoid *P. aeruginosa* sensitive to tobramycin in vitro.

therapeutic interventions has been raised, offering the prospect that the upper respiratory tract may be the proving ground for CF therapies of the future (109).

ACKNOWLEDGMENTS

I thank my Stanford colleagues Jeffrey Wine, Ph.D., Victoria King, M.D., Dale Umetsu M.D., Ph.D., Judy Palmer, M.D., Robert Bocian, M.D., Ph.D., and the late Norman Lewiston, M.D., for many helpful ideas and comments. Dr. King provided many fine photographs illustrating functional endoscopic sinus surgery. I am greatly indebted to Delia Beju, Ph.D., of the Saint Francis Hospital of Tulsa Medical Research Institute in Tulsa, Oklahoma, for generously sharing unpublished electron micrographs detailing the ultrastructure of nasal polyps and data derived from related cytopathologic studies.

REFERENCES

1. Collins FS. Cystic fibrosis: molecular biology and therapeutic implications. Science 1992; 256:774–9.
2. Riordan JR, Rommens JM, Kerem B, Alon N, Rozmahel R, Grzelack Z, Zielenski J, Lok S, Plavsic N, Chou J-L, Drumm M, Iannuzi MC, Collins FS, Tsui L-C. Identification of the cystic fibrosis gene: cloning and characterization of complementary DNA. Science 1989; 245:1066–73.
3. Kerem BS, Rommens JM, Buchanan JA, Markiewicz D, Cox TK, Chakravarti A, Buchwald M, Tsui L-C. Identification of the cystic fibrosis gene: genetic analysis. Science 1989; 245:1073–80.
4. Cutting GR, Kash LM, Rosenstein BJ, Zielenski J, Tsui L-C, Antonarkis SE, Kazazian HH. A cluster of cystic fibrosis mutations in the first nucleotide-binding fold of the cystic fibrosis conductance regulator. Nature 1990; 346:366–9.
5. Lemna WK, Feldman GL, Kerem B, Fernbach SD, Zevkovich EP, O'Brien WE, Collins FS, Tsui L-C, Beaudet AL. Mutation analysis for heterozygote detection and the prenatal diagnosis of cystic fibrosis. N Engl J Med 1990; 322:291–6.
6. Statement from National Institutes of Health Workshop on population screening for the cystic fibrosis gene. N Engl J Med 1990; 323:70–1.
7. Wilfond BS, Fost N. The cystic fibrosis gene: medical and social implications for heterozygote detection. JAMA 1990; 263:2777–83.
8. Tizzano EF, Buchwald M. Cystic fibrosis: beyond the gene to therapy. J Pediatr 1992; 120:337–49.
9. Knowles MR, Gatzy JT, Boucher RC. Increased bioelectric potential difference across respiratory epithelia in cystic fibrosis. N Engl J Med 1981; 305:1489–95.
10. Quinton PM, Bijman J. Higher bioelectric potentials due to decreased chloride absorption in the sweat glands of patients with cystic fibrosis. N Engl J Med 1983; 308:1185–9.
11. Knowles M, Gatzy J, Boucher R. Relative ion permeability of normal and cystic fibrosis nasal epithelium. J Clin Invest 1983; 71:1410–7.
12. Sato K, Sato F. Defective beta adrenergic response of cystic fibrosis sweat glands in vivo and in vitro. J Clin Invest 1984; 73:1763–71.

13. Welsh MJ, Liedtke CM. Chloride and potassium channels in cystic fibrosis airway epithelium. Nature 1986; 322:467–70.
14. Frizzell RA, Rechkemmer G, Shoemaker RL. Altered regulation of airway epithelial cell chloride channels in cystic fibrosis. Science 1986; 233:558–60.
15. Boucher RC, Stutts MJ, Knowles MR, Cantley L, Gatzy JT. Na$^+$ transport in cystic fibrosis respiratory epithelia: abnormal basal rate and response to adenlyate cyclase. J Clin Invest 1986; 78:1245–52.
16. Schoumacher RA, Shoemaker RL, Halm DR, Tallant EA, Wallace RW, Frizell RA. Phosphorylation fails to activate chloride channels from cystic fibrosis airway cells. Nature 1987; 330:752–4.
17. Li M, McCann J, Liedtke C, Nairn A, Greengard P, Welsh M. Cyclic AMP-dependent protein kinase opens chloride channels in normal but not cystic fibrosis airway epithelium. Nature 1988; 331:358–60.
18. Hwang T-C, Lu L, Zeitlin PL, Gruenert DC, Huganir R, Guggino WB, Cl⁻ channels in CF: lack of activation by protein kinase C and cAMP-dependent protein kinase. Science 1989; 244:1351–3.
19. Li M. McCann J, Anderson M, Clancy J, Liedtke C, Nairn A, Greengard P, Welsh M. Regulation of chloride channels by protein kinase C in normal and cystic fibrosis airway epithelia. Science 1989; 244:1353–6.
20. Quinton PM. Cystic fibrosis: a disease in electrolyte transport. FASEB J 1990; 4:2709–17.
21. Welsh MJ. Abnormal regulation of ion channels in cystic fibrosis epithelia. FASEB J 1990; 4:2718–25.
22. Knowles MR, Church NL, Waltner WE, Yankaskas JR, Gilligan P, King M, Edwards LJ, Helms RW, Boucher RC, A pilot study of aerosolized amiloride for the treatment of lung disease in cystic fibrosis. N Engl J Med 1990; 322:1189–94.
23. Knowles MR, Clarke LL, Boucher RC. Activation by extracellular nucleotides of chloride secretion in the airway epithelia of patients with cystic fibrosis. N Engl Med 1991; 325:533–8.
24. Drumm ML, Wilkinson DJ, Smit LS, Worrell RT, Strong TV, Frizell RA, Dawson DC, Collins FS. Chloride conductance expressed by δF508 and other mutant CFTRs in *Xenopus* oocytes. Science 1991; 254:1797–9.
25. Dalemans W, Barbry P, Champigny G, Jallat S, Dott K, Dreyer D, Crystal RG, Pavirani A, Lazdunski M, Lecocq J-P. Altered Cl⁻ channel kinetics associated with major (Delta-F508) cystic fibrosis mutation. Nature 1991; 354:526–8.
26. Drumm ML, Pope H, Cliff WH, Rommens JM, Marvin SA, Tsui L-C, Collins FS, Frizell RA, Wilson JM. Correction of the cystic fibrosis defect *in vitro* by retrovirus-mediated gene transfer. Cell 1990; 62:1227–33.
27. Gregory RJ. Cheng SH, Rich DP, Marshall J, Paul S, Hehir K, Ostedgaard L, Klinger KW, Welsh MJ, Smith AE. Expression and characterization of the cystic fibrosis transmembrane conductance regulator. Nature 1990; 347:382–6.
28. Rich DP, Anderson MP, Gregory RJ, Cheng SH, Paul S, Jefferson DM, McCann JD, Klinger DW, Smith AE, Welsh MJ. Expression of cystic fibrosis transmembrane conductance regulator corrects defective chloride channel regulation in cystic fibrosis airway epithelial cells. Nature 1990; 347:258–65.

29. Cheng SH, Gregory RJ, Marshall J, Paul S, Souza DW, White GA, O'Riordan CT, Smith AE. Defective intracellular transport and processing of CFTR is the molecular basis of most cystic fibrosis. Cell 1990; 63:827–34.

30. Rosenfeld MA, Yoshimura K, Trapnell BC, Yoneyama K, Rosenthal ER, Dalemans W, Fukayama M, Bargon J, Stier LE, Straford-Perricaudet LD, Perricaudet M, Jallat S, Mercenier A, Pavirani A, Lecocq J-P, Guggino WB, Crystal RG. *In vivo* transfer of the human cystic fibrosis gene to the respiratory epithelium. Cell 1992; 68:143–55.

31. Hyde SC, Emsley P, Hasthorn MJ, Mimmack MM, Gileadi U, Pearce SR, Gallagher MP, Gill DR, Hubbard RE, Higgins CF. Structural model of ATP-binding proteins associated with cystic fibrosis, multi-drug resistance and bacterial transport. Nature 1990; 346:362–5.

32. Thomas PJ, Shenbagamurthi P, Ysern X, Pedersen PL. Cystic fibrosis transmembrane conductance regulator: nucleotide binding to synthetic peptide. Science 1991; 251:555–7.

33. Anderson MP, Rich DP, Gregory RJ, Smith AE, Welsh MJ. Generation of cAMP-activated chloride channels by expression of CFTR. Science 1991; 251:679–82.

34. Kartner N, Hanrahan JW, Jensen TJ, Naismith AL, Sun S, Ackenley CA, Reyes EF, Tsui L-C, Rommens RJ, Bear CE, Riordan JR. Expression of the cystic fibrosis gene in nonepithelial invertebrate cells produces a regulated anion conductance. Cell 1991; 64:681–91.

35. Anderson MP, Gregory RJ, Thompson S, et al. Demonstration that CFTR is a chloride channel by alteration of its anion selectivity. Science 1991; 253:202–5.

36. Rich DP, Gregory RJ, Anderson MP, Manavalan R, Smith AE, Welsh MJ. Effect of deleting the R domain on CFTR-generated chloride channels. Science 1991; 253:205–7.

37. Bear CE, Li CH, Kartner N, Bridges RJ, Jensen TJ, Ramjeesingh M, Riordan JR. Purification and functional reconstitution of the cystic fibrosis transmembrane conductance regulator (CFTR). Cell 1992; 68:809–18.

38. Valverde MA, Diaz M, Sepulveda FV, Gill DR, Hyde SC, Higgins CF. Volume-regulated chloride channels associated with the human multidrug-resistance P-glycoprotein. Nature 1992; 355:830–3.

39. Barasch J, Kiss B, Prince A, Saiman L, Gruenert D, Al-Awqati Q. Defective acidification of intracellular organelles in cystic fibrosis. Nature 1991; 352:70–3.

40. Bradbury NA, Jilling T, Berta G, Sorscher EJ, Bridges RJ, Kirk KL. Regulation of plasma membrane recycling by CFTR. Science 1992; 256:530–2.

41. Wilmott RW, Tyson SL, Matthew DJ. Cystic fibrosis survival rates. The influences of allergy and *Pseudomonas aeruginosa*. Am J Dis Child 1985; 139:669–71.

42. Baltimore RS, Christie CDC, Smith GJW. Immunohistologic localization of *Pseudomonas aeruginosa* in lungs from patients with cystic fibrosis. Implications for the pathogenesis of progressive lung deterioration. Am Rev Respir Dis 1989; 140:1650–61.

43. Sorenson RU, Waller, RL, Klinger JD. Infection and immunity to *Pseudomonas*. Clin Rev Allergy 1991; 9:47–74.

44. Greenberg DP, Stutman HR. Infection and immunity to *Staphylococcus aureus* and *Haemophilus influenzae*. Clin Rev Allergy 1991; 9:75–86.
45. Prober CG. The impact of respiratory viral infections in patients with cystic fibrosis. Clin Rev Allergy 1991; 9:87–102.
46. Pribble CG, Black PG, Bosso JA, Turner RB. Clinical manifestations of exacerbations of cystic fibrosis associated with nonbacterial infections. J Pediatr 1990; 117:200–4.
47. Knutsen AP, Slavin RG. Allergic bronchopulmonary aspergillosis in patients with cystic fibrosis. Clin Rev Allergy 1991; 9:103–18.
48. Bodian M (ed). Fibrocystic Disease of the Pancreas: A Congenital Disorder of the Mucus Production–Mucosis. New York: Grune & Stratton, 1952: 130.
49. Pennington CL. Paranasal sinus changes in fibrocystic disease of the pancreas. Arch Otolaryngol 1956; 63:576–79.
50. Lurie MH. Cystic fibrosis of the pancreas and nasal mucosa. Ann Otolaryngol 1959; 68:478–86.
51. Shwachman H, Kulczycki LL, Mueller HL, Flake CG. Nasal polyposis in patients with cystic fibrosis. Pediatrics 1962; 30:389–401.
52. Rulon JT, Brown HA. Nasal polyps and cystic fibrosis of the pancreas. Arch Otolaryngol 1963; 78:192–9.
53. Mendelson RS, Cohen BM. Otorhinolaryngologic aspects of cystic fibrosis. Arch Otolaryngol 1964; 79:312–7.
54. Gharib R, Allen RP, Joos HA, Bravo LR. Paranasal sinuses in cystic fibrosis. Am J Dis Child 1964; 108:499–502.
55. Magid SL, Smith CC, Dolowitz DA. Nasal mucosa in pancreatic cystic fibrosis. Arch Otolaryngol 1967; 86:106–10.
56. Toma GA, Stein GE. Nasal polyposis in cystic fibrosis. J Laryngol Otol 1968; 82:265–8.
57. Baker DC, Smith JT. Nasal symptoms of mucoviscidosis. Otolaryngol Clin North Am 1970; 3:257–64.
58. Singh K, Hampiah M. Nasal polypi and fibro-cystic disease. J Laryngol Otol 1971; 85:185–8.
59. Neely JG, Harrison GM, Jerger JF, Greenberg SD, Presberg J. The otolaryngologic aspects of cystic fibrosis. Trans Am Acad Opnthalmol Otol 1972; 76:313–24.
60. Taylor B, Evans JNG, Hope GA. Upper respiratory tract in cystic fibrosis. Ear-nose-throat survey of 50 children. Arch Dis Child 1974; 49:133–6.
61. Cunningham DG, Gatti WM, Eitenmiller AM, Van Gorder PN. Cystic fibrosis: involvement of the ear, nose, and paranasal sinuses. Illinois Med J 1975; 148:470–4.
62. Bak-Pederson K, Larsen PK. Inflammatory middle ear diseases in patients with cystic fibrosis. Acta Otolaryngol Suppl 1979; 360:138–40.
63. David TJ. Nasal polyposis, opaque paranasal sinuses, and usually normal hearing: the otorhinolaryngological features of cystic fibrosis. J R Soc Med 1986; 79 Suppl 12: 23–6.
64. Cepero R, Smith RJH, Catlin FI, Bressler KL, Furuta GT, Shandera KC. Cystic Fibrosis—an otolaryngologic perspective. Otolaryngol Head Neck Surg 1987; 97: 356–60.

65. Todd NW, Martin WS. Temporal bone pneumatization in cystic fibrosis patients. Laryngoscope 1988; 98:1046–9.

66. Tos M. Distribution of mucus production elements in the respiratory tract: differences between upper and lower airways. Eur J Respir Dis Suppl 1983; 128:269–79.

67. Tos M, Bak-Pederson K. Goblet cell population in the normal middle ear and eustachian tube of children and adults. Ann Otol Rhinol Laryngol 1976; 25:44–50.

68. Berman JM, Colman BH. Nasal aspects of cystic fibrosis in children. J Laryngol Otol 1977; 91:133–9.

69. Tos M, Mogensen C, Thomsen J. Nasal polyps in cystic fibrosis. J Laryngol Otol 1977, 91.827–35.

70. Oppenheimer EH, Rosenstein BJ. Differential pathology of nasal polyps in cystic fibrosis and atopy. Lab Invest 1979; 40:445–9.

71. Boat TF, Kleinerman JI, Carlson DM, Maloney WH, Matthews LM. Human respiratory tract secretions. I. Mucous glycoproteins secreted by cultured nasal polyp epithelium from subjects with allergic rhinitis and cystic fibrosis. Am Rev Respir Dis 1974; 110:428–41.

72. Cheng P-W, Boat TF, Cranfill K, Yankaskas JR, Boucher RC. Increased sulfation of glycoconjugates by cultured nasal epithelial cells from patients with cystic fibrosis. J Clin Invest 1989; 84:68–72.

73. Jahnke V, Theopold H-M. Feinstruktur der Nasenschleimhat bei Mukoviszidose, under besonder Beruksichtigung der Polyposis. Laryng Rhinol (Stuttg) 1977; 56:773–81.

74. Beju D, Knox D, Yates D, Kramer JC, Henley ML. The ultrastructure of nasal polyps in cystic fibrosis [absract]. Pediatr Pulmonol Suppl 6; 1991:316.

75. Ledesma-Medina J, Osman MZ, Girdany BR. Abnormal paranasal sinuses in patients with cystic fibrosis of the pancreas. Pediatr Radiol 1980; 9:61–4.

76. Reilly JS, Kenna MA, Stool SE, Bluestone CD. Nasal surgery in children with cystic fibrosis: complications and risk management. Laryngoscope 1985; 95:1491–3.

77. Zinreich SJ, Kennedy DW, Rosenbaum AE, et al. Paranasal sinuses: CT imaging requirements for endoscopic surgery. Radiology 1987; 163:769–75.

78. Cuyler JP, Monaghan AJ. Cystic fibrosis and sinusitis. J Otolaryngol 1989; 18:173–5.

79. King VV. Upper respiratory disease, sinusitis, and polyposis. Clin Rev Allergy 1991; 9:143–57.

80. Cuyler JP. Follow-up of endoscopic sinus surgery on children with cystic fibrosis. Arch Otolaryngol Head Neck Surg 1992; 118:505–6.

81. Kennedy DW, Loury MC. Nasal and sinus pain: current diagnosis and treatment. Semin Neurol 1988; 8:303–14.

82. Moller NE, Thomsen J. Mucocele of the paranasal sinuses in cystic fibrosis. J Laryngol Otol 1978; 92:1025–7.

83. Guttenplan MD, Wetmore RF. Paranasal sinus mucocele in cystic fibrosis. Clin Pediatr 1989; 28:429–30.

84. Schulte T, Buhr W, Brassel F, Emons D. Mucocele of paranasal sinuses in a young infant with cystic fibrosis. Pediatr Radiol 1990; 20:600.

85. Jaffe BF, Strome M, Khaw K-T, Shwachman H. Nasal polypectomy and sinus surgery for cystic fibrosis—a 10 year review. Otolaryngol Clin North Am 1977; 10:81–90.

86. Crockett DM, McGill TJ, Healy GB, Friedman EM, Salkeld LJ. Nasal and paranasal sinus surgery in children with cystic fibrosis. Ann Otol Rhinol Laryngol 1987; 96:367–72.

87. Stern RC, Boat TF, Wood RE, Matthews LW, Doershuk CF. Treatment and prognosis of nasal polyps in cystic fibrosis. Am J Dis Child 1982; 136:1067–70.

88. Donaldson JD, Gillespie CT. Observations on the efficacy of intranasal beclomethasone dipropionate in cystic fibrosis patients. J Otolaryngol 1988; 17:43–5.

89. Lee ABD, Pitcher-Wilmott RW. The clinical and laboratory correlates of nasal polyps in cystic fibrosis. Int J Pediatr Otorhinolaryngol 1982; 4: 209–14.

90. Duplechain JK, White JA, Miller RH. Pediatric sinusitis. The role of endoscopic sinus surgery in cystic fibrosis and other forms of sinonasal disease. Arch Otolaryngol Head Neck Surg 1991; 117: 422–6.

91. King V, Moss RB. The role of sinus surgery in chronic sinusitis in children. Am J Asthma Allergy Pediatr 1992; 5:203–8.

92. Kennedy DW, Zinreich SJ, Rosenbaum AE, Johns ME. Functional endoscopic sinus surgery: theory and diagnostic evaluation. Arch Otolaryngol Head Neck Surg 1985; 3:576–82.

93. Umetsu DT, Moss RB, King VV, Lewiston NJ. Sinus disease in patients with cystic fibrosis: relation to pulmonary exacerbation. Lancet 1990; 335 (1):1077–8.

94. Lewiston NJ, King V, Umetsu D, Starnes V, Marshall S, Kramer M, Theodore J. Cystic fibrosis patients who have undergone heart-lung transplantation benefit from maxillary sinus antrostomy and repeated sinus lavage. Transplant Proc 1991; 23: 1207–8.

95. Moss RB, Umetsu DT, Wine JJ, King VV. A successful long-term approach to management of sinusitis in cystic fibrosis. Pediatr Pulmonol, 1992; Suppl 8:301–2.

96. Shapiro ED, Milmore GJ, Wald ER, Rodnan JB, Bowen A. Bacteriology of the maxillary sinuses in patients with cystic fibrosis. J Infect Dis 1982; 146:589–93.

97. Plotkowski MC, Chevillard M, Pierrot D, Altemayer D, Pucelle E. Epithelial respiratory cells from cystic fibrosis patients do not possess specific *Pseudomonas aeruginosa*-adhesive properties. J Med Microbiol 1992; 36:104–11.

98. Wong K, Roberts MC, Owens L, Fife M, Smith AL. Selective media for the quantitation of bacteria in cystic fibrosis sputum. J Med Microbiol 1984; 17:113–9.

99. Drake-Lee AB, Morgan DW. Nasal polyps and sinusitis in children with cystic fibrosis. J Laryngol Otol 1989; 103:753–5.

100. Ogle JW, Janda JM, Woods DE, Vasil ML. Characterization and use of a DNA probe as an epidemiological marker for *Pseudomonas aeruginosa*. J Infect Dis 1987; 155:119–26.

101. Knowles MR, Stutts MJ, Spock A, Fischer N, Gatzy JT, Boucher RC. Abnormal ion permeation through cystic fibrsosis respiratory epithelium. Science 1983; 221:1067–70.

102. Wu R, Yankaskas J, Cheng E, Knowles MR, Boucher R. Growth and differentiation of human nasal epithelial cells in culture. Serum-free, hormone-supplemented medium and proteoglycan synthesis. Am Rev Respir Dis 1985; 132:311–20.
103. Bautsch W, Ponelies N, Darnedde T, Fryburg K, Grothues D, Hundreiser J, Miller K, Monajembashi S, Claas A, Gruelich KO, et al. The nasal polyps as a tool for basic research in cystic fibrosis. Scand J Gastroenterol Suppl 1988; 143:5–8.
104. Yankaskas JR, Cotton CU, Knowles MR, Gatzy JT, Boucher RC. Culture of human nasal epithelial cells on collagen matrix supports. A comparison of bioelectric properties of normal and cystic fibrosis epithelia. Am Rev Respir Dis 1985; 132:1281–7.
105. Stutts MJ, Cotton CU, Yankaskas JR, et al. Chloride uptake into cultured airway epithelial cells from cystic fibrosis patients and normal individuals. Proc Natl Acad Sci USA 1985; 82:6677 81.
106. Yankaskas JR, Knowles MR, Gatzy JT, Boucher RC. Persistence of abnormal Cl permeability in cystic fibrosis nasal epithelial cells in heterologous culture. Lancet 1985; 1:954–6.
107. Sauder RA, Chesrown SE, Loughlin GM. Clinical application of transepithelial potential difference measurements in cystic fibrosis. J Pediatr 1987; 111:353–8.
108. Gowen CW, Lawson EE, Gingras-Leatherman J, Gatzy JT, Boucher RC, Knowles MR. Increased nasal potential difference and amiloride sensitivity in neonates with cystic fibrosis. J Pediatr 1986; 108:517–21.
109. Wine JJ, King, VV, Lewiston NJ. Method for rapid evaluation of topically applied agents to cystic fibrosis airways. Am J Physiol 1991; 261 (Lung Cell Mol Physiol 5):L218–21.
110. Di Sant'Agnese PA, Davis PB. Cystic fibrosis in adults: 75 cases and a review of 232 cases in the literature. Am J Med 1979; 66:121–32.
111. Schramm VL, Effron MZ. Nasal polyps in children. Laryngoscope 1980; 90:1489–95.

16

Mucosal and Systemic Immunodeficiency

ALAN P. KNUTSEN
St. Louis University Medical Center
St. Louis, Missouri

In humans, the mucous membranes form the first line of host defense, protecting the internal milieu from environmental pathogens by forming effective mechanical barriers as well as by specific and nonspecific immune mechanisms. Several unique features of the mucosal immune system justify considering it separate although integrated with the systemic immune system. The mucosal immune system is comprised of lymphoid tissue in the mucous membranes of the gastrointestinal, respiratory, urogenital tracts, and mammary gland, forming the mucosa-associated lymphoid tissue (MALT). The lymphocytes in MALT are present diffusely throughout the mucous membranes and also form submucosal aggregates or lymphoid follicles. In the gastrointestinal tract, mucosal lymphocytes and Peyer's patches form the gut-associated lymphoid tissue (GALT) and, in the respiratory tissue, the bronchial-associated lymphoid tissue (BALT). One of the unique features of MALT is that the lymphocytes possess a trafficking pattern such that antigen-specific mucosal lymphocytes are either retained at or home to mucosal sites (1-8). Thus, there are differences of T- and B-cell populations and immunoglobulin isotypes with different antigen specificities in the various mucosal tissues where antigen stimulation initially occurred (9-19). A distinctive characteristic of the mucosal immune system initially reported by Tomasi et al. (20) was that IgA is the predominant immunoglobulin in mucosal secretions. Deficiencies of the immune system affect both mucosal and systemic host defenses. Because the respiratory mucosal membranes are the

283

Table 1   Mucosal Host Defense Mechanisms

Nonspecific
   Mucus secretion
   Mucociliary clearance and peristalsis
   Antimicrobial soluble factors in secretions
   Lactoferrin
   Lysozyme
   Interferon
Immune
   Complement
   Neutrophils, macrophages
Specific
   Immunoglobulins
     sIgA
     sIgM
     IgG
   T lymphocytes

first sites of contact with a multitude of inhaled pathogens, this leads to increased susceptibility to recurrent sinusitis and pulmonary infections as well as systemic infections.

I. NONSPECIFIC HOST DEFENSE MECHANISMS

Since mucous epithelia form a weaker mechanical barrier than skin, a variety of nonspecific mechanisms as well as specific immunity have evolved to augment resistance. As can be seen in Table 1, mucous secretions play a critical role. The respiratory mucosa is comprised of ciliated pseudostratified epithelium coated with a layer of mucus composed of a surface gel layer and a periciliary serous layer. Water constitutes 95–97% of the nasal secretions, with the rest comprised of mucin, electrolytes, and other proteins synthesized locally in the mucosa or derived from plasma (21,22). Mucin is nearly synonymous with the term mucus and is composed of a group of glycoproteins that account for 70–80% of the dry weight of mucus. In addition, mucin constitutes the majority of the physical properties of mucosal secretions, such as the viscoelasticity and pH. There are also several proteins present in nasal secretions that possess antimicrobial activity, such as immunoglobulins, lactoferrin, and lysozyme.

One of the more important nonspecific mechanisms of resistance at mucosal surfaces is the presence of nonpathogenic microbes. The physical properties of mucous secretions (e.g., nutrients, pH, and oxygen tension) influence the bacterial flora present (23). The presence of "normal" bacterial flora limits the growth of more virulent bacteria by competing for nutrients, producing bacteriostatic substances, and inhibiting adherence to epithelial cells. Most bacteria and viruses require direct physical contact with mucosal epithelial cells via specific microbial and host cell surface interactions, which are blocked by mucus (24,25). The mucin glycoproteins bind and coat a variety of bacteria, viruses, and fungi, thus retarding epithelial adherence. In addition, mucous secretions contain a number of proteins, such as antibodies, that increase the entrapment and inactivation of micro-organisms in the secretions. Mucous secretions are increased during inflammatory reactions stimulated by immune reactions of antibody and T cells at mucosal surfaces (26,27). Mechanical clearance further inhibits adherence to epithelial cells and also physically removes trapped micro-organisms. In the respiratory tract this is accomplished by mucociliary clearance and coughing and in the gastrointestinal tract by peristalsis. The importance of proper mucociliary clearance is illustrated in patients with immotile cilia syndrome, in whom this function is abnormal (28). In these patients, proper synchronized cilia beating is abnormal due to defects of cilia structure, such as absence of the dynein arm. Thus, these patients are susceptible to repeated sinopulmonary bacterial infections and may have situs inversus, dextrocardia, and infertility in males. A variety of proteins also secreted by the exocrine seromucous glands into respiratory secretions possess innate antimicrobial properties, such as lactoferrin, lysozyme, and proteases (Table 1). Lactoferrin, an iron-binding protein constituting 2–4% of nasal mucus protein, is bacteriostatic by virtue of depriving bacteria from iron, an important nutrient (29), and IgA antibodies potentiate this effect (30). Lysozyme or muramidase causes lysis of a number of gram-positive bacteria and *Candida* by attacking acetyl-muramic acid in the cell wall of these microbes (31). Lysozyme makes up 15–30% of nasal mucus proteins and is synthesized by serous glands and neutrophils. Its activity may be enhanced by antibodies and complement. In addition, there are other less defined factors in respiratory secretions that inhibit epithelial cell attachment of micro-organisms and proteolytic enzymes in the mucus that degrade antigens. Other innate components of the immune system, such as complement and neutrophils, present in the nasal secretions enhance the antimicrobial activity of antibodies in the secretions. Interferon-alpha is also secreted into nasal secretions and increases following viral infections and immunizations (32).

II. SPECIFIC MUCOSAL IMMUNE SYSTEM

Antigen-specific factors, principally antibodies, are also present in the mucus coat. Early studies demonstrated that antibacterial and antiviral antibodies, subsequently identified as predominantly secretory IgA (sIgA), were present in the secretions (20,33-35). IgA is the most prevalent immunoglobulin in all mucous secretions, with varying amounts of other immunoglobulin isotypes. In the upper airway, IgA predominates, with levels reported to be 84 mg/dl and IgG 30 mg/dl (36). Serum-derived IgG appears to be the major immunoglobulin affording protection in the lower airways (37). IgG is present in nasal secretions, increases during inflammatory reactions, and is also prominent in the tissue (38). Thus, IgG provides significant protection of the upper and lower airways, especially at the tissue level once micro-organisms have invaded the epithelium. In the gut, IgM is the second most prevalent immunoglobulin class. Although IgA makes up only 10–15% of the total immunoglobulin pool, its daily synthesis rate is nearly identical to that of IgG (39). When the amount of sIgA present in secretions is also considered, the total daily synthesis of IgA is the largest of the immunoglobulin isotypes.

A. Secretory IgA

Serum IgA is similar to IgG, consisting principally of monomeric molecules (80–95%) composed of 2 heavy and 2 light chains with a molecular weight of 150 kD. In secretions, IgA is present predominantly in the form of secretory IgA (sIgA), with a molecular weight of approximately 375 kD, consisting of dimers of IgA, but also trimers, plus 2 additional proteins called J chain and secretory component (SC) (20,34,35,40). The J chain, a 15 kD polypeptide, forms disulfide bonds in the Fc portion of polymeric IgA and IgM. Polymers greater than dimers are bound by inter-heavy-chain disulfide bridges. Secretory component binds strongly to IgA in the Fc region, requires the presence of the J chain, and forms both noncovalent forces and disulfide links. Secretory component confers resistance to proteolytic digestion of sIgA in secretion and mediates active transport of IgA into secretions. Two subclasses of IgA are found. IgA1 normally constitutes 90% of the serum IgA whereas IgA2 forms 60–70% of IgA in secretions (41). One of the important biological differences in IgA subclasses is that IgA2 is resistant to bacterial proteases, whereas IgA1 is not (42,43). A number of respiratory pathogens, such as *Streptococcus pneumoniae*, *Neisseria* species, and *Haemophilus influenzae*, produce enzymes that cleave IgA1 molecules at the hinge region, but are not active against IgA2 molecules.

The principal function of sIgA is to bind antigens and micro-organisms, which results in viral neutralization and immune exclusion (44-46). Immune exclusion refers to blockade of macromolecules and micro-organisms from adhering to and invading the epithelial cell layer. Secretory IgA has been demonstrated to coat bacteria, causing agglutination of the bacteria, trapping the organism in the mucus, and inhibiting microbial epithelial cell adherence. Blockade of dietary protein macromolecules also appears to be a function of sIgA as evidenced by increased incidence of serum IgG antibodies to milk proteins in patients with selective IgA deficiency (47). Turk et al. (48) have also suggested that sIgA in nasal secretions may block IgE-mediated reactions. It has been demonstrated that sIgA antibodies have broader specificities than serum IgA, enhancing its role as the first line of defense, especially for newly appearing strains of viruses (49). In addition, antibody specificities in specific mucosal secretions reflect to a degree the site of local antigen stimulation (50). Thus, in the respiratory system, antibodies to a number of respiratory bacteria and viruses are increased compared to other mucosal secretions. This local antibody synthesis is due to a unique lymphoid trafficking pattern.

B. IgG

IgG is found in most mucosal secretions, but unlike sIgA appears to be passively derived from plasma (36). IgG makes up 70–80% of the total immunoglobulin pool and is equally distributed between blood and tissue compartments. Although forming 2–4% of nasal mucus protein secretions, IgG levels increase up to 125-fold during inflammatory reactions and are present in higher concentrations in the nasal tissue (38). Thus, once mucosal barriers have been broached by micro-organisms, IgG plays a significant secondary line of defense. IgG, similarly to IgM, antibodies exhibit strong complement-mediated bacteriolysis and opsonization activities.

C. Secretory IgM

Only small amounts of IgM are normally found in human secretions. IgM is found primarily in the intravascular compartment and is the first isotype to appear after antigenic stimulation. This, combined with its strong opsonic and complement-fixing properties, indicates that IgM is the first line of defense of micro-organisms entering the bloodstream. Usually only small amounts of secretory IgM (sIgM) are found in secretions. However, its levels have been found to be increased during infancy and in individuals with selective IgA deficiency as a compensatory mechanism (51,52). Secretory IgM, similar to serum IgM, is a pentamer connected by a J chain and, like sIgA, also binds with SC (53). Indeed, it binds to SC more strongly than dimeric IgA, suggesting that sIgM may have evolved prior to sIgA. However, sIgM is more sensitive to proteolytic digestion than sIgA. Secretory IgM antibodies, similarly to IgA, are locally synthesized and actively secreted into the secretions. sIgM is functionally similar to sIgA in mediating viral neutralization and immune exclusion, but is much more efficient at mediating opsonophagocytosis and complement-mediated bacteriolysis. In patients with selective lack of IgA, there is a compensatory increase of sIgM in the upper airways that affords some resistance to infection. Secretory IgM plus IgG probably accounts for the milder sinopulmonary infections seen in individuals with selective IgA deficiency than in those with more severe antibody deficiency disorders.

D. Complement and Neutrophils

In host defense mechanisms, especially of polysaccharide-encapsulated bacteria, complement, neutrophils, and macrophages amplify the biological activity of IgG and IgM antibodies. IgG and IgM strongly activate the classic complement pathway, which results in direct bacterial lysis and enhances opsonization and chemotaxis of neutrophils and macrophages. Both neutrophils and macrophages express IgG Fc and complement C3 receptors that mediate opsonization. It is less clear whether IgA can activate complement. Most studies have indicated that monomeric IgA does not activate the classic complement pathway, although there is some evidence that the alternative pathway may be activated by aggregates of IgA (54). In recent years, IgA Fc receptors have been identified on neutrophils and macrophages and show greater binding for dimeric IgA (52).

E. Lymphocytes

In mucosal sites, lymphocytes are present diffusely throughout the mucosal layers and form subepithelial follicles. Development of the mucosal lymphoid system develops early with seeding of Peyer's patches by T and B lymphocytes from bone marrow and thymus by 16–19 weeks gestation (55-57). Subsequently, other mucosal subepithelial follicles develop. At birth, surface membrane IgM B cells (smIgM) predominate in follicles, but over the first 2 years increasing numbers of smIgA B cells appear (58,59). As seen in Table 2, smIgA B cells predominate in all mucosal tissues (60). In the lower respiratory mucosal, smIgG B cells are the second most frequent immunoglobulin-secreting cell, whereas in the gut smIgM B cells are the second most common. There are some interesting patterns of the diffusely distributed lymphocytes found in the mucosal layers of the gastrointestinal tract. In the lamina propria, there are equal numbers or a slight preponderance of T cells compared to B cells. However, in the intraepithelial layer, T cells are almost exclusively found, with a paucity of B cells (16,61,62). Furthermore, CD4+ T cells are found more frequently in the subepithelial lamina propria, whereas CD8+ T cells are more frequent in the intraepithelial layer.

When antigen contacts the gastrointestinal epithelium, it is taken up by specialized cells, microfold (M cells) or follicle-associated epithelium concentrated in epithelium above Peyer's patches (63). M cells are cuboidal cells with short, irregular microvilli. Analogous nonciliated cells have also been described in bronchial, tonsillar, and nasal mucosa (16,64,65). It is not known whether these cells process antigens or merely transfer them to the underlying lymphoid cells. There is a population of nonlymphoid cells resembling dendritic cells located beneath the epithelium and in the T-dependent interfollicular regions that are Ia positive and probably serve as antigen-presenting cells (66). The subepithelial

Table 2 Average Percentage Distribution of Immunoglobulin-Producing Immunocytes in Normal Adult Human Glandular Tissue

Tissue Site	Immunocytes			
	IgA	IgM	IgG	IgD
Lacrimal gland	77	7.2	5.8	9.7
Parotid gland	91	3.0	3.7	2.5
Nasal concha	67	7.8	15.8	9.2
Bronchial mucosa	74	ND	29.0	ND
Gastric body mucosa	73	13.0	14.0	< 1
Gastric antral mucosa	80	8.0	12.0	< 1
Jejunum	81	17.0	2.6	< 1
Ileum	83	11.0	5.0	< 1
Large bowel	90	6.0	4.2	< 1
Lactating mammary gland	68	13.0	16.0	2.4

Source: Ref 60.

tissue resembles lymph nodes: the nodules are comprised of germinal centers
populated with B cells and some cortical T cells and the interstices populated by
T cells.

One of the distinctive characteristics of MALT is the unique migratory pattern that largely separates mucosal lymphoid cells, especially B cells, from the
systemic immune system. This was first described by Craig and Cebra (67), who
demonstrated that irradiating rabbits and reconstituting with cells from Peyer's
patches led to the appearance of IgA immunocytes in the gastrointestinal mucosa and spleen. However, if reconstituted with cells from popliteal lymph
nodes, IgA B cells were not identified in the mucosa and only IgG B cells were
seen in the spleen. Likewise, Rudzik et al. (7) subsequently observed similar
results with bronchial lymph nodes.

From various studies, an overview of MALT lymphoid trafficking can be described (7,10,13,15,16,55,56,60,67-71). Mucosal lymphoid tissue is initially
seeded from primordial lymphoid tissues, such as the bone marrow and thymus,
and localizes within the follicles because of interactions with follicular high-
endothelial venules (55,56). In the mucosal follicles, initial antigen stimulation
induces B- and T-cell proliferation and differentiation (68,69). In the case of B
cells, isotype switching from IgM B cells to IgA B cells occurs as a result of
class-specific switch T cells and cytokines, such as interleukin 5 (IL-5) (70).
Thus, the germinal centers in Peyer's patches and other mucosal follicles become populated predominantly by smIgA B cells, and these cells are the precursors of IgA plasma cells subsequently found in the lamina propria, for

example, the diffusely distributed lymphoid mucosal tissue. Before terminal differentiation, these B cells migrate out of Peyer's patches and other mucosal follicles via afferent lymphatics to regional lymph nodes. For the nose and lungs, this would be the cervical nodes and the bronchial lymph nodes, respectively. There, the B cells acquire the capacity to home selectively to the lamina propria of mucosal surfaces. It is hypothesized that B cell receptors are acquired in the lymph nodes that recognize proteins on the high-endothelial venules (HEV) present in the lamina propria and follicles (69,71). One such protein, a 58–66 kD protein on murine HEV has been identified and shown to be functional in B cell binding and extravasation in mucosal sites. The majority of such migrating B cells are not IgA blast cells, but resting memory B cells. After return to the lamina propria at mucosal sites, these smIgA B cells terminally differentiate into IgA-secreting B plasma cells after additional antigen stimulation and T helper activity. Both helper and suppressor T cells regulate IgA isotype switching and terminal differentiation. Several investigators have identified IgA Fc receptor positive T cells in the lamina propria that express either suppressive or enhancing effects on IgA secretion. In general, the migration of B cells originating from mucosal sites has a propensity to disseminate to multiple mucosal surfaces. Thus, B cells originating from Peyer's patches will populate not only GALT but also BALT, mammary gland, and urogenital lymphoid tissue. However, lymphocytes from bronchial nodes have a greater tendency to return to bronchial mucosa, from cervical nodes to nasal mucosa, and from mesenteric nodes to gastrointestinal mucosa. This trafficking pattern explains the increased antibody titers found in respiratory secretions to organisms that initially stimulate the respiratory mucosa.

Mucosal T cells have a similar migratory pattern to B cells, but also circulate in the systemic immune system to a greater extent, perhaps because T cells bind to HEV less readily than B cells.

F. Transport of sIgA

The transport of sIgA into the mucus secretions is a complex process requiring the synthesis of dimeric IgA and SC, assembly, and transport of the IgA–SC complex to the exterior epithelial surface. IgA plasma cells, upon antigen stimulation and T cell help, are induced to secrete dimeric IgA complexed with J chain (20,35,72,73). Secretory component is synthesized by epithelial cells of mucosal glands and transported and incorporated into the basolateral cell membrane. SC, comprised of both transmembrane and extracellular domains, acts as a receptor for IgA and subsequently binds with J chain. The epithelial cell membrane-bound SC–J–IgA complexes are internalized in endocytic vesicles and migrate through the cytoplasm via the microtubules to the exterior cell surface membranes, where the membrane portion of SC is cleaved, releas-

ing the SC-IgA complex to the exterior cell surface. Secretion of sIgM, but not
IgG or IgE, seems to have a similar transport mechanism to that of sIgA.

III. IMMUNODEFICIENCIES

The importance of normal immune competence in maintaining mucosal integrity
is obvious from the discussion above. In particular, intact opsonophagocytosis
involving antibody, complement, and phagocytic cells (neutrophils and macrophages) is especially important in the defense of respiratory pathogens, such
as *S. pneumoniae*, *H. influenzae* (often nontypable), *M. catarrhalis*, *S. aureus*,
and anaerobes, that cause recurrent sinopulmonary infections. However, other
underlying conditions also predispose children to repeated respiratory infections
(Table 3). The majority of children with repeated sinus and/or pulmonary disease
typically seen in allergy/immunology clinics are atopic (74-76). The allergic patient is more likely to have a family history of atopy, a seasonal pattern of respiratory symptoms consisting of nasal pruritus, ocular allergic symptoms, and/
or wheezing. In addition, atopic dermatitis or food allergy may be present.
Appropriate treatment of the underlying allergic condition often resolves the
susceptibility to secondary sinusitis. In contrast, immunodeficient patients often
have a history of multiple sites of infections: sinusitis, otitis media, pharyngitis,
pneumonia, cellulitis, and perhaps septicemia and meningitis. Isolated sinusitis
is not likely to be on the basis of an underlying immunodeficiency, but is usually
due to anatomical abnormalities, such as adenoidal hyperplasia, mucosal edema
and inflammation, or ostiomeatal obstruction perhaps accompanying allergic
rhinitis. Also, complications from infections are more likely to occur in the immunodeficient patient, such as bronchiectasis, perforated scarred tympanic
membranes, and mastoiditis. Infections in immunodeficient patients are not only
more frequent but also more difficult to eradicate with appropriate medical and
surgical management. In patients with a primary immunodeficiency and repeated sinopulmonary disease, antibody or B cell defects are certainly the most
common (77-79).

The most common primary immunodeficiency is selective IgA deficiency
with a prevalence of 1:500–1:700 in the general population (52). Selective
IgA deficiency is defined by a serum IgA concentration less than 5 mg/dl
without other immune abnormalities. In IgA deficiency, there is usually also
absence of sIgA in the mucous secretions. Deficient sIgA with normal serum
IgA levels has been reported in only a few patients (80). Because of the central role that IgA antibodies play in mucosal host defense, selective IgA deficiency may result in recurrent upper respiratory infections. In selective IgA
deficiency, sIgM levels increase and plasma-derived IgG present in the secretions and tissue afford protection. Thus, patients with this defect tend to have
milder infections than patients with broader antibody defects. Selective IgA

Table 3 Disorders with Increased Susceptibility to Sinopulmonary Infections

Allergic rhinitis
Asthma
Cystic fibrosis
Immotile cilia syndrome
Down syndrome
Secondary immunodeficiency (HIV infection)
Primary humoral immunodeficiencies
  X-linked agammaglobulinemia
  Common variable immunodeficiency
  Hyper-IgM syndrome
  Selective IgA deficiency
  Selective antibody deficiencies with or without IgG subclass deficiency
  Antibody deficiency with normal serum immunoglobulins
  Transient hypogammaglobulinemia of infancy

deficiency is associated with a greater incidence of respiratory allergies and autoimmune disorders (47,52,81). Buckley and Dees (47) reported that in individuals with respiratory allergies the incidence of IgA deficiency was increased to 1:200. The reason for this is not understood, although it has been proposed that there may be greater sensitization with allergens due to loss of IgA-blocking antibodies.

Oxelius et al. (82) first reported that patients with selective IgA deficiency who have increased bacterial sinopulmonary infections are more likely to have other immunoglobulin defects, most notably decreased serum IgG2 subclass deficiency, IgA–IgG2 deficiency. IgG is comprised of four subclasses, identified as IgG1, IgG2, IgG3, and IgG4, differentiated by their different constant gamma heavy chain proteins that confer unique biological activities (83). The normal adult range of serum IgG subclasses is wide, with approximately 65% of the serum IgG made up of IgG1, 20% IgG2, 10% IgG3, and <5% IgG4. Adult IgG1 and IgG3 serum concentrations are attained within the first year of life, but IgG2 levels do not reach adult levels until adolescence. IgG1 and IgG3 strongly activate the classic complement pathway and bind to IgG Fc receptors on monocytes and neutrophils. IgG2, however, only weakly activates the complement pathway and does not bind to Fc receptors on monocytes, although it does on mast cells. Thus, IgG1 and IgG3 antibodies are much more efficient than IgG2 at enhancing bacterial opsonophagocytosis and complement-mediated lysis. IgG antibody responses to protein and polysaccharide antigens reside preferentially within IgG subclasses. In children, most IgG antibody responses to protein antigens, such as bacterial toxoids and viral proteins, are found predominantly within the IgG1 and IgG3 subclasses, and antibody responses to *S. pneu-*

moniae and *H. influenzae* polysaccharide capsular antigens are of the IgG2 subclass (83-86). In children, Siber et al. (86) reported a direct correlation of the serum IgG2 concentrations and antibody responses to polysaccharide antigens. However, asymptomatic individuals with a complete deficiency of IgG2 due to gene deletion of gamma 2 constant gene have been reported (87). This suggests that antibody deficiency to polysaccharide antigens is not due to IgG2 subclass deficiency but rather reflects either abnormal antigen-processing, T- or B cell defect. This is further supported by studies reported by Insel et al. (88) who observed normal antibody responses to conjugated *H. influenzae* polysaccharide antigen but not to unconjugated *H. influenzae* type B (HiB).

Many investigators have subsequently reported in both adult and children selective IgG2 subclass deficiency associated with selective impairment of antibody responses to polysaccharide antigens (89). IgG2 deficiency is also sometimes seen in combination with other IgG subclass deficiencies, especially IgG4. These patients have recurrent sinopulmonary infections and sometimes life-threatening sepsis or meningitis. Ambrosino (90) subsequently observed children who had repeated infections with impaired antibody responses to unconjugated *H. influenzae* polysaccharide antigen but normal IgG subclass levels. Our group (91) has identified approximately 35 children with similar selective antibody deficiency to *S. pneumoniae* and *H. influenzae* type B polysaccharide immunizations and repeated sinopulmonary infections (Table 4). Twenty percent of patients had concomitant IgG2 and 6% had IgA-IgG2 deficiencies. Asthma and atopy were common in this group of children, occurring in 69% and 59% of subjects, respectively. The natural history of this immune disorder is unknown. However, it is suspected that in the majority of children it represents a delayed maturational defect. In others, it may be a permanent defect and in others may herald a more global antibody deficiency disorder, such as common variable immune deficiency (89).

Patients who have a more severe global defect of antibody responses to protein and polysaccharide antigens, often associated with hypogammaglobulinemia, have more severe sinopulmonary infections and potentially fatal infections (Table 3) (77-79). These individuals have chronic sinopulmonary infections and systemic infections with polysaccharide encapsulated organisms, such as *S. pneumoniae*, *H. influenzae*, *M. catarrhalis*, *S. aureus*, and *P. aeruginosa*. These patients are typically not unduly susceptible to infections due to viruses or opportunistic micro-organisms. Often there is a reduction of peripheral lymphoid tissue: lymph nodes are not palpable and tonsillar and adenoid tissue is diminished. Many of these defects are congenital and inherited in an X-linked pattern affecting boys. However, hypogammaglobulinemia may also present during adolescence and adulthood in female subjects as well. The classification of humoral immunodeficiencies is based on the presumed block of B-cell maturation and differentiation.

Table 4 Clinical Characteristics of Children with Selective Antibody Deficiency to Polysaccharide Antigens

Number of patients	35
Gender (male/female)	2:1
Age at diagnosis (yrs)	
Mean ± SD	4.1 ± 2.3
Range	2–10
Onset of symptoms (mos)	
Mean ± SD	7.9 ± 4.9
Symptoms (% of patients)	
Sinusitis	100
Otitis media	94
Pneumonia	72
Pharyngitis	47
Meningitis	6
Surgery (% of patients)	
Adenoidectomy	48
Myringotomy	59
Antrostomy	10
Mastoidectomy	3
Atopy (% of patients)	
Positive skin prick tests	59
Recurrent asthma	69
Allergic rhinitis	59

Mature B cells are derived from bone marrow stem cells. In the bone marrow, the first identifiable cell of B cell lineage is a pre-B cell, defined by the presence of cytoplasmic mu chains (92,93). IgM heavy chains are formed by gene rearrangement of the variable (V), diversity (D), and joining (J) regions of immunoglobulin on chromosome 14 in an antigen-independent process, forming VDJ-Cmu gene complex. Light chain rearrangement occurs likewise. Heavy- and light-chain proteins combine in the endoplasmic reticulum moving through the Golgi apparatus and are transported to the surface membrane, forming surface membrane IgM (smIgM+) immature B cells. smIgD is formed by posttranscriptional translation of germ-line mRNA, identifying smIgM + IgD + mature B cells. Isotype switching to other isotypes occurs by germ-line gene rearrangement using switch recombinase, stimulated by T-helper cell activity. For instance, CD4+ Th2-like T cells synthesize IL-4 that stimulates B cell IgE isotype switching. Mature smIgM + IgD + B cells may also have smIgG or IgA or IgE committed to secreting that immunoglobulin isotype. Differentiation of mature B cells into immunoglobulin secreting immunocytes or plasma cells also is under T-cell regulation, occurring with antigen stimulation. Primary B-cell immunodeficiencies occur due to defects in this normal maturational and differential pathway.

The first congenital B cell immunodeficiency identified was X-linked infantile agammaglobulinemia (XLA) by Colonel Ogden Bruton in 1952 (94). These children have profound hypogammaglobulinemia, with serum IgG levels <100 mg/dl and nondetectable levels of IgA, IgM, and IgE (78,79,95). Antibody titers to infectious organisms and immunizations, such as diphtheria, tetanus, *S. pneumoniae*, and *H. influenzae*, are severely impaired. These patients have recurrent infections beginning after 6 months of age after maternal transplacentally derived IgG is catabolized. Besides sinopulmonary infections, these patients may also have fatal infections due to sepsis and meningitis. As with all severe B-cell defects, repeated pulmonary infections may lead to bronchiectasis and pulmonary failure. Approximately one-third of patients with XLA may also develop polyarthritis that resembles juvenile rheumatoid arthritis, and typically improves with antibody gammaglobulin replacement therapy. Unlike patients with other B-cell immunodeficiencies, patients with XLA are susceptible to infections with echovirus and coxsackievirus, which causes recurrent or chronic meningoencephalitis or dermatomyositis-like illnesses that are frequently fatal (96). In XLA, there is a deficiency of mature B cells, identified by smIgM+ and smIgD+ or by the B-cell-specific monoclonal antibodies CD19 or CD21. However, pre-B cells can be seen in the bone marrow, indicating a maturational defect forming mature B cells. Furthermore, obligate maternal carriers demonstrate complete lyonization of their B cells (97). These studies may be clinically useful to confirm the diagnosis and to determine carrier status of female relatives.

Immunodeficiency with normal IgM (hyper-IgM syndrome) is usually inherited as an X-linked mode but may also occur as an autosomal recessive or dominant trait characterized by decreased serum IgG and IgA concentrations with normal or elevated serum IgM levels (78,79,95,98). IgG antibody responses are markedly abnormal, although IgM antibody titers may be normal, such as isohemagglutinins. Besides increased susceptibility to repeated bacterial infections, these patients also frequently have autoimmune cytopenias, such as cyclic or persistent neutropenia, thrombocytopenia, and hemolytic anemia. Circulating smIgM+IgD+ B cells are present, but IgG- and IgA-bearing lymphocytes are absent. The defect appears to be abnormal B-cell immunoglobulin isotype switching. Mayer et al. (99) have presented evidence that the primary abnormality is decreased "switch" T helper cells that promote isotype switching.

Common variable immune deficiency disorder (CVID) is comprised of a variety of B-cell defects that may be congenital or acquired during adolescence or adulthood (78,79,95,100). The common denominator is hypogammaglobulinemia and deficient antibody responses, although usually not as marked as in XLA. In addition to susceptibility to infections, these patients also have increased incidence of hematologic disorders including hemolytic anemia, thrombocytopenia, neutropenia, and autoimmune diseases, such as alopecia areata, rheumatoid arthritis, systemic lupus erythematosus, and sicca syndrome. Gastrointestinal problems are common, including sprue-like syndrome, disaccharidase deficiencies, intestinal lymphoid nodular hyperplasia, and parasitic infections with *Giardia* and *Helicobacter*. Malignancies are also common, especially non-Hodgkin's lymphoma and gastric, skin, and genital tract carcinomas. Serum IgG levels are typically less than 400 mg/dl but there are usually normal numbers of mature B cells. In the majority of patients, there is defective differentiation of mature B cells into immunoglobulin-secreting immunocytes or plasma cells. T-cell defects with decreased T-helper and increased T-suppressor activities have also been reported (100).

Several investigators have reported adults and children who have symptoms similar to patients with CVID who have normal serum immunoglobulin concentrations but a marked inability to produce normal antibody responses to a variety of protein and polysaccharide antigens, for example, antibody deficiency with normal serum immunoglobulin levels (101,102). The basic defect is an intrinsic B-cell defect to differentiate into immunoglobulin secreting plasma cells.

Transient hypogammaglobulinemia of infancy (THI) needs to be differentiated from the other congenital B-cell defects. In THI, children typically have the onset of increased infections beginning at 6 months of age (78,79). They may have increased number and severity of upper respiratory tract infections and some lower respiratory tract infections. However, they are generally not at increased risk for serious systemic infections. Serum IgG and IgA levels are decreased, mature B cells are present in normal levels, and antibody responses to protein antigens are normal. Siegel et al. (101) reported a transient decrease of T helper activity stimulating B cell IgG synthesis. Serum immunoglobulin levels normalize concomitant with clinical improvement, usually by 3–5 years old. Patients with THI usually do not require gammaglobulin antibody replacement therapy.

IV. GAMMAGLOBULIN ANTIBODY REPLACEMENT THERAPY

The treatment of hypogammaglobulinemia and severe global antibody deficiencies is antibody replacement therapy. This was initially begun in the 1950s with immune serum globulin (ISG), and proved to reduce the risk of severe fatal infection, although patients still tended to have repeated sinopulmonary infections (104). The initial preparation of ISG had to be administered intramuscularly because it contained aggregates of IgG that activate complement, resulting in anaphylactoid reactions if administered intravenously. This limited the amount of ISG antibody replacement. In the early 1980s, an intravenous form of ISG, intravenous immunoglobulin (IVIG), was licensed in the United States. The IgG in IVIG preparation was initially chemically modified so that it did not activate complement. All commercially available IVIG preparations have subsequently contained biologically intact monomeric IgG molecules with varying trace amounts of IgA, IgM, and other serum proteins. IVIG has several advantages compared to ISG. Patients typically prefer IVIG since it is less painful than intramuscularly administered ISG. However, the greatest advantage is that greater amounts of IgG can be administered, achieving near-normal serum trough IgG levels. The initial recommended dosage of IVIG is 300–600 mg/kg given every 4 weeks. Adjustment of dosage is dependent upon clinical response and trough serum IgG concentrations. Several studies comparing higher–dosage regimens that achieve near-normal trough serum IgG levels of 500 mg/dl have demonstrated significant reduction of sinopulmonary infections and improved pulmonary function (105-107). These finding are especially important since the long-term morbidity of patients with severe antibody deficiencies includes bronchiectasis and pulmonary insufficiency.

In patients with selective antibody deficiency to polysaccharide antigens with or without IgG subclass and/or IgA deficiency, the efficacy of IVIG antibody replacement therapy is less clear. Silk et al. (108) have recently reported improvement with IVIG treatment in children who have continued infections despite prophylactic antibiotics. Since the natural history of this immune defect is unknown, periodic discontinuation of IVIG and re-evaluation are required.

REFERENCES

1. Pierce NP, Sack RB. Immune response of the intestinal mucosal to cholera toxoid. J Infect Dis (suppl) 1977; 136:113–7.
2. Husband AJ, Gowans JL. The origin and antigen-dependent distribution of IgA-containing cells in the intestine. J Exp Med 1978; 148:1146–60.
3. Husband AJ, Dunkley ML. Lack of site of origin effects in distribution of IgA-antibody-containing cells. Immunology 1985; 54:215–21.
4. Pierce NF, Cray WC Jr. Determinants of the localization, magnitude and duration of a specific mucosal IgA plasma cell response in enterically immunized rats. J Immunol 1982; 128:1311.
5. Weisz-Carrington P, Roux ME, McWilliams M, Phillips-Quagliata JM, Lamm ME. Organ and isotype distribution of plasma cells producing specific antibody after oral immunization: evidence for a generalized secretory immune system. J Immunol 1979; 123:1705–8.
6. Hall JG, Smith ME. Homing of lymph-borne immunoblasts to the gut. Nature 1970; 226:262–3.
7. Rudzik R, Clancy RL, Perey DYE, Day RB, Bienenstock J. Repopulation with IgA-containing cells of bronchial and intestinal lamina propria after the transfer of homalogous Peyer's patch and bronchial lymphocytes. J Immunol 1975; 114:1599–1604.

8. Dahlgren UIH, Ahlstedt S, Hanson LA. The localization of the antibody response to milk or bile depends on the nature of the antigen. J Immunol 1987; 138:1397–1402.

9. Halstead TE, Hall JG. The homing of lymph-borne immunoblasts to the small gut of neonatal rats. Transplantation 1972; 14:339–346.

10. Guy-Grand D, Griscelli C, Vassali P. The gut associated lymphoid system: nature and properties of the large dividing cells. Eur J Immunol 1974; 4:435–43.

11. McWilliams M, Phillips-Quagliata JM, Lamm ME. Characteristics of mesenteric lymph node cells homing to gut associated lymphoid tissue in syngeneic mice. J Immunol 1975; 115:54–58.

12. McWilliams M, Phillips-Quagliata JM, Lamm ME. Mesenteric lymph node B lymphoblasts which home to the small intestine are precommitted to IgA synthesis. J Exp Med 1977; 145:866–75.

13. McDermott MR, Bienenstock J. Evidence for a common mucosal immunologic system. I. Migration of B immunoblasts into intestinal, respiratory and genital tissues. J Immunol 1979; 122:1892–8.

14. Roux ME, McWilliams M, Phillips-Quagliata JM, Lamm ME. Differentiation pathway of Peyer's patch precursors of IgA plasma cells in the secretory immune system. Cell Immunol 1981; 61:141–53.

15. Bienenstock J, Befus D, McDermott M, Mirski S, Rosenthal K. Regulation of lymphoblast and localization in mucosal tissues, with emphasis on IgA. Fed Proc 1983; 42:3213–7.

16. Kuper CF, Koornstra PJ, Hameleers DMH, Biewenga J, Spit BJ, Duijvestijn AM, Van Breda Vriesman PJC, Sminia T. The role of nasopharyngeal lymphoid tissue. Immunol Today 1992; 13:219–24.

17. Guy-Grand D, Griscelli C, Vassalli P. The mouse gut T lymphocyte, a novel type of T cell. Nature, origin and traffic in mice in normal and graft-versus-host conditions. J Exp Med 1978; 184:1661–77.

18. Lyscom N, Brueton MJ. Intraepithelial, lamina propria and Peyer's patch lymphocytes of the rat small intestine: isolation and characterization in terms of immunoglobulin markers and receptors for monoclonal antibodies. Immunology 1982; 45:775–83.

19. Cahill RNP, Poskitt DC, Frost H, Trnka Z. Two distinct pools of recirculating T lymphocytes: migratory characteristics of nodal and intestinal T lymphocytes. J Exp Med 1977; 145:420–8.

20. Tomasi TB Jr, Bienenstock J. Secretory immunoglobulins. Adv Immunol 1968; 9:1–96.

21. Mygind N. Structure and ultrastructure of the nose. In: Nasal Allergy. Oxford: Blackwell Scientific Publications, 1979: 3–38.

22. Kaliner M, Shelhamer JH, Borson B, Nadel J, Patow C, Marom Z. Human respiratory mucus. Am Rev Respir Dis 1986; 134:612–21.

23. Mackowiak P. The normal microbial flora. N Engl J Med 1982; 307:83–93.

24. Andersson B, Porras 0, Hanson LA, Svanborg Eden C, Leffler H. Non-antibody-containing fractions of breast milk inhibit epithelial attachment of *Streptococcus pneumoniae* and *Haemophilus influenzae*. Lancet 1985; 1:643.

25. Andersson B, Porras 0, Hanson LA, Lagergard T, Svanborg Eden C. Inhibition of attachment of *Streptococcus pneumoniae* and *Haemophilus influenzae* by human milk and receptor oligosaccharides. J Infect Dis 1986; 153:232–7.

26. Lake AM, Bloch KJ, Neutra MR, Walker WA. Intestinal goblet cell mucus release. II. In vivo stimulation by antigen in the immunized rat. J Immunol 1979; 122:834–7.

27. Karlsson G, Hansson H-A, Petruson B, Bjorkander J, Hanson LA. Goblet cell number in the nasal mucosa relates to cell-mediated immunity in patients with antibody deficiency syndrome. Int Arch Allergy Appl Immunol 1985; 78:86–91.

28. Pedersen H, Mygind N. Absence of axonemal arms in nasal mucosa cilia in Kartagener's syndrome. Nature 1976; 262:494–5.

29. Bullen JJ, Rogers HJ, Leigh L. Iron-binding proteins in milk and resistance of *Escherichia coli* infection in infants. Br Med J 1972; 1:69–75.

30. Rogers HJ, Synge C. Bacteriostatic effect of human milk on Escherichia coli: the role of IgA. Immunology 1978; 34:19–28.

31. Hill IR, Porter P. Studies of bactericidal activity to Escherichia coli of porcine serum and colostral immunoglobulins and the role of lysozyme with secretory IgA. Immunology 1974; 26:1239–50.

32. Danielescu G, Barbu C, Sorodoc Y, Cajal N, Sarateanu D, Petrescu A, Motas C, Ganea E. The presence of interferon and type A immunoglobulins in the nasopharyngeal secretions of volunteers immunized with an inactivated influenza vaccine. Acta Virol 1975; 19:245–9.

33. Hanson LA. Comparative immunological studies of the immune globulins of human milk and of blood serum. Int Arch Allergy 1961; 18:241–67.

34. Brandtzaeg P, Baklien K, Bjerke K, Rognum TO, Scott H, Valnes K. Nature and properties of the human gastrointestinal immune system. In: Miller K, Nicklin S, eds. Immunology of the Gastrointestinal Tract. Boca Raton, Fl: CRC Press, 1987:1–85.

35. Mestecky J, McGhee JR. Immunoglobulin A (IgA): molecular and cellular interactions involved in IgA biosynthesis and immune response. Adv Immunol 1987; 40:153–245.

36. Mygind N, Weeke B, Ullman S. Quantitative determination of immunoglobulins in nasal secretions. Int Arch Allergy Appl Immunol 1975; 49:99–107.

37. Newhouse M, Sanchis J, Bienenstock J. Lung defense mechanism. N Engl J Med 1976; 295:1045–52.

38. Kaliner MA. Human nasal host defense and sinusitis. J Allergy Clin Immunol 1992; 90:424–32.

39. Waldmann TA, Strober W. Metabolism of immunoglobulins. Progr Allergy 1969; 13:1–110.

40. Newcomb RW, Normansell D, Stanworth DR. A structural study of human exocrine IgA globulin. J Immunol 1968; 101:905–14.

41. Delacroix DL, Dive C, Rambaud JC, Vaerman JP. IgA subclasses in various secretions and in serum. Immunology 1982; 47:383–5.

42. Kilian M, Mestecky J, Kulhavy R, Tomana M, Butler WT. IgA1 proteases from *Haemophilus influenzae*, *Streptococcus pneumoniae*, *Neisseria meningitidis* and

Streptococcus sanguis: comparative immunochemical studies. J Immunol 1980; 124:2596–600.

43. Mulks MH, Plaut AG. IgA protease production as a characteristic distinguishing pathogenic from harmless Neisseriaceae. N Engl J Med 1978; 299:973–6.
44. Taylor HP, Dimmock NJ. Mechanism of neutralization of influenza virus by secretory IgA is different from that of monomeric IgA or IgG. J Exp Med 1985; 161:198–209.
45. Stokes CR, Soothill JF, Turner MW. Immune exclusion is a function of IgA. Nature 1975; 255:745–6.
46. Walker WA, Wu M, Isselbacher KJ, Bloch KJ. Intestinal uptake of macromolecules. III. Studies on the mechanisms by which immunization interferes with antigen uptake. J Immunol 1975; 115:854–61.
47. Buckley RH, Dees SC. Correlation of milk precipitins with IgA deficiency. N Engl J Med 1969; 281:465–9.
48. Turk A, Lichtenstein LM, Norman PS. Nasal secretory antibody to inhalant allergens in allergic and non-allergic patients. Immunol 1970; 19:85–95. 1970,
49. Shvartzman YS, Agranovskaya EN, Zykov MP. Formation of secretory and circulating antibodies after immunization with live inactivated influenzae virus vaccines. J Infect Dis 1977; 135:697–705.
50. Artenstein MS. Anti-bacterial aspects of local immunity. In: Neter E, Milgrom F, eds. The Immune System and Infectious Diseases. Basel: Karger, 1975: 366–75.
51. Hanson LA, Bjorkander J, Carlsson B, Robertson D, Soderstrom T. The heterogensity of IgA deficiency. J Clin Immunol 1988; 8:159–62.
52. Schaffer FM, Monteiro RC, Volanakis JE, Cooper MD. IgA deficiency. Immunodefic Rev 1991; 3:15–44.
53. Brandtzaeg P. Human secretory immunoglobulin M. An immunochemical and immunohistochemical study. Immunology 1975; 29:559–70.
54. Kerr MA. The structure and function of human IgA. Biochem J 1990; 271:285–96.
55. Howard JC, Hunt SV, Gowans JL. Identification of marrow-derived and thymus-derived small lymphocytes in the lymphoid tissue and thoracic duct lymph of normal rats. J Exp Med 1972; 135:200–19.
56. Waksman BH. The homing pattern of thymus-derived lymphocytes in calf and neonatal mouse Peyer's patches. J Immunol 1973; 111:878–84.
57. Spencer J, MacDonald TT, Finn TT, Isaacson PG. Development of gut associated lymphoid tissue in the terminal ileum of fetal human intestine. Clin Exp Immunol 1986; 64:536–43.
58. Maffei HVL, Kingston D, Hill ID, Shiner M. Histopathologic changes and the immune response within the jejunal mucosa in infants and children. Pediatr Res 1979; 13:733–6.
59. Savilahti E. Immunoglobulin-containing cells in the intestinal mucosa, immunoglobulins in the intestinal juice in children. Clin Exp Immunol 1972; 11:415–25.
60. Hanson LA, Brandtzaeg P. The mucosal immune system. In: Stiehm ER, Fulginiti VA, eds. Immunologic Disorders in Infants and Children. Philadelphia: WB Saunders, 1989; 116–55.

61. Greenwood JH, Austin LL, Dobbins WO III. In vitro characterization of human intestinal intraepithelial lymphocytes. Gastroenterology 1983; 85:1023–35.

62. Cerf-Bensussan N, Schneeberger EE, Bhan AK. Immunohistological and immunoelectron microscopic characterization of the mucosal lymphocytes of human small intestine by the use of monoclonal antibodies. J Immunol 1983; 130:2615–22.

63. Owen RL, Jones AL. Epithelial cell specialization within human Peyer's patches: an ultrastructural study of intestinal lymphoid follicles. Gastroenterology 1974; 66:189–203.

64. Richardson J, Bouchard R, Ferguson CC. Uptake and transport of exogenous proteins by respiratory epithelium. Lab Invest 1976; 35:307–12.

65. McDermott MR, Befus AD, Bienenstock J. The structural basis for immunity in the respiratory tract. Int Rev Exp Pathol 1982; 23:47–112.

66. Richman LK, Graeff AS, Strober W. Antigen presentation by macrophage enriched cells from the mouse Peyer's patch. Cell Immunol 1981; 62:110–8.

67. Craig SW, Cebra JJ. Peyer's patches: an enriched source of precursors for IgA-producing immunocytes in the rabbit. J Exp Med 1971; 134:188–200.

68. Kagnoff MF. Functional characteristics of Peyer's patch lymphoid cells. IV. Effect of antigen feeding on the frequency of antigen-specific B cells. J Immunol 1977; 118:992–7.

69. Butcher EC, Rouse RV, Coffman RL, Nottenburg CN, Hardy RR, Weissman IL. Surface phenotype of Peyer's patch germinal center cells: implications for the role of germinal centers in B cell differentiation. J Immunol 1982; 129:2698–707.

70. Murray PD, McKenzie DT, Swain SL, Kagnoff MF. Interleukin 5 and interleukin 4 produced by Peyer's patch T cells selectively enhance immunoglobulin A expression. J Immunol 1987; 139:2669–74.

71. Streeter PR, Berg EL, Rouse BTN, Bargatze RF, Butcher EC. A tissue-specific endothelial cell molecule involved in lymphocyte homing. Nature 1988; 331:41–6.

72. Brandtzaeg P, Korsrud FR. Significance of different J chain profiles in human tissues: generation of IgA and IgM with binding site for secretory component as related to the J chain expressing capacity of the total local immunocyte population, including IgG and IgD producing cells, and depends on the clinical state of the tissue. Clin Exp Immunol 1984; 58:709–18.

73. Brandtzaeg P. Translocation of immunoglobulins across human epithelia: review of the development of a transport model. Acta Histochem (suppl) 1987; 34:9–32.

74. Shapiro GG, Virant FS, Furukawa CT, Pierson WE, Bierman CW. Immunologic defects in patients with refractory sinusitis. Pediatrics 1991; 87:311–6.

75. Shapiro GG. Sinusitis in children. J Allergy Clin Immunol 1988; 81:1025–7.

76. Polmar SH. The role of the immunologist in sinus disease. J Allergy Clin Immunol 1992; 90:511–5.

77. Hayakawa H, Iwata T, Yata J, Kobayashi N. Primary immunodeficiency syndrome in Japan. I. Overview of a nationwide survey on primary immunodeficiency syndrome. J Clin Immunol 1981; 1:31–9.

78. Rosen FS, Cooper MD, Wedgwood RJP. The primary immunodeficiencies. N Engl J Med 1984; 311:235–242.

79. Rosen FS, Wedgwood RJ, Eibl M, Griscelli JC, Seligmann M, Aiuti F, Kishimoto T, Matsumoto S, Khakhalin LN, Hanson LA, Hitzig WH, Thompson RA, Cooper MD, Good RA, Waldmann TA. Primary immunodeficiency diseases. Report of a WHO scientific group. Immunodefic Rev 1992; 3:195–236.
80. Strober W, Krakauer R, Klaevemen HL, Reynolds HY, Nelson DL. Secretory component deficiency: a disorder of the IgA immune system. N Engl J Med 1976; 294:351–356.
81. Tomasi TB Jr. Human immunoglobulin A. N Engl J Med 1968; 279:1327–1330.
82. Oxelius V-A, Laurell AB, Lindquist B, Golebiowska H, Axelsson V, Bjorkander J, Hanson LA. IgG subclasses in selective IgA deficiency: importance of IgG2-IgA deficiency. N Engl J Med 1981; 304:1476–1477.
83. Shur PH. IgG subclasses—a review. Ann Allergy 1988; 58: 89–99.
84. Spiegelberg HL. Biological activities of immunoglobulins of different classes and subclasses. Adv Immunol 1974; 19:259–94.
85. Stevens R, Dichek D, Keld B, Heiner D. IgGI is the predominant subclass of in vivo- and in vitro-produced anti-tetanus toxoid antibodies and also serves as the membrane IgG molecule for delivering inhibitory signals to anti-tetanus toxoid antibody producing B cells. J Clin Immunol 1983; 3:65–69.
86. Siber GR, Schur PH, Aisenberg AC, Weitzman SA, Schiffman G. Correlation between serum IgG2 concentrations and the antibody response to bacterial polysaccharide antigens. N Engl J Med 1980; 303:178–182.
87. Hammarstrom L, Smith CIE. IgG2 deficiency in a healthy blood donor. Concomitant lack of IgG2, IgA and IgE immunoglobulins and specific anticarbohydrate antibodies. Clin Exp Immunol 1983; 51:600–604.
88. Insel RA, Anderson PW. Response to oligosaccharide-protein conjugate vaccine against Hemophilus influenzae B in two patients with IgG2 deficiency unresponsive to capsular polysaccharide vaccine. N Engl J Med 1986; 315:499–503.
89. Preud'Homme JL, Hanson LA. IgG subclass deficiency. Immunodefic Reviews 1990; 2:129–149.
90. Ambrosino DM, Umetsu DT, Siber GR, Howie G, Goularte TA, Michaels R, Martin P, Schur PH, Noyes J, Schiffman G, Geha RS. Selective defect in the antibody response to Hemophilus influenzae type B in children with recurrent infections and normal serum IgG subclass levels. J Allergy Clin Immunol 1988; 81:1175–1179.
91. Knutsen AP. Patients with IgG subclass and/or selective antibody deficiency to polysaccharide antigens: initiation of a controlled clinical trial of intravenous immune globulin. J Clin Allergy Immunol 1989; 84:640–647.
92. Tonegawa S. Somatic generation of antibody diversity. Nature 1983; 302:575–581.
93. Cooper MD. B lymphocytes. Normal development and function. N Engl J Med 1987; 317:1452–1456.
94. Bruton OC. Agammaglobulinemia. Pediatrics. 1952; 9:722–728.
95. Ochs HD, Wedgwood RJ. Disorders of the B cell system. In: Stiehm ER, ed. Immunologic Disorders in Infants and Children. Philadelphia: WB Saunders, 1989: 226–56.

96. Wilfert CM, Buckley RH, Mohanakumar T, Griffith JF, Katz SL, Whisnant JK, Eggleston PA, Moore M, Treadwell E, Oxman MN, Rosen FS. Persistent and fatal central-nervous-system echovirus infections in patients with agammaglobuline-mia. N Engl J Med 1977; 296:1485–1489.

97. Schwaber J, Rosen FS. X chromosome linked immunodeficiency. Immunodefic Rev 1990; 2:233–251.

98. Notarangelo LN, Duse M, Ugazio AG. Immunodeficiency with hyper-IgM (HIM). Immunodefic Rev 1992; 3:101–121.

99. Mayer L, Kwan SP, Thompson C, Ko HS, Chiorazzi N, Waldamann T, Rosen FS. Evidence for a defect in "switch" T cells in patients with immunodeficiency and hyperimmunoglobulimemia M. N Engl J Med 1986; 314:409–413.

100. Spickett GP, Webster ADB, Farrant J. Cellular abnormalities in common variable immunodeficiency. Immunodeficiency Reviews 1990; 2:199–219.

101. Knutsen AP, O'Connor DM. Antibody deficiency with normal immunoglobulins in a child with hypoplastic anema. Clin Immunol Immunopathol 1985; 36:330–7.

102. Saxon A, Kobayashi RH, Stevens RH, Singer AD, Stiehm ER, Siegel SC. In vitro analysis of humoral immunity in antibody deficiency with normal immunoglobu-lins. Clin Immunol Immunopathol 1980; 17:235–244.

103. Siegal RL, Issekutz T, Schwaber J, Rosen FS, Geha RS. Deficiency of T helper cells in transient hypogammaglobulinmia of infancy. N Engl J Med 1981; 305:1307–13.

104. Eibl MM, Wedgwood RJ. Intravenous immunoglobulin: a review. Immunodefic Rev 1989; 1:1–42.

105. Cunningham-Rundles C, Siegal FP, Smithwick EM, Lion-Boule A, Cunningham-Rundles S, O'Malley J, Barandun S, Good RA. Efficacy of intravenous immu-noglobulin in primary immunodeficiency disease. Ann Intern Med 1984; 101:435–9.

106. Ochs HD, Fischer SH, Wedgwood RJ, Wara DW, Cowan MJ, Ammann AJ, Saxon A, Budinger MD, Allred RU, Rousell RH. Comparison of high-dose and low-dose intravenous immunoglobulin therapy in patients with primary immunodeficiency diseases. Am J Med 1984; 76:78–82 (suppl).

107. Roifman CM, Levison H, Gelfand EW. High-dose versus low-dose intravenous immunoglobulin in hypogammaglobulinaemia and chronic lung disease. Lancet 1987; 1:1075–7.

108. Silk HJ, Ambrosino D, Geha RS. Effect of intravenous gammaglobulin therapy in IgG2 deficient and IgG2 sufficient children with recurrent infections and poor re-sponse to immunization with Hemophilus influenzae type B capsular polysaccha-ride antigen. Ann Allergy 1990; 64:21–5.

17

Fulminant Sinusitis

JAMES H. BOYD and JOHN H. GLADNEY
Saint Louis University School of Medicine
St. Louis, Missouri

I. INTRODUCTION

Fulminant sinusitis describes a clinical picture of dramatic rapid progression of the common symptoms of sinusitis. The specific symptoms are dependent on the sinus or sinuses involved. Before antibiotics were available, a high proportion of patients' conditions progressed to involvement of surrounding structures. Pain is the most common complaint of people with fulminant sinusitis. The location of the pain will usually identify the source of involvement. Occasionally the patient will be able to localize the side involved by the amount of discharge.

The clinical appearance of fulminant sinusitis is similar to that seen with lesser forms of acute sinusitis. This includes preceding viral upper respiratory infection, allergic rhinitis, or worsening or quiescent chronic sinusitis. It has been shown that the sinus cavity is not normally sterile, but instead contains normal flora of both aerobes and anaerobes (1). It has been estimated that 0.5% of common colds are complicated by sinus infection. The average adult has two or three colds per year, in comparison to children's six to eight colds per year. The combination of sinus obstruction with a virulent organism results in a progressive infection. The addition of antibiotics to which the organism is sensitive often will reverse the progression over 24 hr. Relief of the obstruction will likewise allow decompression of the sepsis into the nasal passage rather than the surrounding tissues.

Predisposing factors to the progression of simple acute sinusitis into fulminant sinusitis are unclear. Anatomical abnormalities, such as the paradoxical middle turbinate and concha bullosa air cells, have been implicated in an increased incidence of acute and chronic bacterial sinusitis (2). Excessive aeration of agger nasi cells may also be instrumental in the development of frontal sinusitis (3). Significant immunocompromise will increase the likelihood of rapid progression of sinusitis. This occurs in patients with acquired immunodeficiency syndrome (AIDS), chemotherapeutically induced immune deficiency, or other debilitating diseases such as diabetes (4). Patients with defects of antibody response are much more likely to experience fulminant progression of infections by pyogenic bacteria with polysaccharide capsules (i.e., *Streptococcus pneumoniae*, *Haemophilus influenzae*, or *Pseudomonas* species). Patients who have undergone splenectomy, as well as those with lymphoma, chronic lymphocytic leukemia, or who have received myelosuppressive chemotherapy are included in this group (5).

The goal of treating fulminant sinusitis is resolution of the inflammatory process and prevention of intracranial or orbital complication. The most common intracranial complication of sinusitis is meningitis. It should be understood that meningitis of an otitic source is much more common than that from the sinuses. Meningitis from sinusitis or an otitic source is more common in children than adults. In the era before antibiotics, meningitis was the most common source of death from sinusitis (6). The source of sinus-induced meningitis is most commonly the frontal sinus followed by the sphenoid, ethmoid, and maxillary sinuses, in that order (7). The most common organisms involved with meningitis are *Streptococcus pneumoniae*, staphylococcal species, other streptococcal species, and *Hemophilus influenzae*. Orbital complications are not uncommon and usually result from frontal sinusitis in adults and ethmoid sinusitis in children. Before the development of adequate antibiotics, the ability to manage patients surgically to prevent these complications was limited by the common development of osteomyelitis postoperatively. With adequate antibiotics, early surgical intervention is now feasible and often prevents severe intracranial or intraorbital complications.

II. CONSERVATIVE MANAGEMENT

A. Decongestant and Mucolytic Therapy

The conservative management of sinusitis deserves a brief mention since this treatment prevents the progression of acute sinusitis to fulminant sinusitis. The use of decongestants in acute sinusitis is well accepted. Intranasal spray preparations of oxymetazoline or phenylephrine are efficacious in providing a significant reduction of nasal congestion. Their use is generally limited to a few days to prevent rebound nasal congestion. Systemic decongestants are also effective in reducing vascular nasal congestion to promote drainage. Their systemic delivery may provide decongestant effects at sites an intranasal spray would not reach. Attention should be paid to the cardiovascular and central nervous system stimulating side effects of both pseudoephedrine and phenylpropanolamine.

Mucoevacuant therapy may provide some improvement in drainage during acute sinusitis. The two most commonly utilized compounds are guaifenesin and iodinated glycerol. These are often provided in combination with a decongestant medication. Their role in chronic sinusitis with inspissated mucus is probably more significant than in acute or fulminant sinusitis.

Steroid therapy has been suggested during acute sinusitis to assist in relief of nasal inflammation. Only rarely is systemic steroid administration warranted in acute sinusitis. More commonly, topical steroids may be of benefit in the setting of nasal allergies that have contributed to the development of an acute sinusitis.

B. Antimicrobial Therapy

The mainstay of treatment of acute sinusitis is antibiotic therapy. Numerous medications are currently available to combat acute sinusitis. The choice of which particular antibiotic will depend in part on the severity of the condition. In fulminant sinusitis or impending involvement of surrounding tissues, a broad-spectrum antibiotic that covers beta-lactamase-producing organisms is recommended. If any concern regarding the adequacy of an oral preparation exists, hospital admission with intravenous antibiotic therapy is indicated. This provides close observation of the response to antibiotics and allow for early management of orbital or intracranial complications.

III. FULMINANT FRONTAL SINUSITIS

A. Diagnosis and Early Management

Before the modern age of antibiotic therapy, acute sinusitis developed into fulminant sinusitis with involvement of surrounding tissues with regularity. The surgical management of acute sinusitis is currently rarely necessary. With the institution of endoscopic sinus surgery, occasionally less invasive techniques can be utilized to decompress suppurative sinuses. Surgery is only indicated in the situation of progression on adequate antibiotic therapy and impending orbital or neurologic complication.

Acute frontal sinusitis is usually due to secondary contamination and obstruction from an infected homolateral ethmoid sinusitis. Occasionally, there will be anatomical abnormalities in the long course of the frontal duct that can contribute to stasis and infection of the frontal sinus. Even more rarely, tumors such as

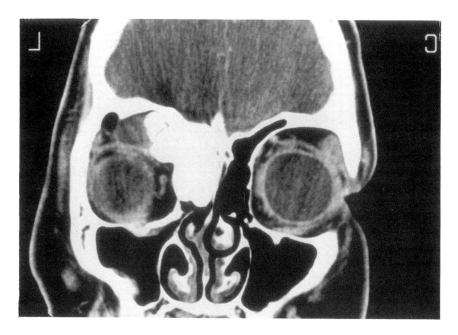

Figure 1 Frontoethmoid osteoma with secondary frontal sinusitis/mucopyocele.

an osteoma, an inverting papilloma, or an adenocarcinoma of the ethmoid sinus region will obstruct the frontal recess. This usually produces chronic sinusitis or mucocele formation in the obstructed sinus. After bacterial seeding occurs, acute fulminant sinusitis may ensue (Fig. 1).

Acute frontal sinusitis should be easily recognized. The patient will most often complain of ipsilateral supraorbital pain. Pressure upon the forehead or orbital roof will elicit worsening pain. Occasionally the skin of the forehead will be warm and erythematous. Edema of the upper eyelid or forehead should imply impending extension of the disease beyond the confines of the sinus. Orbital complications are most often the results of extension from the frontal sinus in adults, as opposed to the ethmoid sinuses in children. Inspection of the nasal cavity will often reveal mucopurulent material in the anterior extent of the middle meatus (frontal recess). Fever and systemic toxicity are common when significant obstruction of purulent outflow exists.

The proximity of the frontal sinus to the cranial vault mandates aggressive management of fulminant frontal sinusitis. Before modern antibiotics, suppurative complications were common. Bois discussed the pathogenesis of these complications in regard to the surgical management (8). Pressure, from the suppuration in the bony confines of the obstructed sinus, can result in necrosis of

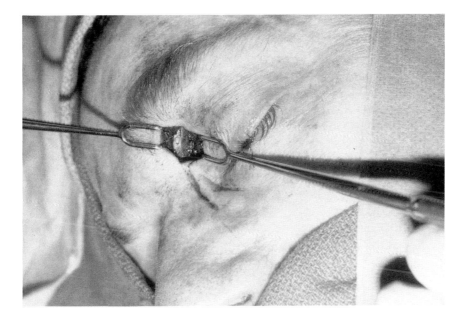

Figure 2 Surgical approach for frontal sinus trephination.

the sinus mucosa and thrombosis of the valveless communicating veins between the sinuses and surrounding structures. The subsequent septic thrombophlebitis may progress via the diploic system of the frontal bone to intracranial or orbital tissues. Osteomyelitis of the frontal bone (Pott's puffy tumor) was not uncommon in the preantibiotic era and was often attributed to surgical contamination of the diploic space. Prevention of this condition is achieved by early institution of aggressive antimicrobial therapy. In addition, trephination through the floor of the frontal sinus, rather than the anterior wall, prevents exposure of significant diploic cancellous bone to the suppurative process (Fig. 2). If antibiotic therapy is not rapidly effective, the management should proceed to surgical therapy prior to complication. It should be added that the frontal sinus disease is usually secondary to extension from the ethmoid sinuses, which must be dealt with appropriately as well.

B. Surgical Therapy

1. Intranasal Frontal Sinus Decompression

Surgical therapy of the frontal sinus may be classified into four basic categories: intranasal relief of frontal recess (duct) obstruction, external relief of frontal recess obstruction, external drainage of suppurative material (trephination), or ablation of the sinus cavity. Resection of the anterior ethmoid cells and anterior middle turbinate to improve drainage of the infected frontal sinus has long been proposed as the appropriate initial treatment of frontal sinusitis (9). With the advent of endoscopic sinus surgery, the safety and feasibility of intranasal frontal sinus drainage have improved. Despite this, in fulminant frontal sinusitis the acute inflammation in the anterior ethmoid sinuses may produce excessive bleeding, with subsequent increased risk of complication and decreased adequacy of drainage even with the improved visualization offered with the endoscopic approach. One advantage of the endoscopic approach is the eradication of disease in the anterior ethmoid sinuses simultaneously. Another advantage is the lack of external scars associated with the other approaches. If this approach is utilized, close follow-up is mandatory postoperatively to ensure patency of the nasofrontal duct.

2. External Frontoethmoidectomy

The external frontoethmoidectomy is a well-recognized procedure for drainage of both the ethmoid and frontal system. Initially described by Lynch, it provides adequate exposure to drain the frontal sinus and remove the anterior ethmoid cells that may block the frontal duct (10). The disadvantages include late stenosis of the frontal duct and an external scar. The details of the surgery are beyond the scope of this chapter.

3. Frontal Sinus Trephination

A much simpler version of the external frontoethmoidectomy is the frontal sinus trephine. Trephination of the frontal sinus is more commonly utilized in fulminant frontal sinusitis than the external frontoethmoidectomy. In a patient with frontal pain, fever, erythema, upper eyelid edema, but no obvious orbital complications, an initial 24 hr trial of intravenous antibiotics should be given. If there is clear progression of the inflammation or a lack of defervescence after this period, operative drainage should be considered.

Frontal sinus trephination is completed through a small incision at the medial orbital roof that corresponds to the floor of the frontal sinus (Fig. 2). Care is taken to place this medially to avoid the supraorbital nerve and vessels. The incision is taken down to bone at the margin of the orbital rim. A small cutting burr may be utilized to fenestrate the medial floor of the frontal sinus. After evacuation and culture of the mucopurulent material, the sinus cavity should be vigorously irrigated. A single-/ or double-catheter system may be placed through the incision for postoperative irrigation with antibiotics and or steroids. The incision is closed around the drainage system (Fig. 3). Irrigations through the sinus should continue three to four times daily until the return is clear and/or there is free flow into the nose. The catheter is removed and the patient maintained on oral antibiotics until definitive surgery can be performed.

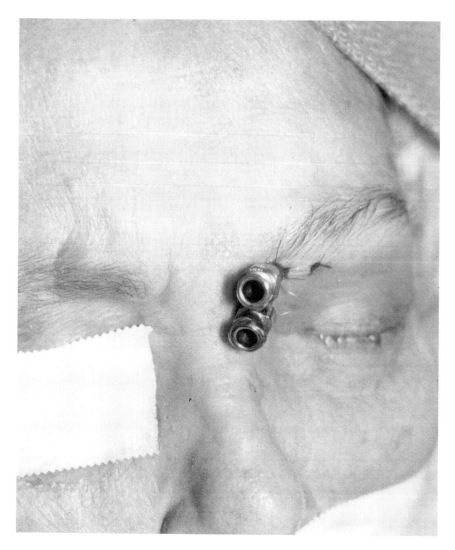

Figure 3 Dual angiocatheter irrigation system after frontal sinus trephination.

4. Osteoplastic Flap Frontal Sinus Obliteration

The workhorse of the otolaryngologist for treatment of chronic frontal sinusitis is the osteoplastic flap. It entails elevation of the anterior wall of the frontal sinus hinged on the pericranium/periorbital tissues inferiorly. The mucosa is meticulously removed, the frontal duct is obstructed with fascia, and the sinus is filled with fat for obliteration. Although this procedure is very efficacious in the treatment of chronic frontal sinusitis and mucocele, it has a very limited role in the treatment of acute frontal sinusitis due to the significant risk of frontal bone osteomyelitis.

IV. FULMINANT ETHMOID SINUSITIS

A. Diagnosis and Early Management

Much of any discussion of fulminant ethmoid sinusitis necessarily revolves around its extension to other structures, namely the orbital contents. It should be emphasized that the early involvement of an ophthalmologist is both medically and medicolegally imperative. Orbital extension of sinusitis is more common in children than adults. Although this is discussed at length in other chapters, it is appropriate to reiterate this here. Chandler's classification of orbital extension of ethmoid sinusitis remains the basis of management of fulminant ethmoid sinusitis (11). He classified these patients into six groups dependent on the clinical and radiologic findings. The first group involved preseptal inflammatory edema of the periorbital tissues. This is characteristically not tender and is located over the frontal process of the maxilla just above the medial canthal tendon. No proptosis is present in this group.

The second group described has orbital cellulitis. These patients possess some degree of proptosis, tenderness of orbital contents, and edema. Visual acuity may begin to decrease in this group. On histologic examination they exhibit diffuse edema of the orbital contents with inflammatory cells and bacteria. No localized accumulation of purulence can be demonstrated. These first two groups of patients should be managed expectantly with intravenous antibiotics, topical and systemic decongestants, and mucolytic therapy. There is no role for aspiration of the orbital contents for culture and sensitivity (12). Any sign of progression, such as return of fever, or a decrease in either ocular mobility or visual acuity, should prompt swift surgical intervention.

The third group are those with a subperiosteal abscess. These patients have a well-localized accumulation of purulence between the lamina papyracea and the periorbita. Computed tomography reliably demonstrates the location and extent of the abscess cavity. B-mode ultrasound reveals most abscesses but may miss those at the orbital apex due to shielding by the globe (12). With a subperiosteal abscess, the globe is slightly proptotic and displaced laterally and inferiorly.

The fourth group described were patients with an orbital abscess, that is, frank accumulation of purulence within the periorbita. They will show significant proptosis, chemosis, as well as ophthalmoplegia. Visual acuity may be decreased due to optic neuritis or retinal artery occlusion. The fifth group are those whose infection has progressed to the cavernous sinus with subsequent septic thrombosis. This is often associated with concomitant meningitis. Progression of unilateral eye findings to the opposite eye is considered nearly pathognomonic of this entity.

B. Surgical Therapy

As mentioned, the first two groups of patients with fulminate ethmoid sinusitis may be managed without emergency surgery. The last three groups often must be treated both medically as well as surgically to a minimize morbidity and prevent mortality.

1. External Ethmoidectomy

External ethmoidectomy, combined with some degree of orbital drainage, is recommended for patients with subperiosteal abscess or orbital abscess. Via a standard Lynch incision the medial canthal tendon is identified. The periorbita is elevated from the lamina papyracea. In the case of a periorbital abscess, some would recommend simple drainage of the abscess while others would perform an ethmoidectomy as well. A Penrose or other type of drain should be left in the wound to prevent reaccumulation of pus. The drain is left intact until the patient is afebrile and the drainage has subsided. The degree of orbital exploration necessary depends upon the location and volume of the abscess. If an orbital abscess has been identified on the preoperative evaluation, the orbital exploration should be done by, or in conjunction with, an ophthalmologist. Usually the inflammatory edema of the eye regresses significantly over the first 24 hr postoperatively. The scar is usually minimal even when the wound heals secondarily after removal of the drain.

2. Intranasal Ethmoidectomy

Although intranasal endoscopic or traditional ethmoidectomy is efficacious in the management of chronic ethmoid sinusitis, it plays a very limited role in the management of acute sinusitis. Bleeding of the acutely inflamed tissues often prevents good visualization and can result in operative complications. Endoscopic ethmoidectomy has been reported for the treatment of acute sinusitis with orbital cellulitis, but many surgeons would not agree with this approach to management (13). Inadequate drainage may result in progression of the process with subsequent visual or intracranial complication.

V. FULMINANT SPHENOID SINUSITIS

A. Diagnosis and Early Management

The sphenoid sinus is often overlooked as a source of acute progressive sinusitis. Periodically, it is brought to the clinician's attention secondary to reports of involvement of surrounding structures. Since antibiotics have been available, the overall morbidity from infectious processes in the sphenoid sinus has decreased dramatically (6). The position of the sphenoid sinus ostium high in the sphenoethmoid recess prevents easy visualization of purulent drainage or other pathologic processes by anterior rhinoscopy (Fig. 3). The drainage also most commonly does not present as anterior rhinorrhea, but instead as posterior nasal drainage.

Most acute sphenoid sinusitis will present with headache as the major complaint (14, 15). Most patients will complain of severe retro-orbital pain, although localization to the vertex, frontal, or temporal regions has been reported (16). The pain is usually worse in the early morning and exacerbated by position changes. Despite these clues, the sphenoid sinus is not high on the differential diagnosis list for most physicians. Involvement of cranial nerves will clearly raise the index of suspicion and accelerate the work-up of the headache. It is fortunate that cranial neuropathies are much less common in inflammatory lesions of the sphenoid than with neoplastic processes (17). When cranial neuropathies do occur secondary to inflammatory sinus disease, the sphenoid is the most common source. Of the cranial nerves involved, the abducens is most common. This is explained by its medial position in the cavernous sinus and hence is juxtaposed to the lateral sphenoid sinus wall. The aeration of the sinus has an inverse relationship to the thickness of the sinus bony wall (18). This thinness or occasional dehiscence of the lateral wall will place intracranial structures at increased risk from acute sphenoid sinusitis. In addition, the thickness of the sinus wall must be kept in mind if irrigation of the sinus is performed.

The microbiological colonization of acute sphenoid sinusitis includes *Staphylococcus aureus*, *Streptococcus pneumoniae*, and other streptococcal species. Multiple organisms are seen with much less frequency in acute sphenoid sinusitis than with chronic sinusitis. The incidence of anaerobic organisms is likewise lower with acute sphenoid infection than with chronic sinusitis. When there is extension to the central nervous system from sphenoid sinusitis, the same organism is usually isolated from both the sphenoid and the cerebrospinal fluid (15).

There is often an unfortunate and significant delay between the onset of symptoms and presentation to the otolaryngologist. Isolated sphenoid sinus infection is relatively rare. When a patient presents with severe headache, fever, and systemic toxemia, sinus films may be helpful. If sphenoid sinusitis is a consideration, a submentovertex view should be included, in addition to the standard lateral, Water's, and Caldwell's views. Even with the addition of the submentovertex view, a significant number of patients with sphenoid sinusitis will be missed if computed tomography is not done (15). If isolated sphenoid sinusitis is suspected from the x-rays, the patient should be managed as a medical emergency. Institution of intravenous antibiotics, topical decongestants, and close observation for progression should be maintained. Occasionally irrigation of the sphenoid sinus will facilitate clearance of the infection (Fig. 4). Failure of the patient to defervescence, either persistence or worsening of the headache, or evidence of extension to the surrounding structures should be an indication for emergency surgical therapy.

Development of diplopia and photophobia may be premonitory symptoms of cavernous sinus thrombosis (19). Progression of unilateral orbital findings to the contralateral side should be considered pathognomonic for septic cavernous sinus thrombosis. Only 15% of septic cavernous sinus thrombosis cases are the result of sinusitis. The vast majority of the others arise from minor infections of the skin of the midface (16). This may account for the high predominance of staphylococcal species as the causative agents in the majority of cavernous sinus phlebitides. With the improvement in antibiotic therapy, the mortality from this entity has been reduced from 80 to 13% (20). Whether anticoagulative therapy or high-dosage steroids are of benefit in this disease remains highly controversial.

B. Surgical Therapy

1. Sphenoidotomy

Surgical approaches to the sphenoid include simple cannulation and irrigation, external sphenoethmoidectomy, transantral sphenoethmoidectomy, intranasal sphenoidotomy, or endoscopic intranasal sphenoidotomy. Selection of the surgical technique should depend on the complex of sinuses involved. If isolated sphenoid sinusitis is being managed on an emergency basis, endoscopic sphenoidotomy is probably the procedure of choice, if the operator has experience in this approach. Since local anesthesia works poorly in the acidotic environment of acute inflammation, most procedures in this setting should be performed under general anesthesia.

As with all endoscopic procedures, a full coronal computed tomogram should be obtained preoperatively. Occasionally both axial and coronal images are of assistance in the evaluation of the sphenoid. The computed tomogram will ensure the need for operative management, provide information regarding involvement of other sinuses or adjacent tissue, and detail the subtleties of the patient's skull base anatomy. After adequate local or general anesthesia is obtained, topical vasoconstriction should be achieved using cocaine or phenylephrine. Additional vasoconstriction may be gained by local injection of epinephrine solution in a concentration of 1:100,000. In the case of isolated sphenoid sinusitis, the sphenoethmoid recess should be identified. The ostium of the sphenoid is located just medially in the groove between the septum and the superior turbinate at an angle of 25–30 degrees from the nasal floor (Fig. 5). If the ostium is accessible, cannulation with a suction will confirm its location. The distance to the

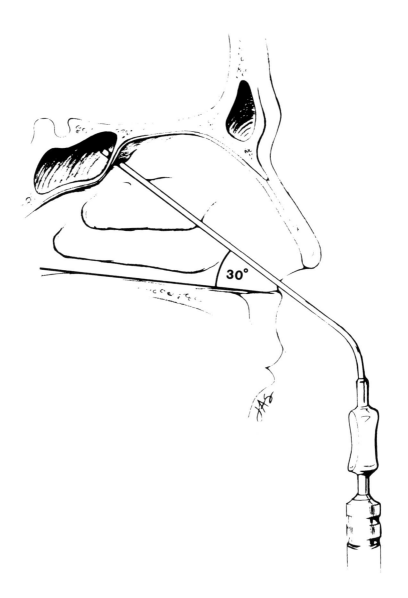

Figure 4   Location of the sphenoid os in the frontoethmoid recess at an angle of 25–30 degrees from the nasal floor.

opening of the sphenoid is usually 7 cm from the anterior choana. Once the sphenoid rostrum is identified, the posterior end of the middle turbinate may be removed with turbinate scissors or straight polyp forceps. This will open access to the sphenoethmoid recess for subsequent enlargement of the ostia. Removal of part of the superior turbinate may also facilitate this. If the sinus ostia is evident, a fine Kerrison rongeur may be utilized to enlarge the opening downward. In rare cases, the ostia cannot be cannulated and entry into the sinus may be achieved with the suction or a small osteotome in the inferiomedial extent of the sphenoid face. After entry, specimens should be taken for aerobic, anaerobic, and fungal cultures. Irrigation of the sinus with saline should be performed for optimal removal of inspissated secretions or mucopurulent materials. Bleeding from the branches of the sphenopalatine artery will occasionally be profuse enough to require bipolar cautery. If bleeding is persistent, a Merocel sponge may be placed in the region and removed the following day. One should avoid packing the nose, if possible, to promote continued drainage from the region.

C. Combined Approaches

If ocular complications are present due to concomitant ethmoid sinus disease or orbital apex extension from sphenoid infection exists, one should utilize an external approach. This would provide improved control of the orbital contents while ensuring adequate drainage. If concomitant maxillary disease is present, the transantral approach may afford an advantage. It should be kept in mind that only when a complication is anticipated from the involved sinus should that sinus be included in the emergency management of the problem. If the patient's condition fails to improve promptly after surgical drainage and continued intravenous antibiotics, the evaluation for intracranial or orbital extension should be repeated (i.e., computed tomography and lumbar puncture). In particular, progression of a unilateral ocular process to the contralateral eye should be considered diagnostic for septic cavernous sinus thrombosis. With adequate antibiotic therapy the mortality from this entity has improved dramatically, but still warrants very aggressive management.

VI. FULMINANT MAXILLARY SINUSITIS

A. Diagnosis and Early Management

Acute inflammation in the maxillary antrum is often a result of continuing inflammation in the anterior ethmoid cells and ostiomeatal complex. Despite this, patients will often present with isolated symptoms of maxillary or dental pain and toxemia due to fulminant progression of the maxillary sinus infection. Those patients will generally have facial edema and erythema, maxillary or dental pain to percussion, purulent rhinorrhea, fever, and general malaise. Although older children will be able to provide a reliable history of initial facial pain, young children will have a less obvious complex of symptoms of acute maxillary sinusitis, (i.e., fetid breath, cough, nasal discharge, and fever) (21).

A scenario commonly encountered by the otolaryngologist is acute maxillary sinusitis in the nasotracheally intubated patient. In this setting, the most important therapeutic maneuver is removal of all nasal tubes. Aspiration and irrigation of the involved sinus will often reveal an infecting organism despite broad-spectrum antibiotic administration. The organisms responsible in the hospital setting often include *Staphylococcus aureus*, *Pseudomonas* sp., *Enterobacteria*, and *Bacteroides* species. Polymicrobial infections exist in nearly one-half of these patients (22). This should be contrasted with routine acute maxillary sinusitis, with a high preponderance of *Streptococcus pneumoniae* and *Hemophilus influenzae*. Anaerobes are often seen in acute maxillary sinusitis when the cause involves extension of a dental infection (23).

B. Surgical Therapy

The vast majority of patients with maxillary sinus infections can be managed with oral antibiotics, topical or systemic decongestants, and pain medication, if necessary. Occasionally, the toxemia of the sinusitis can be severe enough to warrant antral puncture and irrigation. Since this can be performed in an outpatient setting with little risk or morbidity, most otolaryngologists would prefer this before hospitalization and intravenous antibiotics. The risk of osteomyelitis of the maxillary bone is very small due to its abundant blood supply, in addition to the relative paucity of marrow space in the medial sinus wall. The membranous fontanelle of the medial maxillary sinus walls have much less resistance to rupture than the bony confines of the frontal or sphenoid sinus. Accessory ostia of the maxillary sinus are commonly found on the lateral nasal wall and considered by many to be due to this suppurative process.

If acute fulminant maxillary sinusitis develops despite adequate antibiotic coverage, antral puncture is easily performed and provides a representative sample for culture (Fig. 5). Concomitant irrigation of the sinus may also assist the sinus in clearing the infectious process more rapidly. Often the ultimate resolution is dependent on clearing the ethmoid sinuses of persistent disease. Cultures of nasal secretions from the middle or inferior meatus have shown poor correlation with the antral irrigation specimens and are therefore of little value (24, 25). The culture obtained properly will reliably predict the efficacy of antibiotic therapy if the organism is found to be sensitive on in vitro testing (25).

Antral puncture is best achieved under the inferior turbinate. The bone of the maxilla just below the root of the inferior turbinate is thin and allows easier penetration (Fig. 5). Placement of a pledget of 10% cocaine solution on the inferior turbinate and inferior meatus will provide local anesthesia and vasoconstriction.

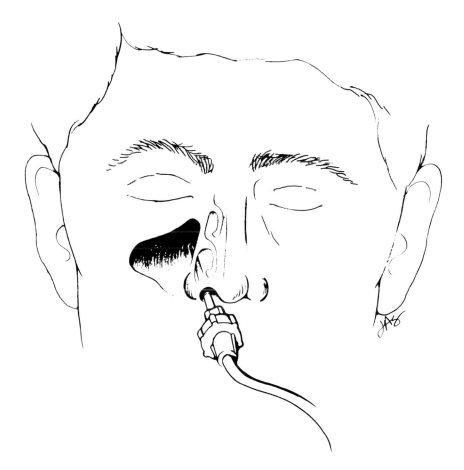

Figure 5 Approach for maxillary sinus irrigation and culture.

Swabbing the region with a iodine antiseptic paint will avoid contamination from nasal organisms. The antral trocar attached to a stopcock valve and a 20 ml syringe allows closed aspiration of maxillary sinus contents as well as instillation of sterile normal saline irrigation. The physician would usually like to see aspiration of purulent material or air prior to irrigation. The sinus should not be irrigated with extreme force, since tip placement in a thickened mucous membrane would result in extreme pain to the patient. Irrigation, alternating with aspiration, should continue until the effluent is clear.

Most well-designed studies evaluating the organisms found in acute maxillary sinusitis have revealed *Streptococcus pneumoniae*, *Haemophilus influenzae*, and *Branhamella catarrhalis* to be the most common (26). In comparison, studies that did not adequately prepare the nasal vestibule and inferior meatus with povidone–iodine (Betadine) had a preponderance of staphylococcal contaminants. (27)

REFERENCES

1. Brook I. Aerobic and anaerobic bacterial flora of normal maxillary sinuses. Laryngoscope 1981; 91:372–6.
2. Stammberger H. Endoscopic endonasal surgery—concepts in treatment of recurring rhinosinusitis. Part I. Anatomic and pathophysiologic considerations. Otolaryngol Head Neck Surg 1986; 94:143–7.
3. Kuhn FA, Bolger WE, Tisdal RG. The agger nasi cell in frontal recess obstruction: an anatomic, radiologic and clinical correlation. Operative techniques. Otolaryngol Head Neck Surg 1991; 2:226–31.
4. Jackson RM, Rice DH. Acute bacterial sinusitis and diabetes mellitus. Otolaryngol Head Neck Surg 1987: 97:469–73.
5. Rybak LP. Medical treatment of chronic sinusitis in the immunocompetent and immunosuppressed patient: a review. Otolaryngol Head Neck Surg 1982; 90:534–9.
6. Teed RW. Meningitis from the sphenoid sinus. Arch Otolaryngol Head Neck Surg 1938; 28:589–619.
7. Quick CA, Payne E. Complicate acute sinusitis. Laryngoscope 1972; 82:1248–63.
8. Bois LR. Acute frontal sinusitis: the trephine operation for selected cases. Laryngoscope 1942; 52:458–68.
9. Lothrop. HA. Frontal sinus suppuration. Ann Surg 1912; 59:937–57.
10. Lynch RC. The technique of a radical frontal sinus operation which has given me the best results. Laryngoscope 1921; 31:1–5.
11. Chandler JR, Langenbrummer DJ, Stevens ER. The pathogenesis of orbital complication in acute sinusitis. Laryngoscope 1970; 80:1414–28.
12. Schram VL, Curtin HD, Kennerdell JS. Evaluation of orbital cellulitis and results in treatment. Laryngoscope 1982; 92:732–8.
13. Stammberger H. Endoscopic endonasal surgery—concepts in treatment of recurring rhinosinusitis. Part II. Surgical techniques. Otolaryngol Head Neck Surg 1986; 94:147–56.
14. Pearlman SJ, Steven J, Lawson W, Biller HF, Freidman WH, Potter GD. Isolated sphenoid sinus disease. Laryngoscope 1989; 99:716–20.
15. Lew, D, Southwick FS, Montgomery WW, Weber AL, Baker AS. Sphenoid sinusitis: a review of 30 cases. N Engl J Med 1983; 309:1149–54.
16. Sofferman RA. Cavernous sinus thrombophlebitis secondary to sphenoid sinusitis. Laryngoscope 1983; 93:797–800.
17. Weisberger EL, Dedo HH. Cranial neuropathies in sinus disease. Laryngoscope 1977; 87:357–93.
18. Tremble GE. Irrigation of the sphenoid sinus. Ann Otol Rhinol Laryngol 1970; 79:840–843.
19. Pascarelli E, Lemlich A. Diplopia and photophobia as premonitory symptoms in cavernous sinus thrombosis. Ann Otol Rhinol Laryngol 1964; 73:210–217.

20. Yarrington CT. Cavernous sinus thrombosis revisited. Proc R Soc Lond 1977; 70:456–9.

21. Wald ER, Milmoe GJ, Bowen A, Ledesma-Medina J, Salamon N, Blustone CD. Acute maxillary sinusitis in children. N Engl J Med 1981; 304:749–54.

22. Linden BE, Aguilar EA, Allen SJ. Sinusitis in nasotracheally intubated patients. Arch Otolaryngol Head Neck Surg 1988; 144:860–1.

23. Axelson A, Brorson JE. The correlation between bacteriological findings in the nose nad maxillary sinus in acute maxillary sinusitis. Laryngoscope 1973; 83:2003–11.

24. Gwaltney JM, Syndor A, Sande MA. Etiology and antimicrobial treatment of acute sinusitis. Ann Otol Rhinol Laryngol 1981; 90:68–71

25. Evans FO, Syndor JB, Moore WEC, Moore GR, Manwaring JL, Brill AH, Jackson RT, Hanna S, Skaar JS, Holdeman LV, Fitz-Hugh GS, Sande MA, Gwaltney JM. Sinusitis of the maxillary antrum. N Engl J Med 1975; 293:735–9.

26. Hamory BH, Sande MA, Snydor A, Seale DL, Gwaltney JM. Etiology and antimicrobial therapy of acute maxillary sinusitis. J Infect Dis 1979; 139:197–202.

27. Catlin FI, Leighton EC, Reynolds RC. The bacteriology of acute and chronic sinusitis. South Med J 1965; 58:1498–502.

Index

Axon response 28
Azelastine 99
Azithromycin 75, 98

Bacillus catarrhalis (*see Moraxella catarrhalis*)
Bacillus fragilis 49
Bacillus melaniogenecus 49
Bacteria (*see also* individual species) 42
  anaerobic 21, 31, 45, 46, 50, 96, 98, 162, 191, 198, 268, 291
  cocci gram positive 45
  diphtheroids 43, 267
  gram negative 43, 46, 49
Bacterial adherence 26
Bacterial infection 177
Bacterial infection, secondary 42
Bacteroides spp. 31, 45, 49, 98, 162, 318
Basal lamella 7, 117
Basal lamina 8, 15
Basement membrane 20
Beclomethasone 74, 75, 77, 199, 265
Beta-adrenergic responsiveness 165
Beta-lactamase 96, 97
Bleeding 82, 310
Blindness 147, 149, 179
Blood dyscrasia 49
Blood flow, mucosal 24, 28
Bone 62
  erosion 60
  ethmoid 5, 6, 7, 9
  frontal 5, 6, 10, 179
  lacrimal 5, 7
  maxilla 5, 7
  nasal 5, 6, 7
  palatine 5, 6, 7
  sphenoid 5, 6, 7, 10
  sphenoid lesser wing 17
Bradykinin 26, 27, 33
Brain 3
Bromhexine 79
Bronchi 20, 24, 159
Bronchial associated lymphoid tissue (BALT) 283, 290

Bronchiectasis 291, 295
Bronchiolitis 44
Bronchitis 3, 78, 255
Bronchitis, chronic 256
Bronchoconstriction 28, 159
Bronchospasm 160, 167, 168, 242
Budesonide 77
Bulla ethmoidalis 112
Burns 49

C3b-opsonization 31
Calcitonin gene-related peptide 27
Caldwell-Luc procedure 58, 124, 135, 136, 166, 168, 265
Candida 162, 285
Candidin 32
Canine fossa 134, 135
Capillaries, fenestrated 20
Capsaicin 26, 28
Carcinoma 296
Carcinoma, squamous cell 23, 58, 64
Cavernous sinus thrombosis 1, 175, 179, 180, 194, 315
Cefaclor 51, 75, 97
Cefadroxil 98
Cefalexin 77
Cefixime 98
Cefpodoxime 77
Cefprozil 77, 98
Cefuroxime axetil 51, 75, 98, 138, 197, 199
Cell
  antigen presenting 21, 186, 288
  basal 20
  epithelial 20, 255
  goblet 20, 255, 256, 257
  goblet hyperplasia 24, 32
  leukocyte 31
  lymphocyte 21, 126, 256
  lymphocyte B 32, 189, 288, 289, 294, 295
  lymphocyte T 32, 163, 285, 288, 289, 290
  lymphocyte T CD20+ 32
  lymphocyte T CD3+ 32

Platelets 168
Pneumococcal antigen 7 22
Pneumocystis carinii 185, 197
Pneumonia 3, 44, 187, 266, 291
Pollen 94, 240
  exposure 33
  grass 33
  ragweed 33, 79, 164
Polyarthritis 295
Polypectomy 168, 240, 252, 264
Polypoid mucosa 119
Polyposis (*see* polyps, nasal)
Polyps, nasal 22, 34, 68, 78, 80, 82,
    110, 111, 112, 113, 114, 126,
    165, 166, 167, 176, 178,
    247, 263
Polytomography 61
Postcapillary venules 20
Postnasal drainage 2, 74, 108,
    159, 162, 193, 262, 263,
    266, 314
Potassium iodide 79
Pott's puffy tumor 179, 309
Prednisone 78, 266
Prenatal diagnosis 28
Pressure 74
Prophylaxis 199
Proptosis 121, 149, 180, 312
Prostaglandin 27, 44
Prostaglandin PGD2 33
Protease 24, 285
Proteoglycans 24
Proteus mirabilis 49
Pseudallescheriasis 49
Pseudoephedrine 75, 197, 199, 307
Pseudomembranous enterocolitis 98
Pseudomonas aeruginosa 46, 49,
    96, 191, 192, 198, 250,
    252, 266, 267, 268, 269,
    270, 271, 293
Pseudomonas boydii 192
Pseudomonas spp. 31, 32, 125, 268,
    306, 318
Pterygoid fossa 18
Pterygoid process 10

Pterygopalatine fossa 8, 11, 135
Puberty 10
Puncture
  maxillary anterior 196
  maxillary antral 194
Pus 31, 73, 77, 160

Radioallergosorbent test (RAST) 177
Radiograph
  Caldwell view 194, 314
  lateral view 194, 314
  plain 2, 44, 50, 60, 79, 93, 137,
    160, 194, 195, 262, 314
  submentovertex view 314
  Waters view 60, 194, 284, 314
Radiographic evaluation 60
Radiographic opacification 195, 251, 254
Radionuclide 163
Receptor, cold 27
Receptor, muscarinic M1 and M3 28
Receptor, warm 27
Reflex
  nasobronchial 28, 164, 165
  neurogenic 44
  parasympathetic 20, 28, 33
  rhinosinobronchial 242
  sinobronchial 28, 102
Renal glomerulus 20
Resistant organisms 77
Respiratory syncytial virus 43, 44
Reticular formation 164
Retrobulbar hemorrhage 147, 149
Retropharyngeal lymph nodes 11
Reye's syndrome 80
Rheumatoid arthritis 296
Rhinitis
  allergic 3, 23, 33, 78, 88, 89, 90,
    91, 94, 99, 100, 101, 108, 164,
    165, 176, 177, 305
  atrophic 178
  chronic 176
  chronic cholinergic 28
  medicamentosa 29, 77, 78
  nonallergic 23, 28, 178
  nonallergic eosinophilic 91

About the Editor

HOWARD M. DRUCE is Associate Director of Therapeutic Research at Hoffmann-La Roche Inc., Nutley, New Jersey, and Clinical Associate Professor of Medicine in the Division of Allergy and Immunology at the University of Medicine and Dentistry of New Jersey, New Jersey Medical School, Newark. The author or coauthor of more than 70 professional papers that reflect his research interests in the pathogenesis of chronic sinusitis, nasal pathophysiology, and the control of nasal microcirculation, he is a Fellow of the American College of Physicians, the American Academy of Allergy and Immunology, and the American College of Allergy and Immunology, and a member of the British Society for Immunology and the American Federation for Clinical Research, among other organizations. Dr. Druce received the B.A. degree (1974) in physiology from the University of Oxford, England, and the M.B., B.S. degree (1977) from the University of London, England. He is a licentiate of the Royal College of Physicians of England and a diplomate of the American Board of Internal Medicine and the American Board of Allergy and Immunology.